COMMUNITY RESEARCH IN ENVIRONMENTAL HEALTH

Dedicated to

Ruth Virginia Sherlog Brugge (1923–1989) and David Martin Brugge (DB)

and

*For my community partners who have become friends and colleagues.
With gratitude for what I have learned from you and respect for your
committed and vital work. (HPH)*

Community Research in Environmental Health

Studies in Science, Advocacy and Ethics

DISCARD

Edited by
DOUG BRUGGE
Tufts University School of Medicine
H. PATRICIA HYNES
Boston University School of Public Health

ASHGATE

Published by
Ashgate Publishing Limited
Gower House
Croft Road
Aldershot
Hants GU11 3HR
England

Ashgate Publishing Company
Suite 420
101 Cherry Street
Burlington
VT 05401-4405
USA

Ashgate website: http://www.ashgate.com

British Library Cataloguing in Publication Data
Community research in environmental health : studies in
    science, advocacy and ethics
    1. Environmental health - Research - Citizen participation
    2. Health risk assessment - Citizen participation
    I. Brugge, Doug II. Hynes, H. Patricia
    363.7'057'072

Library of Congress Cataloging-in-Publication Data
Community research in environmental health : studies in science, advocacy and ethics/
    [edited] by Doug Brugge and H. Patricia Hynes.
        p. ; cm.
    Includes bibliographical references and index.
    ISBN 0-7546-4176-7
        1. Environmental health--Research--United States. 2. Environmental protection--
United States. 3. Urban health--United States.
I. Brugge, Doug. II. Hynes, H. Patricia.
[DNLM: 1. Environmental Health--Boston. 2. Urban Health--Boston. 3. Cross-
Sectional Studies--Boston. 4. Public Housing--Boston. WA 380 C734 2004]

    RA566.3.C65 2004
    362.196'98--dc22

                                                                2004020997

    ISBN 0 7546 4176 7

Typeset by IML Typographers, Birkenhead, Merseyside and Printed in Great Britain
by Athenaeum Press, Tyne and Wear

Contents

List of Figures

List of Tables

List of Contributors

Maneesha Aggarwal is with the Division of Environmental Health Sciences, Joseph L. Mailman School of Public Health at Columbia University.

Julian Agyeman is with the Urban and Environmental Policy and Planning, Tufts University.

Katherine Alaimo is with the Michigan State University Department of Food Science and Human Nutrition.

Carol Allen is with Public Health – Seattle and King County and Seattle Partners for Healthy Communities.

Ashley E. Atkinson is with Greening of Detroit.

Abigail Averbach is with the Massachusetts Department of Public Health.

Doug Brugge is with the Department of Family Medicine and Community Health at Tufts University School of Medicine.

Dale Bryan is with the Urban and Environmental Policy and Planning, Tufts University.

Paul Carroll is with the New England Regional Laboratory, US Environmental Protection Agency.

Sanders Chai is with the University of Washington School of Public Health and Community Medicine and the University of Washington School Medicine.

Fu Mei Cheung is with the Boston Chinatown Neighborhood Center.

Philip Dickey is with Washington Toxics Coalition.

Patricia George is with the Citizen Alert Native American Program.

Robert Goble is with the Center for Technology, Environment, and Development, Clark University.

Dan Handy is with Landmark College.

Christina Hill is a recent graduate of Tufts University.

Pete Hutchison is with the First Presbyterian Church, Flint, Michigan.

H. Patricia Hynes is with the Department of Environmental Health at Boston University School of Public Health.

Nicole A.H. Janssen is with the Department of Environmental Sciences, Environmental and Occupational Health Group, University of Wageningen.

Carol Kawecki is with the National Center for Healthy Housing.

Patrick L. Kinney is with the Division of Environmental Health Sciences, Joseph L. Mailman School of Public Health at Columbia University.

James Krieger is with Public Health Department – Seattle and King County, the University of Washington School of Public Health and Community Medicine, the University of Washington School Medicine, and Seattle Partners for Healthy Communities.

Zenobia Lai is with Greater Boston Legal Services.

Jody Lally is with the University of Massachusetts Lowell.

Andrew Leong is with the Law Center, University of Massachusetts Boston and the Campaign to Protect Chinatown.

Jill S. Litt is with the Department of Preventive Medicine and Biometrics, University of Colorado Health Sciences Center.

Robert Maxfield is with the New England Regional Laboratory, US Environmental Protection Agency.

Pat McLaine is with the National Center for Healthy Housing.

Rachel Morello-Frosch is with Brown University.

Mary E. Northridge is with the Division of Environmental Health Sciences, Joseph L. Mailman School of Public Health at Columbia University and the Harlem Center for Health Promotion and Disease Prevention.

Manuel Pastor Jr. is with the Center for Justice, Tolerance and Community, University of California.

Carlos Porras is with Communities for a Better Environment.

Dianne Quigley is with the Religion Department, Syracuse University.

William Rand is with the Department of Family Medicine and Community Health at Tufts University School of Medicine.

Thomas M. Reischl is with the Prevention Research Center of Michigan, University of Michigan, School of Public Health.

James Sadd is with Environmental Sciences, Occidental College.

Virginia Sanchez is with the Citizen Alert Native American Program.

Peggy Shepard is with West Harlem Environmental Action, Inc.

Lin Song is with Public Health – Seattle and King County.

Tim K. Takaro is with the University of Washington School of Public Health and Community Medicine and the University of Washington School Medicine.

Julie Watts is with the Massachusetts Department of Public Health.

Marcia Weaver is with the University of Washington School of Public Health and Community Medicine.

Steve Wing is with the Department of Epidemiology, School of Public Health, University of North Carolina.

Introduction

Science with the People

Doug Brugge and H. Patricia Hynes

Background

In recent years there has been a growing interest in community research. While much of this work has been in other fields, the area of environmental health has seen its own burgeoning interest in research conducted at the community level with active participation by members of the community. We believe that this trend has been driven by the emergence of the environmental justice movement. Our experience and that of our colleagues who have engaged in multiple community collaborations is the basis for this book.

We have worked both together and on separate projects. The topical areas of the studies that we have done include lead contaminated soil, asthma and housing conditions, traffic injuries, the impact of development on environmental health, and the impact of radiation hazards on Native Americans. Several of the chapters herein report in detail on our work. Others are the work of colleagues we have met through our work who are engaged in similar collaborations and whose topics include local and regional air pollution, urban community gardens, urban rivers and industrial hog production. We make no claim that the work presented here is fully representative of the broader range of community-based environmental health projects. We do feel that there are multiple lessons that we and other researchers in the book have learned in the process and that these lessons will be of interest and instructive to students, researchers, community members and government agencies. Further, we feel that they are consistent with lessons put forward by others (Minkler and Wallerstein, 2003).

Indeed, we see in our students a constant demand for education about how to engage in the type of work that we do. Our students are both attracted to community research and perplexed by the seemingly steep challenges to such endeavors. Our students are particularly enthusiastic with our classes because we use real world, project based methods that give them opportunities to actually engage with communities in solution-oriented learning. The fact that community-collaborative research appears to enhance education and the student experience is a notable ancillary benefit to the original impulse that motivates such collaborations.

We find that the basic force driving change in the way that research is done in communities comes from the communities themselves. More and more, in our experience, communities demand that research that is relevant to their interests be conducted in such a way that they have input into the research process. They want to help set the research questions or hypotheses that will be tested. They want to participate in the research process by being hired on as staff. They want to be in the room when decisions that affect the analysis of the data are made. They want to have funding shared with them and research conducted that directly benefits them. And they absolutely insist that the results be reported back to them and that they have a chance to present *their* interpretation of the findings.

Given our interest over many years in forming research collaborations that are as equitable as possible with communities, we welcome the changes that we see around us. But even so, we have to acknowledge that there are innumerable challenges and that our students are correct to find navigation of the terrain of community research daunting. Our hope in publishing in one place this series of case studies is that they will be useful to persons engaged in community research, who are seeking more insight into their work, and to people just starting out, like our students.

Science for the People

Today's landscape is a sharp contrast to 20-30 years ago when the dominant paradigm among progressive academics in science was slanted more toward addressing the politics of the scientific process and the political role of scientists in conducting basic research than toward engaging in research with communities. In this modality, science was done "for" the people, rather than in collaboration "with" the community. A 1975 pamphlet put out by Science for the People reads in part:

> Science for the People means recognizing the political nature of science; it means access for all people to useful human knowledge; it means the organizing of women and men in science to struggle along with other communities aimed at fundamental social change.
>
> We are Science for the People.
>
> We are scientists, engineers, students, teachers, technicians and many others brought together by the common experience of frustration in our attempts to be socially productive human beings. We see the dehumanization and alienation of people as part of a social order of exploitation, racism, sexism and war. We seek to uncover the roots of the diseased social and economic order which [sic] fragments work and our lives. But our purpose is not merely to understand this system: it is to change it.
>
> Join us! You and we are part of the people science should be for.
> (Personal communication, Charles Schwartz, Professor Emeritus, Department of Physics, University of California, Berkeley)

Besides the more explicitly political tone of the times, the statement speaks to scientists in a more ideological (largely Marxist) framework than today's community-collaborative initiatives. It is about organizing scientists to join with and support the dominant movements of the time, the anti-war movement, the woman's movement, the Black power movement and the labor movement. The word "community" does come up, but it is not clear that it in any way refers to what today would be considered community-collaborative research.

In his autobiography, the Harvard University geneticist and long-time activist with Science for the People, Jon Beckwith, frames the choice he and others faced as either staying in science and addressing the social consequences of science or leaving science (Beckwith, 2002). While Beckwith reports having been involved in some community organizing, most notably with respect to Harvard's expansion into the adjacent Mission Hill community, such organizing was not connected to his research.

We believe that the work included in this book represents a third choice. The editors and contributors to this volume practice applied science, a path not explored by Beckwith. In many ways applied science is a satisfying solution for those desiring to bring social and political values to their work, but wanting to remain active researchers. In the realm of applied science, the real world impact of research is more immediate and the researcher has greater influence over how research findings are used in policy setting.

Today's Climate

Today's growth of interest in community research takes place at a time when the prevailing political winds are not so progressive and protest on campus and among academicians and scientists about global and national concerns is more muted than in the 1960s and 1970s. Indeed, recent analysis by Sheldon Krimsky highlights the fact that the academic enterprise is being pulled increasingly into for-profit ventures with negative impacts on the traditional role of the campus as a place for public interest research (Krimsky, 2003). It is interesting that the corporatization of the academy is on the rise at the same time that community-collaborative research is growing.

Nonetheless, outside of the universities, there has been a 20-fold surge of non-governmental organizations over the past 50 years as a civilian response to the political monocultures and monopolies of government and business (Runyan, 1999). From this strikingly heterogeneous "third sector," many unprecedented expressions of environmentalism have emerged. These include an environmentalism distinctly and popularly expressed in developing countries, as well as the environmental justice movement among urban and rural poor, blue collar communities and people of color in the United States. Both of these socially conscious expressions of environmentalism have arisen within the structural contexts of worldwide urbanization, industrial and economic globalization, and the proliferation of inexpensive telecommunications.[1]

Environmental Justice

The environmental justice movement in the United States has been a driving impetus for the expansion of community participation in environmental research because it has a strong community orientation. The environmental justice movement has goals that are not as all encompassing or as ideologically framed as those envisioned by Science for the People; but because the environmental justice movement emerged from the grassroots and continues to this day to be grounded in popular and local struggles, its unit of identity is largely the community and its goal is to remove the disproportionate burden of pollution on low-income communities and communities of color. Because addressing environmental problems easily leads into a thicket of technical details, and low-income communities rarely have the expertise to grapple with these technicalities, there emerge opportunities for collaboration between environmental justice communities and academic researchers.

While environmental justice has almost certainly been an issue for centuries (think of the early encounters between Native Americans and Europeans, for example), the conscious self-described environmental justice movement has more recent origins. Two activist struggles and two publications stand out as seminal markers of the emergence of the movement. In 1978 Lois Gibbs organized, with other blue-collar housewives and mothers, a successful protest to have families relocated from a neighborhood in Love Canal that had been built adjacent to a mile-long trench filled with industrial waste. Their action launched modern grassroots environmentalism based on "popular science," citizen protest, and making links between health and environmental pollution. In 1982 an African-American community in Warren County, North Carolina protested EPA's siting of a national landfill for the disposal of polychlorinated biphenyls (PCBs) in their community. The event sparked a sequence of studies and protests against the deliberate siting of waste facilities and "dirty" industries in poor communities of color, identifying the practice as *environmental racism.*

Toxic Wastes and Race in the United States, issued by the United Church of Christ in 1987 (United Church of Christ Commission for Racial Justice, 1987) and *Dumping in Dixie: Race, Class, and Environmental Quality*, written by Robert Bullard and published in 1990 (Bullard, 1990) were instrumental in forging a nationwide and cohesive movement out of what had been localized activist struggles largely invisible to much of the public, university researchers included. In 1991 hundreds of delegates from every state in the United States attended the first People of Color Environmental Leadership Summit in Washington, D.C. The conference created a national visibility for the issue of environmental justice and culminated with a set of principles of environmental justice that have been the cornerstone of environmental justice work. In 1994, President Clinton issued Executive Order 12898 which directed each federal agency to make the achievement of environmental justice a part of its mission, a measure of the immense impact of the movement on federal government consciousness.

In subsequent years the issue of environmental justice has gained wide recognition and grown in strength. The idea of organizing low income communities and/or communities of color around environmental issues has even changed the conception of what is the environment in many circles. No longer is environment seen as only or primarily rain forests and whales. Nor is environment so tied to the traditional media-based approach of air, water and soil employed by government agencies. The impact of the urban center and the lived environment on human beings has been brought to the fore. Housing and school building conditions, roadway construction, trashy vacant lots and traffic emerge as critical problems alongside toxic waste dumps and polluting factories. It is the social environment, the lived environment, the built environment as well as the physical environment about which environmental justice is most often concerned.

Communities taking up the call for environmental justice build on the activist tradition of the civil rights movement of the 1950s and 1960s. Thus, this is not a sterile demand for technical solutions. Rather, it is a broad call for justice emphasizing the empowerment of the people affected, the re-distribution of resources, and the principle that all people – regardless of race, class and gender – have equal right to a safe and healthful environment. Environmental justice strains at the boundaries of what is "environment" because there are so many pressing issues in these communities. And these activists are not likely to sit back and let the "experts" frame the problem and determine the solution. Expert is, in their eyes, often a questionable designation in the first place since it emanates from the very sources of power that they see as oppressive. Too often environmental justice communities find that the traditional experts are wrong or on the wrong side. They don't trust the experts and, at a minimum, want to engage researchers and other professionals on an equal footing. Thus, when such communities see the need for research or see value in a proposed study that is brought to them, they are motivated to negotiate terms that fall into one or another of the various forms of community collaboration.

Such arrangements can be as simple as research on issues of interest to the community, which is traditional in most respects, but which stems from the community's request/demand that their problem be studied, to more fully participatory research. The chapters in this book result from projects that fall at various points along what we regard as a continuum of community-collaborative research. While some may argue that one end of the spectrum is superior to the other, we regard each community and each study included here as valuable community-collaborative research with the possibility that differing models of collaboration may be appropriate in different settings. To us, the bottom line is a shift from serving the people (a client model or science "for the people") to the community as partner or *science with the people*.

Who is the Community?

The intense interest in community research has at times leapt ahead of a clear notion of what does or does not constitute a community. This superficially simple point is actually not so easy to answer. Below we list a few definitions that we have found:

> Com-mu-ni-ty\ ke-my-net-e\ n, pl –ties [ME comunete, fr. MF comunete, fr. L communitat-, communitas, fr. Communis] 1: a unified body of individuals: as a: STATE COMMONWEALTH b: the people with common interests living in a particular area; broadly: the area itself <the problems of a large~> c: an interacting population of various kinds of individuals (as species) in a common location d: a group of people with a common characteristic or interest living together within a larger society < a~ of retired persons> e: a group linked by a common policy f: a body of persons or nations having a common history or common social, economic, and political interests < the international ~> g: a body of persons of common and esp. professional interests scattered through a larger society <the academic~> 2: society at large 3 a: joint ownership or participation <~of goods> b: common character: likeness <~of interest> c: social activity: FELLOWSHIP d: a social state or condition.
>
> (Webster's Ninth New Collegiate Dictionary, 1984)

> Community refers to populations that may be defined by geography, race, ethnicity, gender, sexual orientation, common interest or cause, such as health or service agencies and organizations, practitioners, policy makers, or lay public groups with public health concerns.
>
> (CDC- Notice of Availability of Funds 2002)

Community-based research is research that is conducted by, with, or for communities (e.g., with civic, grassroots, or worker groups throughout civil society). This research differs from the bulk of the research and development (R&D) conducted in the United States, most of which – at a total cost of about $170 billion per year – is performed on behalf of business, the military, the federal government, or in pursuit of the scientific and academic communities' intellectual interests.

    (Loka Institute http://www.loka.org/CRN/execsumm.pdf. accessed 12/18/03)

The results of our analysis point to a core definition of community as *a group of people with diverse characteristics who are linked by social ties, share common perspectives, and engage in joint action in geographical locations or settings.*

    (MacQueen et al., 2001)

We like the last definition. All of the communities with which we work have had some aspect of geographic boundaries, even if not all the community members lived within the boundary. Likewise, we feel that social ties and joint action are necessary to forge a community out of people who would otherwise simply be living and working in proximity to each other. More problematic is the issue of shared perspectives and who speaks for the community. We have tended to work with community-based organizations that meet the above definition and that speak at least for a prominent sector of the community, but that may or may not speak for all members of the community, if that is even possible. Finally, while environmental justice communities may share common perspectives on environmental insults and environmental goals, they may diverge on other social issues or political strategies.

Science with the People

With the growth of environmental justice and community participation in research, both within and beyond the environmental health area, has come increasing respectability. While it is true that participatory research is by no means the dominant approach, and while it is also true that environmental justice research is still a fraction of environmental research, there has been substantial progress. The change is reflected in the literature. Recently the journal *Science* carried an article on protecting communities (as opposed to the prevailing notion that one protects individuals) in biomedical research (Weijer and Emanuel, 2000). A whole issue of the federal government published journal, *Public Health Reports* (2000), was devoted to partnerships with communities. The first issue of the new CDC journal, *Preventing Chronic Disease*, featured a number of articles on community-based research. And numerous other authors have written articles that begin to set a theoretical and methodological basis for a community role in research collaborations (Israel et al, 1998; Baker et al., 1999; Schensul, 1999).

    Funding for community collaborative research, environmental justice and the two combined increased throughout the 1990s. Today there is a steady stream of requests for proposals from the National Institutes of Health, the Environmental Protection Agency and the Centers for Disease Control and Prevention that *requires* the proponent to have community partners. The annual National Institute of Environmental Health Sciences RFA for environmental justice community collaborations is a prime example of this trend in environmental science (O'Fallon et al., 2003; Minkler and Wallerstein, 2003).

Another example, albeit one that is broader than environment or environmental justice, is the Community-Campus Partnerships for Health at the University of California, San Francisco that describes itself thus:

> ... a nonprofit organization that promotes health through partnerships between communities and higher educational institutions. In just five years, we have grown to a network of over 1000 communities and campuses that are collaborating to promote health through service-learning, community-based research, community service and other partnership strategies. These partnerships are powerful tools for improving health professional education, civic responsibility and the overall health of communities.
> (http://www.futurehealth.ucsf.edu/ccph.html, accessed 3/6/02)

Further, college and graduate classes that focus on community collaboration or environmental justice abound. We cannot quantify their growth because they have not been cataloged as such (although this should be researched). Besides teaching such classes ourselves and seeing first hand the interest and demand among students for such classes, we have many colleagues doing the same on other campuses. One of the co-authors recently received the national Delta Omega Award for Innovative Curriculum from the public health honor society for her community-collaborative and project-based course, Urban Environmental Health, a testament to the timeliness and relevance of our book's topic.[2] In short, the time is ripe for introspection and analysis, for assessing and promoting community research in a variety of ways. We hope this book will be one of those ways.

Summary of the Book

This volume is a compilation of case studies that we have either personally been involved in or that we have invited from our colleagues. The cases examine the nature and form that the community collaboration took, the scientific design and findings from the work and the ethical issues that had to be dealt with. Many of the chapters were previously published in the peer reviewed public health literature. A few are published here for the first time.

We divide the book into four topical areas: housing, open space, urban development, and transportation, and environmental exposure. About half of the chapters report findings from studies, the other half are concerned more with reporting on the process and/or methods used. Most of the studies in this volume involved providing funding to the community and an active role in decision-making. The main exception is chapter 10, a regional study of air pollution in California that, while responding to community determined research question, did not engage a small geographical community in the way that the other studies did.

Most of the chapters report on studies that engaged in community-based participatory research. We chose deliberately, however, not to limit the volume to such studies. In our experience, there are non-participatory forms of research with communities that are also valid, and in some cases, most appropriate. The traffic injury study of Boston Chinatown (Chapter 8) is such an example. It is better described as research commissioned by community partners who were busy and understaffed and preferred to have the work done for them, somewhat as a company or city agency might hire a consultant.

Most of the studies reported here were conducted in response to community requests or demands. However, we do not think that all good community-collaborations have to start with the community approaching the researchers. In our experience, there are instances where university partners first raised the idea of the study that led to solid and mutually beneficial collaborations. A case in point is our Healthy Public Housing Initiative. In HPHI there was activity and interest both in the community and at local universities, but it was the editors of this volume, the university partners, who first brought the idea of a research partnership to the community and to city agencies.

Community collaborations may be with either community-based agencies, such as community health centers and service agencies or with more grassroots entities, such as resident associations and small advocacy groups. This distinction is not commented on in most of the literature on community collaborative research. Several of the studies reported here, included grassroots partners and trained and employed residents (as opposed to activists or agency staff) in their research. These include the pilot study to the Healthy Public Housing Initiative described in Chapter 1, the study of diesel exhaust in East Harlem described in Chapter 9 and the work with Native American tribes downwind from the US nuclear test site in Nevada, which is described in Chapter 11.

Many of the studies reported had substantial regional and federal funding from the US National Institutes of Environmental Health Sciences or the US Environmental Protection Agency. These include the survey research in public housing (Chapter 1), research ethics study of HPHI (Chapter 2), the Seattle Healthy Homes project (Chapter 3), the lead safe yards project (Chapter 5), the Harlem study of diesel exhaust (Chapter 9), the regional air pollution study (Chapter 10), the nuclear risk management for Native Communities project (Chapter 11), and the hog production study (Chapter 12). Some of the studies managed to produce results published in peer-reviewed journals with only limited funds from small grants (Chapters 7 and 8). Some of the chapters would best be described as pilot studies leading to larger follow-up studies. Chapter 1 is a pilot study that helped create the Healthy Public Housing Initiative, a large multi-year intervention study. The most significant outcome of one of the studies of Boston Chinatown, Chapters 7, was that it developed methods for conducting survey research in that community. Chapter 4 is a narrative description of the early stages of developing a university-community partnership.

It is also notable that the chapters fall into several research methodologies. Some utilized interviews (Chapter 2, 11), observation (Chapter 4), and/or survey questionnaires (Chapters 1, 6, 7, 11). Others collected physical measurements of environmental parameters (Chapters 3, 5, 9). Still others analyzed existing databases (Chapters 8, 10). Two of the chapters describe early stages of intervention studies (Chapters 2, 3).

Chapters 2 and 12 address the topic of the ethics of community-collaborative research. Chapter 2 is a qualitative study of perceptions of research ethics within the Healthy Public Housing Initiative that we co-direct. Chapter 12 is a narrative telling of an ethical conflict encountered by a community participatory study of hog production in North Carolina. Over the last 25 years, grassroots environmental organizations and the environmental justice movement have challenged the federal and state governments and university researchers to conduct research that is relevant, transparent, accountable and collaborative. Communities have pushed to have the evidence of their lived experience taken into consideration. Numerous models of community collaborative research have arisen, ranging from scientists working with the research questions of the community to scientists training community members as researchers. The studies assembled in this book span this continuum and offer insights into how to do environmental and public health research that engages the community as partner. The rise of community research, variably called community-based and community-based participatory research, gives scientists the opportunity to integrate social justice with sound science.

Notes

1   In these national and international community-based movements, women are often a plurality of members, leaders, and strategists, an undoubted consequence of the global women's movement over the past 30 years (Hynes 1998). An international survey of public attitudes about the environment, commissioned by the United Nations Environment Programme, found that women across the world, in industrial and developing countries alike, express more concern over the state of the environment than do men. They also favor more stringent environmental laws and more public spending for environmental protection than do men (Seager 1993). Some of the emergent NGOs are nationwide environmental organizations. The Natural Resources Defense Council is a good example of one that is activist and relatively prominent. But the NRDC and its fellow environmental organizations are not about fundamental social change in the way that Science for the People was. These are reform organizations that seek to improve the system often by addressing single-issue causes. Further, they are less interested in grassroots organizing than they are in policy analysis and Washington DC level politics. There is a role for academic researchers with the national environmental organizations as technical advisors, but not usually as research partners with communities.
2   The 2003 award was given to H. Patricia Hynes and Russ Lopez (course instructors) and Rob Schadt (course advisor in educational technology).

Acknowledgments

We would like to thank Hassanatu Blake, Chris Chinn and Mahrukh Mohiuddin for assistance with preparing the manuscript. Doug Brugge's effort was partially supported by a faculty fellowship from the University College for Citizenship and Public Service at Tufts University.

References

Baker, E.A., Homan, S., Schonhoff, R., Kreuter, M. (1999), "Principles of practice for academic/practice/community research partnerships," *American Journal of Preventive Medicine*, **16**, 86–93.
Beckwith, J. (2002), *Making genes making waves: A social activist in science*, Cambridge: Harvard University Press.

Bullard, R. (1990), *Dumping in Dixie: Race, class, and environmental quality*, Boulder: Westview Press.

Hynes, H.P. (1998), "The many and the few", in Mankiller, W., Mink, G., Navarro, M., Smith, B. and Steinem, G. (eds), *The Reader's companion to U.S. women's history*, Boston: Houghton Mifflin.

Israel, B.A., Schulz, A.J., Parker, E.A. (1998), "Review of community-based research: Assessing partnership approaches to improve public health," *Annual Review of Public Health*, **19**, 173–202.

Krimsky, S. (2003), *Science in the private interest: Has the lure of profits corrupted biomedical research?* New York: Rowman & Littlefield Publishers, Inc.

MacQueen, K.M., McLellan, E., Metzger, D.S., Kegeles, S., Strauss, R.P., Scotti, R., Blanchard, L., Trotter, R.T. (2001), "What is community? An evidence-based definition for participatory public health," *American Journal of Public Health*, **91**, 1929–38.

Minkler, M. and Wallerstein, N. (eds) (2003), Community-based participatory research for health, San Francisco, CA: Jossey-Bass, a Wiley Imprint.

O'Fallon, L.R., Wolfle, G.M., Brown, D., Dearry, A., Olden, K. (2003), "Strategies for setting a national research agenda that is responsive to community needs," *Environmental Health Perspectives*, **111**, 1855–60.

Runyan, C. (1999), "Action on the front lines", *WorldWatch*, Nov/Dec: 12–21.

Schensul, J.J. (1999), "Organizing community research partnerships in the struggle against AIDS," *Health Education and Behavior*, **26**, 266–83.

Seager, J. (1993), *Earth follies: Coming to feminist terms with the global environmental crisis*, New York: Routledge.

United Church of Christ Commission for Racial Justice (1987), *Toxic wastes and race in the United States: a national study of racial and socioeconomic characteristics of communities with hazardous waste sites*, New York: United Church of Christ.

Weijer, C., Emanuel, E.J. (2000), "Protecting communities in biomedical research," *Science*, **289**, 1142–44.

SECTION A:
HOUSING

Chapter 1

Public Health and the Physical Environment in Boston Public Housing: A Community-Based Survey and Action Agenda

H. Patricia Hynes, Doug Brugge, Julie Watts and Jody Lally

Give me a million pounds for the care of my patients, and I would spend it on improving their housing.
(Dr. Jarman, GP in the Paddington area, London, cited in Ambrose and Hill, *Bad Housing: Counting the Cost*)

Introduction

Health in its many kindred forms – the health of people and families; community health; healthy homes; and clean, secure neighborhoods – has proven to be a unifying ideal and organizing issue, particularly in urban communities, for more than a century. The acute conditions of 19th century tenements and factory neighborhoods, which catalyzed public health and housing reform measures, have been eliminated from U.S. cities. However, a confluence of economic and social forces has siphoned off resources and opportunities from older center cities: the exodus of white middle and working class to suburbs; corporate relocation away from center cities to suburban office parks and developing countries; "redlining" of urban neighborhoods; and federal cutbacks in aid to cities (Drier, 1992). Consequently, during the latter half of this century, the urban poor have been concentrated and ghetto-ized in substandard housing in inner cities, without a secure employment base and adequate public services.

We are witnessing today a resurgence of engagement in the ideals of healthy cities and healthy communities, precipitated in part by a new social movement – environmental justice – which has expanded the parameters of environmental health to include the physical, social and built environments of inner-city neighborhoods. Environmental justice arose in the 1980s and 1990s as a new archetype of environmental protection. While using conventional tools of environmental analysis (such as sampling and measuring of contaminants, exposure assessment and comparative risk assessment) and the force of environmental law, environmental justice introduces new dimensions to older environmental frameworks. These dimensions include bringing a consciousness of race, class and gender – with a strong emphasis on the needs of low-income communities of color – to environmental analysis research, remedial action and resource allocation (Capek, 1993).

Additionally environmental justice adds a *place-based* and community-based focus to the traditional locus of environmental protection in the media of air, water and soil. Redressing environmental injustice, then, includes economic and political empowerment as well as environmental protection for communities inequitably burdened by poverty and pollution. The integration of social justice and community well-being with mainstream environmental protection and public health goals has altered structurally the progressive environmental health agenda: improving the living conditions of poor people in urban areas has gained equal standing with watershed protection and the provision of safe drinking water.

Historically those working in the fields of public health, urban planning and environmental health found common cause in the human health crises of the urban poor because their daily living conditions were primary determinants of their health. Late nineteenth and early twentieth century reforms brought sanitation, central water supply, building code, fresh air through ventilation in buildings and central parks to urban areas. Federally-funded public housing was first built in the late 1930s, following more than two decades of housing activism, to provide "decent, safe and sanitary dwellings for families of low income ..." because private market forces failed to do so (Ladner Birch, 1978). Thanks to the talented and unremitting work of Catherine Bauer and Edith Elmer Wood (pioneers of publicly-supported housing for those who could not afford decent market housing), lofty and comprehensive principles of neighborhood design informed the early policy and construction of public housing. These included: A minimum of street traffic; an abundance of open space, playgrounds and parks; buildings for community activities; and proximity to work. Building a neighborhood community, not merely individual housing units, was the guiding design principle, as prescribed by Bauer and Wood, for the first 300 projects constructed between 1937 and 1941.

However, in the majority of cities today (and Boston has been no exception), the image, reputation and reality of public housing has fallen from the founding standard of the Wagner-Steagall Act – "decent, safe, and sanitary dwellings" – to that of an unsafe, unhealthful and undesirable living environment. Often isolated by siting, cheaply built, usually ugly and chronically ill-maintained (all opposites of the original physical and social blueprint for public housing), public housing has, in many cases, become a contributor to bad health by its poor physical conditions; its cluster of social ills that arise in a culture of concentrated, no-exit poverty; and its resultant stigma.[1]

This study, *Public Health in Boston Public Housing*, was undertaken to document the public health status of public housing and its residents for two compelling reasons. First, the alarming rise in asthma incidence, particularly in inner city neighborhoods, is victimizing children and families already struggling with other environmental health issues, including lead poisoning, and social crises such as poverty and lack of affordable housing and health care. Like lead poisoning, asthma provokes questions about the nexus of health and housing conditions. Second, public housing can be a locus of action and intervention for a number of strategic reasons. Located near community health centers, having tenant task forces, and centrally administered and financed by a housing authority responsible for building maintenance and renovation, public housing holds the potential for collaborative projects whose goal is to improve the health of low-income people through improving their housing.

Health and Housing: The Nexus

In February 1998 the Doc4Kids Project at the Boston Medical Center released their report *Not Safe at Home: How America's Housing Crisis Threatens the Health of Its Children* (Doc4Kids, 1998). Based on clinical experience and an extensive search of medical literature, pediatricians documented the links between unsafe and unhealthy homes, homelessness, and poor children's health crises, namely asthma and respiratory diseases, lead poisoning, injuries and malnutrition. Extrapolating from smaller studies where large data sets were lacking, the authors estimate the cumulative impact of inadequate housing on children's health in the United States. Three housing-related health conditions most relevant for our study are:

Asthma
- Hospitalizations per year for asthma among inner-city children ages 4–9 attributable to cockroach infestation – 17 849

Injuries
- Burns to children from exposed radiators per year – 1485

Lead Poisoning
- Approximate number of IQ points that will be lost to lead poisoning among children ages 1-5 in the United States – 2.5 million

Injuries

The overall findings of *Not Safe at Home* support public health studies which have systematically demonstrated that poorly maintained housing is strongly linked with childhood injuries and lead poisoning, and that damp, mouldy, indoor environments are associated with increased respiratory disease and asthma. A 1974 study of injuries to children associated with consumer products, for example, estimated that two out of three childhood injuries take place in the home. Ninety-one percent of injuries to children under 5 years of age occurred at home. Residential building conditions and design, including structural elements and defects such as faulty fire detection systems, windows without screens and window guards, steam radiators without covers, high-temperature hot water, missing balusters and insufficient lighting were strong determinants of injuries (Gallagher et al., 1985). In analyzing surveillance data on lead poisoning, the Centers for Disease Control has identified the key housing-related criteria in high-risk neighborhoods: pre-1950 housing that is in poor condition (*Screening Young Children for Lead Poisoning*, 1997).

Dampness and Respiratory Health

Dampness is linked to health consequences because of its potential to increase moulds and dust mites, both of which are allergenic. Numerous studies have examined the relationship between dampness and mould in the home and respiratory health. The majority has focused on children because of the confounding effects on adult respiratory health of active smoking and occupational exposures.

The results of a health and housing questionnaire mailed to teachers for distribution to parents and guardians of 600 school-age children in 24 communities in the United States and Canada revealed the prevalence of dampness conditions in homes to be between 40 and 60 percent. The study found that increased respiratory conditions are associated with dampness and mould (Spengler et al., 1994a). The same principal investigator found a significant association between upper respiratory and bronchitic symptoms and home dampness in a questionnaire administered through teachers to 9000 school age children in West Virginia (Spengler et al., 1994b). A case-control study conducted among Dutch children found significantly increased sensitization to dust mites and/or moulds among children living in damp housing when compared to children in non-damp housing (Verhoeff et al., 1995). Other investigators report that wheeze, cough, bronchitis and other chest illnesses in children are associated with damp housing whether or not mould is visible (Brunekreef et al., 1989). In a parent-administered questionnaire that included parental as well as childhood respiratory symptoms, Brunekreef found that the association between home dampness and respiratory symptoms reported for children also applies to adults (Brunekreef, 1992).

Chemical Exposures in Home Environment

Recent focus on the indoor environment has expanded the scope of environmental health protection to include the home environment as well as the workplace and ecosystems, based on the amount of time people spend indoors as well as the degraded conditions of housing for the poor. According to the U.S. Environmental Protection Agency, people in industrial countries spend about 90 percent of their time indoors, with infants, the elderly and those with chronic illnesses staying inside even more. Contaminants found in the indoor environment range from environmental tobacco smoke and other combustion products to biologicals such as dust mites and moulds; volatile organic compounds; and lead, asbestos and radon. Poor ventilation and lack of fresh air exchange result in indoor air that concentrates particles, moisture, microbes and chemical vapors that commonly harm the respiratory system and lung (American Lung Association et al., 1994).

Building materials used in the indoor environment have been found to be detrimental to health. Danish researchers investigated the question of whether particle board impacted children's health. The results of a questionnaire sent to more than 1000 households showed that children living in a home with a large amount of particle board had higher risk of headache, irritation of the throat, and the need for daily antiasthmatic medication than those with low or no particle board (Daugbjerg, 1988).

Between 1980 and 1990, the U.S. EPA undertook a series of studies, known as the TEAM studies, to measure human exposure in indoor and outdoor air, food and drinking water to a set of common pollutants. With the results from a probabilistic sample of 3000 persons in a dozen geographical areas, they concluded that "the most important sources of pollution are small and close to the person" (Wallace, 1995). Benzene is a case in point: although atmospheric benzene is produced by auto combustion (82 percent of total), petrochemical refineries and plants (14 percent), with the remaining sources being personal and home products (3 percent) and cigarettes (0.1 percent), the TEAM studies found that almost half of people's exposure to benzene, a known carcinogen, came from smoking, due to the small volume of air close to the source.

With the TEAM findings, EPA concluded that sources in the home – such as dry-cleaned clothes, household deodorizers and pesticides, cigarette smoke, contaminated dust tracked in from outside, chloroform from chlorinated hot shower and cooking water, PAHs from cooking – can result in greater human exposure than industrial and outdoor sources because of "efficiency of delivery" and the small volume of air in the home coupled with lack of indoor ventilation. The TEAM studies calculated upper-bound lifetime cancer risks from 33 carcinogenic chemicals and pesticides commonly found in the homes studied and found that "indoor exposures account for about 85 percent of the total cancer risk" (Wallace, 1995).

Many involved in researching and improving the indoor environment have noted that environmental regulations have, to date, regulated pollutants discharged to outdoor air, water and soil; but that the same pollutants entering or emitted in the indoor home (and office) environment are, for the most part, unregulated. Indoor environment problems may result from inferior building design, dirty or malfunctioning heating and cooling systems, and inadequate building maintenance; from home furnishings and consumer products which are regulated at the time of manufacturing but which, nonetheless, may pose a health hazard when used in the home; and from occupant activities, such as smoking and tracking in dirt and dust. The findings of the TEAM studies have suggested measures that people can take to reduce the risks in homes:

- Eliminate smoking indoors
- Avoid home deodorizer products
- Minimize dry cleaning and air dry-cleaned clothing out of doors
- Replace household cleaners with less toxic brands
- Take off shoes entering the home or install a walk-in mat; and
- Employ exhaust fans in kitchens and bathrooms.[2]

Public Housing and Health

"Bad Housing" and Health

In a project entitled *Health Gains in Housing*, Dr. Peter Ambrose, director of urban regional research at University of Sussex, compared "sickness episodes" in residents of high-quality public housing in West London with those of residents in low-quality public housing in East London. "Sickness episodes" among those in better quality housing were 1/7 of those in poor quality housing. Damp, poor heating and pest infestations were associated with more illness days among residents in low-quality housing (*Home Is Where the Hurt Is*, 1997). In a subsequent position paper on the cost-effectiveness of safe, well-maintained public housing, Ambrose and co-author Stephen Hill present a typology of costs, including housing repair; health, police and emergency services; drug, crime and other social ills, which are associated with bad housing. They argue that the costs of failing to provide decent homes in stable environments to families – in the forms of ill health, under achievement, crime and vandalism – will far exceed the investment in adequate maintenance and repair of housing (Ambrose and Hill, 1996).

Dampness and Mould

One of the strongest study designs of the relationship between dampness and mould growth and symptomatic ill health among residents in public housing is a cross-sectional study of households with children that was conducted in public housing in Glasgow, Edinburgh and London (Platt et al., 1989). Separate and independent assessments of housing and health were carried out by trained housing and health researchers, minimizing respondent and interviewer bias. Adults and children alike living in damp and mouldy dwellings reported more symptoms overall, including nausea, vomiting, wheeze, sore throat, runny nose and headaches. The number of symptoms was positively associated with increasing severity of damp and mould, and a dose-response relationship was found. All of these associations persisted after possible confounding conditions, such as household income, smoking, unemployment and overcrowding, were controlled for.

Heat

Uncontrollable heat and high heat sources, such as steam radiators, are potential health risks in public housing. Radiator-related burns among children in Chicago public housing were reported in a 1996 case series report (Quinlan, 1996). After clinicians who treated the children alerted the Chicago Housing Authority and tenants' association, units were inspected and radiator covers were installed. The inspection revealed that only 14 percent of radiators had proper covers.

While heat stress-related disorders have been studied in the workplace, no studies were found on the effect of overheating in public housing. However, a number of heat-related studies are suggestive of potential health impacts, such as fatigue, of chronic overheating in the home. One experimental study measuring the effect of high heat on sleep found that heat caused restless and less efficient sleeping (Di Nisi et al., 1989). In a surveillance study, the CDC constructed dot maps showing clustering of heat-related deaths among elderly persons. Some, but not all of the risk factors, include relative poverty and highly urbanized settings (Martinez et al., 1989). Overheating in winter, combined with low relative humidity, causes drying and irritation of the mucous membranes which encourages rhinitis and respiratory infections (Lowry, 1989).

In searching the health and housing literature for studies on health in public housing, one researcher concludes that, with a few exceptions, notably British research, "studies of public housing are largely confined to those that look at health behaviors and mental illness" (Souza, 1997). Yet, even with the handful of studies cited here, what is unequivocally clear is that a "clinical" response – whether doctor diagnosing a patient illness, or a master home environmentalist advising a tenant as *consumer* and indoor *occupant* – is insufficient for public housing residents. The nexus of health and housing calls for structural and interdisciplinary solutions. The documented human impacts of poor housing and poverty, such as depression, high number of sick days, chronic respiratory illness and so on, do require medical attention. But the enduring solution – "safe, secure, and sanitary housing" – requires a collaborative response from housing, public health and urban planning institutions, a response which begins with a systematic survey of housing and health conditions.

Project Overview

Studies of health and housing, in the United States and Great Britain, have consistently demonstrated associations between poorly maintained housing, contaminated indoor air and ill health. The *Public Health in Boston Public Housing* project focuses on indoor environmental health in West Broadway Housing in South Boston, one of three housing developments in that neighborhood and one of 68 public housing developments managed by the Boston Housing Authority (BHA). The overall goal of this project is to develop a model survey and plan of action, based on the principles of successful university-community partnerships, with the aim of public housing improvement and community environmental health promotion. Once demonstrated in West Broadway Housing, the model can be adapted to other housing developments.[3]

The partners involved in this program are Boston University School of Public Health, West Broadway Tenant Task Force, South Boston Neighborhood Health Center and Tufts University School of Medicine. The Boston Housing Authority has supported the project through providing access to records and demographic data and agreeing to participate in the Advisory Board. The project was supported by funding from the U.S. Environmental Protection Agency Region I and grows out of Boston University School of Public Health's Urban Environmental Health Initiative.

Specific components of the Public Health in Public Housing project include:

1   Training teams of public housing tenants and health center staff in environmental health issues of the indoor environment and in the use of an indoor environment survey tool.
2   Documenting conditions in a representative sample of West Broadway Housing units by using the survey tool, to be carried out by the tenant-health center teams.
3   Analyzing the survey data, using statistical software, and incorporating relevant elements of the state housing code and childhood injury prevention guidelines into the analysis.
4   Developing a plan of action, based on survey results, for indoor environment improvements and improved maintenance by the BHA in West Broadway Housing.
5   Designing and implementing participatory methods of educating and involving tenants in environmental health promotion and informing them of the range of

medical, social and educational services available through the South Boston Neighborhood Health Center.

Methods

This cross-sectional study of the indoor environment at West Broadway Housing builds on an education project consisting of a 15-hour course for West Broadway tenants and health center staff conducted in 1997. The course included instruction on physical, chemical and biological indoor contaminants and hazards, a walk-through of tenants' apartments, and the development of an indoor environment survey instrument and elementary mapping tool. We piloted the survey with the tenants and health center staff in order to receive their feedback on the survey questions and parameters and also to train them in conducting the survey.

Community-Based Research

Throughout the training of tenants and health workers, their conducting of surveys, and the resultant community health promotion program that is currently in process, we have employed principles of community-based research. These principles include a receptivity toward the knowledge and "local theory" of community and health center participants; sharing of skills and knowledge; just compensation to community members for work done on the project; gathering data for the purposes of education, action and social change; the inclusion of social and environmental determinants of health as well as behavioral ones; and sharing results with the tenants and health center staff. (Israel et al., 1998).

Tenants' knowledge and experience living in West Broadway influenced the survey: discussions with the residents, during our training and the walkthrough of their apartments, resulted in our adding questions in a number of categories, including heating, appliances and building maintenance. A recommendation from one health worker resulted in our including the section of questions on child safety. Skills and knowledge were shared in the spirit of demystifying principles of indoor environment and to enable tenants to conduct the surveys in as professional a manner as possible. They, in turn, gave feedback during the trainings and after the surveys were completed about survey questions which were ambiguous or awkwardly constructed. Our survey is clearer and more reliable, as a consequence. We reimbursed tenants for their participation with a fair market hourly wage, in recognition of their skilled work for the project. Finally, from the onset we clarified that the goal of the project was to generate representative data for the purpose of improving the conditions of buildings and building maintenance for the sake of improved health – in other words, knowledge for the sake of positive community action. We helped build the capacity in the health center to win funding for follow-up education and action programs with interested tenants participating, thus strengthening the collaboration among partners. (These programs are described in the final section.)

The Public Health in Public Housing survey has 19 categories with 142 questions. The categories encompass the commonly researched and surveyed aspects of indoor environment relating to ill health, including asthma triggers and factors associated with other respiratory illnesses, as well as those building conditions most linked with injury and illness. We included a set of questions on maintenance staff and maintenance history and also the tenant task force to ascertain the tenants' experience with and evaluation of each.

Survey Population

We chose West Broadway Housing in South Boston as the site for the pilot training and survey for a series of reasons. Over 25 percent of South Boston residents live in public housing; and the majority of housing residents use the South Boston Neighborhood Health Center. Thus our work in West Broadway Housing could be replicated in the other South Boston housing developments in collaboration with the health center and BHA tenant task forces. Another determining factor was the timing of the new community-based health initiatives in South Boston. The South Boston Neighborhood Health Center was launching a Public Health Initiative that could serve as an umbrella and, eventually, proponent of this project. Further, the Tobacco Control Project of the Public Health Initiative had previously worked with a cohort of West Broadway tenants in an asthma education training and has an innovative, community-wide campaign around smoking which would link naturally with this project. We were also advised by the Boston Housing Authority that the West Broadway Tenant Task Force was active and would most likely take great interest in the project.

In October 1994, *U.S. News and World Report* named the census tracts containing the South Boston housing developments as one of 15 "white underclass" neighborhoods in the United States ("The White Underclass"), where "white underclass neighborhood" was defined as an urban area comprising at least two contiguous census tracts in which a majority of residents were white non-Hispanic, 40 or more percent were living in poverty, and more than 300 white, female-heads of households lived with their children. Since the early 1990s the developments have been rapidly integrated by the BHA, as a result of a class action lawsuit against the authority. Today, the 7500 residents of the three housing developments are approximately 49 percent white, 25 percent African-American, 15 percent Latino, and 11 percent Asian. Like public housing overall, the majority heads-of-household are women, due to the greater poverty of poor women with children.

In the year we initiated this project, many of the themes that plague public housing – social alienation, social tension and victimization – erupted in South Boston. A number of white teenage males committed suicide in West Broadway and Old Colony Housing. About the same time, newspapers reported crackdowns on organized drug trafficking in the same projects. In response to racist incidents against Latino families at Old Colony Housing, the Boston Housing Authority evicted families of the young white men responsible for the incidents. This decisive action followed a protracted series of complaints by Latinas in Old Colony Housing of harassment on the part of white residents there (Abraham, 1997). In July 1999, the BHA agreed to pay $1.5 million in a settlement with minority tenant plaintiffs in South Boston and Charlestown public housing who had filed a federal class action lawsuit citing assault and harassment in the BHA developments (Flint 1999).

While newspapers covered the "negatives," we found notable assets in West Broadway Housing. The Tenant Task Force was highly interested in the survey and lent full support to the effort, promoting it by word of mouth. Social networks among women residents enabled us to survey a representative sample of 50 residents easily and rapidly. In the serial community meetings now taking place for follow-up health programs to address smoking and asthma, attendance by West Broadway residents has been large, enthusiastic and sustained.

Survey Sample

West Broadway Housing consists of 691 apartment units in 27 buildings. Built in the late-1940s, at a period of cost-cutting in public housing, they are repetitious, three-story (for the most part) brick "boxes" which resemble – and may have been – temporary military housing built after World War II. Renovations of most of the buildings have been done in stages, with each stage differing in the extent of work. Some of the renovations have added attractive cosmetic touches, such as rooflines and overhangs that relieve the boxiness, two-toned exterior paint, and grounds improvements. Buildings that have not yet been renovated are either closed or sparsely inhabited. Currently 540 housing units are occupied.

Using a random number function in Microsoft Excel, we generated a simple random sample of 80 residential units. A mailing, in multiple languages (English, Spanish, Vietnamese and Chinese), to the 80 units resulted in two respondents for the survey. The survey teams then contacted the residents in the sample by knocking on doors. Once 50 residents from the sample agreed to participate, they terminated the outreach effort.

Each survey was conducted by a team of two, one from the health center and the other from West Broadway Housing. In two cases, a student from BU School of Public Health conducted the survey in Spanish. The team verified certain responses (such as size of cracks and water stains) through visual inspection and also marked a simple map to indicate the floor and room in which structural problems occurred. Health conditions were self-reported by the respondent.

Survey Results

Survey data was stored at BU School of Public Health in Epi Info, a software package developed by the Centers for Disease Control and Prevention, and transferred to SAS for statistical analysis. Descriptive statistical analysis presented in Table 1.1 summarizes the public health problems that cluster primarily around the physical conditions of the building and apartments: water leaks, moisture and mould; uncontrolled heating and surfaces that burn the skin; insufficient ventilation; lead paint remaining in some apartments; and sanitation in public areas.

Table 1.1   Summary of key physical environment concerns

Leaks, Moisture and Mould	64%	Leaks from ceiling, wall, radiators, toilet, tub or sink
	20%	Mould growth
Ventilation and Heating	46%	Not enough fresh air in apartment
	72%	No exhaust fan in bathroom or fan is not working
	66%	Apartment is too hot in winter
	82%	Leave window open in winter
	32%	Use oven to heat apartment
	26%	Air conditioning and heat on in winter
Sanitation and Infestation	48%	Visible indications of cockroaches in the building
	35%	Visible indications of mice/rats around building
	48%	Dumpsters collected after they overflow
	24%	Can smell dumpsters from apartment
Lead Paint	34%	Chipping or peeling paints in apartment
	66%	Was not notified about the lead content of paint

Other findings summarized in Table 1.2 suggest vital areas for tenant health education and advocacy, such as child safety programs, smoking cessation programs and asthma education.

Table 1.2   Summary of key health and safety findings

Child Health and Safety	25%	Wall/floor steam pipes hot enough to burn
	40%	Radiator surface can burn
	57%	Lives above the first floor and has no window guards*
	27%	Has children who do not know what to do in event of a fire*
	30%	Does not keep medicines out of reach of children*
	74%	Unused electrical outlets not covered*
	68%	Does not have emergency numbers posted*
	32%	Does not keep lighters and matches out of reach*
	13%	Leaves children unattended in bathtub*
	56%	Tap water too hot*
Smoking	49%	Respondent smokes
	23%	Ever prohibit smoking in apartment
Asthma	26%	Respondent reports being diagnosed with asthma
Symptoms in Last Month	56%	Headaches
	50%	Sore or dry throat
	46%	Coughing
	40%	Excessive tiredness
	32%	Respiratory problems

*Only families with children under 10 years old responded, 22 families.

Discussion

What is New Here? And for Whom?

From the researchers' perspective, the dominance of physical and structural problems, which may contribute to poor air quality and indoor biological contaminants, over hazardous chemical sources in the indoor environment was an important finding. Eight-two percent of residents' surveyed report leaving their windows open in winter because of overheating, while 24 percent use their oven at times to heat the apartment. Fifty-eight percent report that the air is stuffy, and 46 percent report not enough fresh air. The composite picture is one of uncontrollable heating and stagnant air: year-round overheating for most, underheating for a smaller group, thermostats not functioning, windows open in winter as well as summer, and stuffy air.

Responses to questions about use and storage of hazardous materials and chemicals reveal that residents of West Broadway store few consumer chemicals, most typically a can of pesticide, cleanser and oven cleaner, and a bottle of bleach. Few work in hazardous jobs where they would bring home chemical contaminants on clothes; virtually none has home hobbies that use hazardous chemicals. As for outdoor sources of pollution, the fumes and odors from nearby buses, trucks and cars appeared to equal the proximity of autobody shops, gasoline stations, dry cleaners and a factory as dominant local pollution sources of concern to residents.

Neither the tenants nor the housing authority are surprised with the findings about leaks and moisture, overheating, lack of ventilation and conditions of cleanliness. What is new for the BHA is the systematized survey of housing-related problems. While the housing authority has plenty of work order records, annual inspection reports, and anecdotal information about building-related problems, they have not undertaken a representative study of their housing to document the most common repairs requested and conducted, and the most common housing problems identified in annual unit inspections.

As for the tenants, upon hearing the survey findings, they responded that we are documenting what they already know because they have lived with it. Almost 100 percent report knowing the system of submitting a work order for problems in need of repair; and 72 percent report that the maintenance staff is responsive. The issue, as they indicated in the survey, is that repairs are often short-term and inadequate. Fifty percent made repeated requests for the same problem. From the data on water leaks, for example, we found that the two main reported sources of leaks are plumbing-related (in the apartment or the upstairs apartment) and wet weather-related (suggesting leaks in roof and/or exterior wall). Both of these are a function of building maintenance and repair.

A major limitation in public housing design is lack of cross-ventilation. More than half report that their apartment is stuffy and the majority report exhaust fans in bathrooms and kitchens to be not working or non-existent. On the issue of lead, public housing authorities have historically undertaken some level of de-leading of apartments. However, we found that many tenants were uninformed about the extent of de-leading at West Broadway, although Massachusetts state law requires a landlord to notify tenants whether the apartment has been de-leaded or not. The majority (66 percent) report that they have not been notified by the BHA as to whether their apartment has been de-leaded.

We have noted that the rates reported for headaches, sore or dry throat, coughing, excessive tiredness and respiratory problems in the previous month are high. All of these health symptoms are associated in the literature cited earlier with either indoor moisture and dampness or with overheating. The prevalence rate of medically-diagnosed asthma among the adult respondents, 26 percent, exceeds the national average by a factor of four to five. We documented a 49 percent prevalence rate of smoking – a key non-allergenic asthma trigger, as well as a 20 percent prevalence rate of visible mould, and a high rate of leaks or moisture conditions (64 percent) which would contribute to allergenic sources such as dust mites, mould and fungi.

Correlational Analysis

We calculated unadjusted prevalence odds ratios for various combinations of reported environmental problems and health symptoms in the last month. Table 1.3 displays the results for those associations tested which have a 95 percent confidence level. Overall, we found that 74 percent (26 out of 35) of the associations were positive (increasing exposure correlated with increasing symptoms). It is worth noting that some of the exposure variables are associated with each other. Moisture was positively correlated with mould, and mould was positively correlated with cockroaches and with overheating.

Table 1.3   Association of symptoms and environmental conditions reported as crude prevalence odds ratios (95% confidence interval)

	Moisture	Mould growth	Overheating	Cockroaches	Smoke
Dizziness	1.85 (0.33, 10.28)	1.42 (0.24, 8.37)	0.60* (0.46, 0.76)	0.60 (0.13, 2.84)	1.05 (0.23, 4.78)
Coughing	3.34 (0.96, 11.62)	6.67* (1.25, 35.65)	2.88 (0.83, 10.03)	1.36 (0.45, 4.16)	4.29* (1.29, 14.26)
Tiredness	2.30 (0.66, 7.95)	1.00 (0.24, 4.11)	4.96* (1.20, 20.55)	1.14 (0.37, 3.55)	2.57 (0.79, 8.40)
Nosebleeds	6.65 (0.77, 57.62)	1.00 (0.18, 5.56)	1.26 (0.28, 5.63)	3.16 (0.71, 14.02)	0.19 (0.04, 1.03)
Sneezing	1.39 (0.43, 4.49)	0.47 (0.11, 2.10)	2.55 (0.73, 8.87)	0.83 (0.27, 2.55)	1.08 (0.35, 3.32)
Wheezing	0.82 (0.25, 2.72)	3.50 (0.83, 14.69)	2.40 (0.64, 8.93)	3.33 (0.99, 11.22)	2.68 (0.79, 9.07)
Sore/dry throat	4.33* (1.24, 15.21)	5.41* (1.02, 28.79)	3.69* (1.05, 12.96)	1.00 (0.33, 3.03)	2.50 (0.79, 7.90)

* $p < 0.05$

We found that there were statistically significant associations between a number of health symptoms in the last month before the survey and environmental factors. It is important to qualify this finding. The survey that we conducted was cross-sectional in nature, which means that it is inherently unable to determine causality. Thus we can only say that certain symptoms were associated with certain environmental conditions. Further both the symptoms and the environmental conditions were self reported and not confirmed in any way. While self-reporting may be accurate it also contains the possibility that bias on the part of the person interviewed could creep in (i.e., that someone with asthma responds to the cockroach question differently because they are more aware of cockroaches).

Despite the limitations of our study, we feel that the statistically significant associations that we observed are largely (but not entirely) in agreement with the scientific literature about the environment and its impact on health. Sore/dry throat and coughing were, for example, associated with moisture and mould (just missing statistical significance in the case of coughing and moisture). Both are associated with asthma and respiratory illness in the literature (Brunekreef et al., 1989). Cockroaches were associated with wheezing, which is also a well-documented association (Rosenstreich et al., 1997). Coughing was associated with smoking. Tiredness was associated with overheating, a plausible association based on loss of sleep (Di Nisi et al., 1989). Furthermore, because our small sample size limits our statistical power to observe correlation between parameters, it is striking that we found any.

Sample Population

The sample population surveyed was not fully representative of the racial composition of West Broadway Housing. No Asians were surveyed, although the list of 80 from which respondents were drawn had six Asian names. Blacks were sampled at close to the rate in the list of 80 (12 percent compared to 9.8 percent), while Hispanics were under sampled (12 percent to 19.5 percent). This most likely resulted from the method in which we achieved participation in the survey. Having few responses to the mailing, the survey team resorted to knocking on doors and explaining the survey and its purpose. Post survey discussions with the survey team revealed that they contacted first those tenants on the randomized list whom they knew or whose names they recognized, and then those on the list with nearby addresses. They contacted 65 of the 80 units before getting 50 willing to be interviewed. Of the 15 who were not interviewed, ten were not home, and five declined.

The survey team, with the exception of a Latina who is BUSPH student, was white, non-Hispanic and English-speaking only. The Asian, Hispanic and African-American tenants at West Broadway are recent residents there, while those members of the survey team from West Broadway are, like the Tenant Task Force as a whole, longtime white residents. In addition to cultural, linguistic and racial barriers presented by a primarily white survey team, new residents to West Broadway Housing may be more reticent to participate in a survey (even anonymously) which asked critical questions about housing conditions. However, one immediate way to ensure that the project benefits all tenants is to design the follow-up plans of action, such as building improvements, smoking cessation and child safety programs, so that they reach as many tenants as possible.

Plans of Action and Ongoing Work

Public Housing developments should take the lead by assessing the health needs of their families around such areas as asthma prevention, injuries and lead poisoning. Health care institutions, which often have significant resources, should collaborate with public housing organizations to identify the health needs of their families.

A number of coordinated follow-up activities are being undertaken in West Broadway Housing by various partners in this project. Some are being done in response to our survey findings; others are independently initiated but are corroborated and supported by our findings.

South Boston Community Health Center with West Broadway Residents

The Public Health Initiative of the South Boston Neighborhood Health Center has received funding from the USEPA Region I to undertake a "train the trainer" program at West Broadway Housing for educating residents in indoor environment triggers and techniques to reduce their exposure to contaminants and allergens. Called the Indoor Air Quality Initiative, this program was planned with the Tenant Task Force in order to have the maximum reach to West Broadway residents. Thus far, two groups of residents (15 in all) have received educational training in indoor air quality, asthma and tobacco. Called Indoor Air Advocates, each group was responsible for designing a public health outreach project around the issues they studied. One developed a brochure on the environmental causes of certain health problems and distributed the brochure at community events and within West Broadway. The other has channeled their education and activism around smoking into forming a "non-smoking" group in which they will devise and determine what social and personal methods work best for themselves and for other tenants, like themselves, in public housing. A third group is being recruited among the Spanish-speaking residents at West Broadway. All participants are paid a stipend, and the project uses pre- and post-testing for evaluation knowledge learned. Thus far, the first two groups had 100 percent attendance.

Boston Medical Center

The Boston Medical Center will conduct a pilot project to assess the indoor and local outdoor air environments of a sample of 26 residents of West Broadway with asthma, including the 13 residents who reported being diagnosed with asthma in our survey. The project will measure temperature, humidity, important indoor allergens in settled dust, airborne fungal spores, environmental tobacco smoke and fine and coarse airborne particles at baseline and 12 months later. A second aim of the project is the measure asthma severity of residents in the sample homes. This will be measured by means of an asthma-specific quality-of-life questionnaire and 2 weeks of monitoring daily FEV1, symptoms and medication use. The relation of asthma severity to the environmental measurements will be examined. The specific indoor and outdoor parameters to be measured reflect primary sources of poor indoor air at West Broadway identified in our survey: overheating, high prevalence of moisture, smoking and combustion fumes from local traffic.

Boston Housing Authority

In winter 1999, the BHA will commence a complete replacement of the present central steam heating system at West Broadway Housing with a gas-fired system in each building that will give individual apartment dwellers control over their heating. Concurrently, water-efficient toilets will be installed. This structural change was in the conceptual phase as our study began; but our findings confirm that overheating was the major environmental complaint at West Broadway Housing.

Energy, Health and Housing Collaborative

As we were completing our survey in West Broadway Housing, we were invited to join our model with another proposal on energy, health and housing that was also targeting Boston public housing. A collaborative has now formed, including the three public health schools of Boston, Citizens Energy Corporation, the Committee for Boston Public Housing and the Boston Housing Authority, for the purpose of coordinating a 5-year effort to reduce indoor environmental hazards, improve energy efficiency and improve residents' health in Boston public housing. The project goal is to identify and evaluate residential environmental problems contributing to increased health risks and to implement corrective action. Such measures will improve resident health while also addressing urgent repair and energy conservation needs. Savings in health care and energy conservation will offset the expenditures for corrective action and better maintenance. The net result of this effort would be a national model for codes and standards of practice that could improve the health of public housing residents throughout the country.

Essential elements of the proposal include direct measures of exposure and health risks during the assessment and implementation phase of the project; training programs for BHA staff and residents to give them the skills to assess and evaluate current environmental conditions; and implementation of mitigation measures such as physical building improvements and education programs. Through economic analysis of health, energy and mitigation measures, we hope to demonstrate that savings in energy costs and health expenditures for treating respiratory ailments exceed the costs of implementing education and mitigation programs, so that the project can be extended and become self-sustaining and replicable for other public housing authorities. Thus far, the collaborative has submitted proposals for funding to a number of national foundations.

RARE Grant

Tufts University School of Medicine, in collaboration with the Committee for Boston Public Housing, Harvard University School of Public Health and Boston Medical Center, did a follow-up study funded by the U.S. EPA to evaluate an asthma intervention program in the Franklin Hill public housing development.

Student Projects

In spring 1999, students in the Master's in Public Health program at Boston University School of Public Health undertook a series of community-based projects at West Broadway Housing on child safety and safe pesticide and rodent control programs which arise from the survey findings. Working with the community organizer at West Broadway Housing and using materials from the City of Boston's Childhood Injury Prevention Program, they designed a child safety program, which could be implemented by tenants trained in principles of child injury prevention. Students researched the pesticide and rodent control programs at West Broadway Housing and assessed safety issues, especially for children. After investigating Integrated Pest Management, they made public health recommendations concerning the current practices used by the Boston Housing Authority at West Broadway Housing. From results of the survey on tenants' use of pesticides, students designed an educational program for tenants about safe pest control that could be implemented by the Tenant Task Force and the South Boston Neighborhood Health Center.

Public health is an applied field in which scholarship includes not only the discovery of knowledge but also (and equally) the integration, communication and application of knowledge (Richardson and Field, 1995). From its incipience, the *Public Health in Public Housing* project was intended to be holistic, in the sense that health and housing problems revealed through the survey would be presented and discussed publicly and addressed in follow-up plans of corrective action. Thanks to the participatory, community-based and goal-driven nature of this pilot survey, the project has a transparency which has attracted numerous partners – including housing residents, the housing authority, community health centers and other key Boston-based institutions – for extending and expanding this work.

Notes

1   And yet, there are waiting lists for public housing. Nationally people wait an average of 1 ½ years to get into public housing (Doc4Kids). The Boston Housing Authority manages about 15 500 family and elderly units in public housing and has almost the same number of families on their waiting list for those housing developments. The national and local shortage of subsidized housing means that for nearly every family living in public housing, or in a subsidized variant called Section 8 housing, another family lives in overcrowded conditions, or pays most of their income for rent and teeters on the edge of homelessness, or is homeless. Thus public housing today, *no matter what its conditions*, is a refuge from choosing between rent and food for one's children, and from homelessness.

2   However, this "personal" and "consumerist" approach to improving the indoor environment, with its emphasis on individual behavior, is of limited use for many. It assumes a level of resources and control of one's building and housing environment which are rarely available to renters, people on fixed incomes and residents of public housing. What do they do about particle board widely used in low-cost construction and cabinets? Or living in a building in which a drycleaners operates? Furthermore, the few health studies of residents in public housing suggest (as do our own findings in the West Broadway survey) that building-related problems – such as dampness and poor ventilation – are at least as egregious as indoor smoking, and substantially more so than consumer products, in health problems reported. We found minimal cleaning products and

home pesticides in West Broadway apartments, for reasons of income; and dry-cleaning would be a luxury consumer practice. Further, an environmentalism based on consumer choice has the potential to let the producer – whether lawn and garden pesticide manufacturers or home deodorizer manufacturers and also the mass marketing industry – off the hook.
3   We have trained residents of Franklin Hill Housing in Dorchester who subsequently conducted the survey in their housing development. We are currently analyzing the results.

Acknowledgments

The authors would like to acknowledge the residents of West Broadway Housing and the staff of the Public Health Initiative of the South Boston Community Health Center for their contribution to this project.

References

Abraham, Y. (1997), "Colonial unrest", *The Boston Phoenix*, 24 January, 16–18.
Ambrose, P., and Hill, S. (1996), "Bad housing: Counting the cost", *The Housing Policy Context*, 20–33.
American Lung Association, United States Environmental Protection Agency, Consumer Safety Product Commission, and American Medical Association (1994), *Indoor Air Pollution: An Introduction for Health Professionals*, U.S. Government Printing Office, 1994-523-217/81322.
Birch, E.L. (1978), "Woman-made America: The case of early public housing policy", *AIP Journal*, April, 132.
Brunekreef, B., Dockery, D.W., Speizer, F.E., Ware, J.H., Spengler, J.D. and Ferris, B.G. (1989), "Home dampness and respiratory morbidity in children", *American Review of Respiratory Disease*, **140**, 1363–7.
Brunekreef, B. (1992), "Damp housing and adult respiratory symptoms", *Allergy*, **45**, 498–502.
Capek, S. (1993), "The environmental justice frame: A conceptual discussion and an application", *Social Problems*, **40**, 5–24.
Centers for Disease Control and Prevention (1997), *Screening Young Children for Lead Poisoning: Guidance for State and Local Officials*, Atlanta: Centers for Disease Control and Prevention.
Daugbjerg, P. (1989), "Is particle board in the home detrimental to health?", *Environmental Research*, **48**, 154–63.
Di Nisi, J., Erhart, J., Galeou, M. and Libert, J.P. (1989), "Influence on repeated passive body heating on subsequent night sleep in humans", *European Journal of Applied Physiology and Occupational Physiology*, **59**, 138–45.
Doc4Kids Project (1998), *Not Safe at Home: How America's Housing Crisis Threatens the Health of Its Children*, Boston: Boston Medical Center. Also available from doc4kids@bu.edu.
Dreier, P. (1992), "Bush to cities: Drop dead", *The Progressive*, July, 20–23.
Flint, A., Davis, R. (1999), "BHA will pay $1.5m to settle rights suit", *The Boston Globe*, 27 July, A10.
Gallagher, S., Hunter, P. and Guyer, B. (1985), "A home injury prevention program for children", *Pediatric Clinics of North America*, **32**, 95–112.
"Home is where the hurt is" (1997) *Nursing Times*, **93** (32).

Israel, B., Schulz, A., Parker, E. and Becker, A. (1998), "Review of community-based research: Assessing partnership approaches to improve public health", *Annual Review of Public Health*, **19**, 173–202.

Lowry, S. (1989), "Temperature and humidity", *British Medical Journal*, **299**, 1326–8.

Martinez, B.F., Annest, J.L., Kilbourne, E.M., Kirk, M.L., Lui, K.J. and Smith, S.M. (1989), "Geographic distribution of heat-related injuries among elderly persons", *Journal of the American Medical Association*, **262**, 2246–50.

McCarthy, P., Byrne, D., Harrison, S. and Keithley, J. (1985), "Respiratory conditions: Effect of housing and other factors", *Journal of Epidemiology and Community Health*, **39**, 15–19.

Platt, S.D., Martin, C.J., Hunt, S.M. and Lewis, C.W. (1989), "Damp housing, mould growth, and symptomatic health state", *British Medical Journal*, **298**, 1673–8.

Quinlan, K. (1996), "Injury Control in practice: Home radiator burns in inner-city children", *Archives of Pediatric and Adolescent Medicine*, **150**, 954–7.

Richardson, W.C. and Fields, P.M. (1995), "The role of the university in urban health", in Richardson and Fields (eds), *The University in the Urban Community: Responsibility for Public Health*, Washington: Association of Academic Health Centers.

Rosenstreich, D.L., Eggleson, P., Kattan, M., Baker, D., Slavin, R.G., Gergen, P., Mitchell, H., McNiff-Mortimer, K., Lynn, H., Ownby, D., Malveaux, F. (1997), "The role of cockroach allergy and exposure to cockroach allergen in causing morbidity among inner-city children with asthma", *New England Journal of Medicine*, **336**, 1356–63.

Souza, K. (1997), "Public health and housing: A review", unpublished paper, Boston University School of Public Health.

Spengler, J., Neas, L., Satoshi, N., Dockery, D., Speizer, F., Wane, J. and Raizenne, M. (1994a), "Respiratory symptoms and housing characteristics", *Indoor Air*, April, 72–82.

Spengler, J., Nakai, S., Özkaynak, H. and Schwab, M. (1994b), "Housing factors and respiratory health symptoms: Kanawha Valley, West Virginia", paper presented at the International Workshop, *Indoor Air – An Integrated Approach,* Gold Coast, Australia, 27 November–1 December 1994.

"The white underclass" (1994), *U.S. News & World Report*, October, 40–48, 53.

Verhoeff, A.P., van Strien, R.T., van Wijnen, J.H. and Brunekreef, B. (1995), "Damp housing and child respiratory symptoms: The role of sensitization to dust mites and molds", *American Journal of Epidemiology*, **141**, 103–10.

Wallace, L.A. (1995), "Human exposure to environmental pollutants: A decade of exposure", *Clinical and Experimental Allergy*, **25**, 4.

Chapter 2

A Case Study of Community-Based Participatory Research Ethics: The Healthy Public Housing Initiative

Doug Brugge and Alison Kole

Introduction

There is growing interest in community-based participatory research (Baker et al., 1999; Israel et al., 1998; Schensul, 1999; Sullivan, 2001; Minkler and Wallerstein, 2003) as well as community impacts of more traditional biomedical research (Weijer and Emanuel, 2000). We are interested in the ethics of community-based participatory research because we suspect that this type of research has some distinct ethical dimensions associated with its collaborative framework and the active involvement of the community in the research process.

Current Institutional Review Board standards represent a commitment on the part of the U.S. Government to protect the autonomy and rights of *individuals* participating in clinical and behavioral research studies. For example, the *Belmont Report* of 1979, the foundation upon which current ethics guidelines is built, has three tenets: respect for persons, beneficence, and justice, all of which are framed with regard to individuals participating in research (The National Commission for the Protection of Human Subjects of Biomedical and Behavioral Research, 1979). Within a Western social construct, ethical consideration of the rights of persons is a natural extension of a society in which the dominant philosophy is one of individualism. Robert Levine comments on the *Belmont Report*: "It is usually quite appropriate to view investigator-subject relationships as relationships between strangers. Thus, in general an individualistic ethics is appropriate" (Levine, 1988).

Individually based ethical frameworks are not necessarily beneficial for the community with which individuals are affiliated, however. Drawing from biomedical community research (that is not participatory), Charles Weijer pointed to studies of Tay-Sachs disease that found that the mutation was more common among Ashkenazi Jewish populations (Weijer, 1999). Because all identifying information had been removed from the databank, the National Institutes of Health (NIH) Office of Human Subjects Review did not require individual informed consent, as it considered the identities of individuals to be already protected. While this protects individuals, on a population level such findings could lead to discrimination against Jews (Lehrman, 1997).

Another problem with such a framework is that the United States is composed of a diverse array of ethnicities that do not all adhere to individualistic philosophies. According to Jillian Inouye, for example, Asian Americans often incorporate "kinship solidarity", which is "the view that the individual is subservient to the kinship-based group or family" (Inouye, 1999). John Casken writes: "In contrast to all the Pacific Islander jurisdictions, the United States is basically a classical liberal society" devoid of the traditional community-oriented belief system inherent to Pacific Islander tradition (Casken, 1999). Hispanic Americans also maintain a similar tradition, familism, which, helps explain why Hispanics may include family members in joint decisions about medical treatment or preventive care (Suarez and Ramirez, 1999).

Within an international context, there is literature exploring the ethics of randomized clinical trials in developing nations having different cultural values than the United States (Christakis, 1988; Angell, 1997). Recently questions have been raised about fairness and availability of benefits to countries that host human research. Relevant to this study is the idea that international research should engage the affected population in developing, evaluating and benefiting from research (Anonymous, 2002).

Within both US and international contexts, there are numerous studies on the ethics of conducting research in communities unified by ethnicity, who therefore share common beliefs, values, and/or politics (Christakis, 1988; Angell, 1997; Anonymous, 2002; Ryan, 2002; and Brown, 1985). However, we found no literature on the ethics of conducting research, participatory or otherwise, within US communities that are ethnically and culturally diverse, but are united by a common thread of poverty, such as those in the public housing that were a part of the study described below.

Communities within Public Housing

Black and Hispanic populations have historically had the highest rates of poverty in the United States (US Bureau of the Census, 2001 and 2000). However, there are poor families of all backgrounds and there are large numbers of poor whites. Accordingly, while some public housing developments are predominantly Black and/or Hispanic, families from many populations are frequently brought together in such developments (El-Asarki et al., 1998). A community is created in public housing that depends on personal relationships to an extent unfamiliar to most professionals today in the US (Bradley, 2001). The community is further shaped by the distinctive ethnic composition of residents, their needs, and their interaction with city and development authorities.

Lorna Ryan commented on the impact of power differences (Ryan, 2002):

... those studied are often in relatively powerless positions, lacking cultural and/or institutional power ... the researcher is generally not a member of the community, she or he is generally qualified, with specialized technical language and she or he has the final say about the content of a research report and the dissemination of research findings (largely through the medium of print).

Thus, at a minimum, the relationship between researchers and residents of public housing poses ethical dilemmas due to the unequal power dynamic between socio-economically and educationally 'wealthy' researchers and underprivileged residents.

Our goal in this study was to generate ideas and hypotheses that would inform future research into the ethics of community-based participatory research with diverse, low-income US populations. Results of a similar approach to examining community-based research methods in Seattle, without the emphasis on ethics, have recently been published (Sullivan et al., 2001).

Methods

The Healthy Public Housing Initiative

This study explores perceptions of research ethics among participants in the Healthy Public Housing Initiative (HPHI). Several pilot studies preceded the establishment of the HPHI. The pilot studies, like the full study employed community-participatory research methods, in that community organizations were partners in the work. Community organization staff and residents of public housing were hired to work on the research (Hynes et al., 2000), were frequently co-authors on the resulting publications (Brugge et al., 2001; Brugge et al., 2003) and exerted considerable influence on decision-making. Unlike some participatory research that links only agency staff with universities, HPHI hired grassroots residents following intensive job training and included city agencies as full partners as well.

The HPHI began in January 2000 using focus groups, surveys and a longitudinal intervention study to assess childhood asthma among public housing residents. Boston and Harvard University Schools of Public Health, and Tufts University School of Medicine led the HPHI. At the time of this investigation the community partners were the Committee for Boston Public Housing (CBPH) and the South Boston Community Health Center (SBCHC), and the West Broadway and Franklin Hill tenant associations. Two city agencies, the Boston Housing Authority and the Boston Public Health Commission were members of the collaborative, as were two consultants, Peregrine Energy and Urban Habitat Initiatives.

Interviews

Key informant interviews were conducted with 14 individuals who were staff or students at the 11 organizational partners to the Healthy Public Housing Initiative during the summer of 2001, when the HPHI was in its start-up phase. The interviews covered about one-half of the active individuals working on the project. Given the scale of the study, we could not attempt to assess how representative interviewees were of their community, city agency or university.

Interviewees were recruited such that they provided representation from academic researchers, community partners, the city partners and consultants to the project. Two of the interviews were excluded from further analysis. One excluded interview was with a staff person at a community partner who did not have enough direct experience with the project at the time to comment on most of the questions, the other was a student who also had limited contact with the project and likewise declined to comment on most questions.

The interviews consisted of four demographic questions and 12 questions pertaining to ethics of community-based research (Table 2.1). In keeping with the exploratory nature of our study, questions were open-ended and did not prompt respondents. All interviews were conducted by one of us (AK) either at Tufts University School of Medicine or in the community. Each person interviewed signed a consent form that assured him or her that their name would not be associated with their comments. Interviews were audio taped and transcribed verbatim by two undergraduate students who received training in research ethics prior to listening to the interviews. The Tufts University School of Medicine IRB approved the protocol.

Analysis

One of us (DB) did a content analysis after names had been removed from the transcripts. The attempt at blinding did not entirely work because of the author's involvement in the project and knowledge of the participants. His knowledge of the project, however, likely helped in identifying some themes that might be obscure to someone with no association with the work. The analysis coded themes from the interviews with the goal of generating ideas that could be the basis for future research. All themes raised for each question for each interviewee were coded. Themes that were raised multiple times by the same interviewee to the same question were collapsed and counted as one theme. This approach was designed to allow richness and complexity to emerge from the interviews.

Table 2.1　Interview questions

1. Sector (community, city, research, consultant)
2. Number of years in research
3. Number of years in community-based research
4. Number of years involved in the community
1. What are the three main benefits to the community which can be gained from community-based research which make this type of research unique compared to other types of research?
2. According to the IRB, the principle of protecting research participants is defined as beneficence. Beneficence is upheld by researchers who follow two general rules: "do no harm" and "maximize possible benefits and minimize risks" (The National Commission for the Protection of Human Subjects of Biomedical and Behavioral Research, 1979). How do researchers protect the participants in community-based research from harm and secure the wellbeing of their participants?

3. Informed consent represents a trust, between researcher and participant, that the participant has been honestly informed of all the risks and benefits of the study. How do you think the concept of trust and honesty can be expanded to encompass the relationship between researcher and community?
4. When thinking about the ethics regarding the publication of data, what are the main considerations researchers must think about when doing community-based research which are different from doing other types of research?
5. What are the ethical responsibilities of researchers involved in community-based research that are different from clinical or behavioral researchers, for example?
6. What are the ethical responsibilities of community partners involved in community-based research?
7. What are the ethical responsibilities of the city partners involved in community-based research?
8. What does the term "good science" mean from a community-based research perspective?
9. From an ethical standpoint, what defines success in a community-based research study, with respect to study outcomes?
10. Describe how you feel about what defines the appropriate relationship between researchers and participants? What defines the appropriate relationship between researchers and the community?
11. Thinking about the IRB training you completed, name three amendments you would like to see added to the text, which would educate readers on the ethics of doing community-based research?
12. What is the appropriate ethical approach to a situation in which a tenant participating in a research project is found to be engaging in activities considered to be in violation of their contract with the landlords? What if the researcher witnesses evidence of intentional injury to a child from a participating apartment?

Themes accepted for coding ranged from a single word to longer discussions of an idea. Comments that were designated as one theme were deemed the same based on professional judgment. If there was uncertainty, the default was to keep themes distinct. All themes that were coded are reported in the results section organized by question. Those raised by more than one interviewee are reported with the number of times that they were raised. Quotes were extracted and reprinted in the results when they added nuance or detail to the theme in the judgment of the coder. The interviewer (author AC) reviewed and approved the summation of the coded themes. Drafts of the findings and the manuscript were circulated to all interviewees to allow comment both on content and to assure that they were comfortable with the level of confidentiality the quotes provided. The approach used was consistent with methods described elsewhere (Glesne and Peshkin, 1992; Siedman, 1991).

Results

Demographics of Interviewees

Interviewed were five people who were from the community partners, two from the city agencies, two who were consultants to the project and three who were researchers. Ten of the 12 interviewees were white. The average years in any type of research was 8.54 (SD 6.79) with a minimum of 0 years and a maximum of 20 years. Interestingly, the interviewees with the most years in research were a consultant and a community person. This was perhaps because none of the project directors were interviewed due to scheduling limitations. The average years in community-based research were lower, 5.00 years (SD 6.19) with a range of 0 to 20 years. Average years involved in the community outside of research was 16.25 (SD 11.69) with a range of 0 to 40 years. The community interviewees had substantially more years of involvement in community work (average for community interviewees was 24.40 years; SD 13.32).

Emergent Themes

Question 1. *What are the three main benefits to the community which can be gained from community-based research which make this type of research unique compared to other types of research?*
There was broad agreement among those interviewed about the benefits to the community. The most frequently cited benefit was bringing added resources (including money, skills and knowledge) to the community. Another frequently cited benefit was that the research could provide the community with data that it needs to advocate for itself. This was stated as, "confirmation that certain conditions cause certain health problems" by one community interviewee. Also noted were the possibilities that the researchers would ask better questions because they understood the community and that the community would understand the research process better for their participation. Mentioned as benefits by single interviewees was more emphasis on qualitative information and learning about community assets (instead of community problems).

Question 2. *According to the IRB, the principle of protecting research participants is defined as beneficence. Beneficence is upheld by researchers who follow two general rules: "do no harm" and "maximize possible benefits and minimize risks" (The National Commission for the Protection of Human Subjects of Biomedical and Behavioral Research, 1979). How do researchers protect the participants in community-based research from harm and secure the well-being of their participants?*
Most interviewees thought that there were distinct ethical concerns in community-based research that did not exist in other types of research. However a small number of interviewees (two community members and one researcher) either thought there was no difference or listed only concerns (i.e., informed consent) that apply to traditional research as well. Stated most strongly the researcher said, "I think this is no different than any other type of research." A couple of other interviewees listed

common concerns, such as dangers of going door to door and obtaining informed consent, as well as concerns distinct to community-based studies.

Three interviewees thought that active involvement of community members/ organizations would lead these groups to defend the community and protect their interests. Others stated a related theme that seemed to be based on the same concern. They said that 1) there needed to be equality between researchers and the community; 2) that the community needs to have a voice and be involved as much as possible; 3) that two-way communication was important. One community member suggested that involving the participants might result in them being more truthful with researchers and also thought that the results needed to be reported back to the community. Two interviewees, a consultant to the project and a community member, used the phrase "lab rats" to describe what the community must *not* be in the research process.

Three interviewees pointed out that there were methodological issues with respect to having community members survey their own community. A community member and a consultant to the project both indicated that privacy might be more important and problematic because the interviewers and interviewees know each other. A city staff person said that research methodology is at odds with what makes sense to the community, that is, confidentiality is the opposite of what you need if you are doing organizing.

One community member discussed the problem of "unflattering data" and "blaming the victim". But this person went on to say that, "on the other hand, I think one of the important strengths of the communities themselves no matter what the sources are, whether they are institutional racism, or cultural, historical forces or whatever, people can begin to feel better if they uncover the data, if they're asking the questions." This same person also commented on the need to ask the right questions and the ability of the community to contribute to formulating such questions.

The risk of not meeting expectations was raised by a city staff person and two interviewees pointed to the need for tangible benefits to the community to come out of the research.

Question 3. Informed consent represents a trust, between researcher and participant, that the participant has been honestly informed of all the risks and benefits of the study. How do you think the concept of trust and honesty can be expanded to encompass the relationship between researcher and community?
Three interviewees raised a concern about defining what is the community and how can it have trust in the research process. "I am not sure that the community is an entity that can have trust," stated the researcher who thought informed consent should be with individuals. A consultant observed that, "a community ... is very broadly defined and is a very nebulous thing in most cases." A community member wondered, "how would you know what the community thinks about us [the project]. I mean would you take a poll? ... Would you let elected officials speak for the community?"

Three interviewees pointed to involvement of community organizations as key and one community member noted that that "didn't happen in the Healthy Public Housing" until, "community oriented people stuck to their guns and insisted on the involvement of community groups." Four interviewees raised relationship building in one fashion or another. One consultant spoke of "breaking bread" together. A city agency staff person talked of the years of smaller scale projects that were needed to lay the basis for the current project, saying, "it took [two of the project directors] a while to get in, they had to talk to the right people at [the agency] who were willing to put aside their fears ... of headlines about them."

One community member suggested that it would have been helpful if the universities had a greater presence in the communities, "offering classes" prior to requesting a partnership around research. Four interviewees, two researchers and two from the community thought that honest (even brutally honest) clarity about what researchers want to do is needed. Also raised were 1) the need for the community to get something back from the research; 2) being willing to "stand down" from ideas you think are right in order to get to a middle ground; 3) the need for recognition that the researchers do not necessarily know about community problems; 4) that monetary payments as the sole incentive do not work and 5) the need to allow for the possibility of little ideas "dinging up" out of people's lived experience.

Question 4. *When thinking about the ethics regarding the publication of data, what are the main considerations researchers must think about when doing community-based research which are different from doing other types of research?*
Six interviewees expressed concern about privacy or confidentiality. One city staff person restated the contrast between research anonymity and the need for openness in an organizing model, saying, "in a community benefits model you want people to identify themselves." A researcher, concerned about small sample sizes said that, "if you are publishing a study of 100 households in a single [public housing] development it is possible for people to see who was involved."

Two interviewees, community and city agency persons, thought the key to publishing data was sharing it in an accessible way with the community. Six interviewees, however, expressed concern that results showing that housing conditions were negatively affecting resident's health could be used in the policy arena to divert support away from public housing rather than to fix it up. Said a researcher, "the community has been concerned that politicians seeing the research would say that they should take their money out of public housing because it is just making kids sick."

The conclusion that five interviewees came to was that there was a need to "take a political stand" or present data with "a positive spin" instead of simply stating findings and walking away. Interestingly, only one of the persons stating this position was from the community, the rest being, two researchers, a consultant and a city staff person. Other issues raised by single interviewees were: which partners own the data produced by the study, the need to focus on interventions rather than simply documenting problems, being careful not to "embellish" data, the value of publishing this type of research in medical journals alongside clinical trials, considering where money is going in the budget and acknowledging participants, "who actually worked hard in the process".

Question 5. *What are the ethical responsibilities of researchers involved in community-based research that are different from clinical or behavioral researchers, for example?*
Four interviewees, each from a different sector, noted the need for adherence to traditional ethical frameworks, such as informed consent, confidentiality and doing

no harm. Four interviewees raised questions about how the research would benefit the community. One community member compared community-based research to clinical medicine in that, "you get some obligations over time" and observed that service and research may both be a part of community-based projects.

Two interviewees, one a researcher and the other a community member, brought up concerns about the influence of money given to research participants who are poor. The community member said, "say that we are doing the survey and you are not clear as researchers what are their motivations. Say that we are paying them to do the research, how do we know the information we get is really valid? Or the people are just in it for the money because they are poor." This person went on to suggest that respondents might also slant their answers in either direction, depending on their motivation. Two researchers emphasized the need for adherence to conventional research methods. One pointed out the need not to give away the hypothesis in certain situations. The other stressed that the data had to be "correct and objective" and that you have to be sure that "no information is being fudged".

Other points raised included a comment by one of the consultants that, "this is so unique and the fact that all these people are around the table on an issue. A lot of these people have not been around the table on an issue before and it just amazes me on a daily basis to see some of those individuals at each other's throats in various fashions trying to work things out. It has not been easy."

One community interviewee thought that more anecdotal information from focus groups was important. Another community member thought there should be a support group for researchers doing community-based research. This same person asked that researchers behave as allies to the community, that they check their defensiveness at the door and that they not pretend that they have no agenda. A different community interviewee thought that the main thing was getting to know the community because, "it [can] actually turn out to be very different than what you thought".

Question 6. *What are the ethical responsibilities of community partners involved in community-based research?*

There was strong sentiment expressed by seven interviewees from all sectors of the project that the participants from the community should protect the community and represent its interests to the project. But most interviewees did not leave it at that. Balancing the other roles of the community partner was expressed as also obtaining valid answers and serving as a liaison between the community and researchers.

Two community interviewees explicitly addressed the limits placed on them by forming a partnership. One noted that, "you can't both accept to work with the university and then be mad when the university acts like a university." The other told of having to "water down" a public statement because of being in the collaboration with the city agencies who were nervous about lawsuits and observed that while it made sense to make the trade-off, there was a "price to pay". This person thought the community had to ask, "When is it a good time to collaborate?" Three other interviewees mentioned partnership issues, but not in as much detail.

Two interviewees, both with the city, thought that funding arrangements with the community raised ethical issues. One said, "funding drives a lot of things, but I would hope that people don't just sit at the table and look at the immediate funding needs and resources."

Other points included the need for community partners to make sure that 1) the right questions are asked; 2) researchers follow the data where it leads; 3) as partners they recognize and honor their responsibilities for the commitment they have made; 4) they serve as a source of information and data; 5) they are honest about their own agenda; 6) they learn about what the researchers are doing and about the research process; and 7) they think about how the research might be used. One community member thought that the first Policy Advisory Council meeting of the project was too research focused and did not focus adequately on the community.

Question 7. *What are the ethical responsibilities of the city partners involved in community-based research?*
Both city agency staff that were interviewed expressed strongly and with some detail the idea that it was the responsibility of their agencies to, in the words of one, "effect policy changes based on research." One of these interviewees went on to point out that the universities do not have the power or mandate to implement such changes. Two other interviewees, both researchers, also noted, with less emphasis, that the city is the place where policy changes would happen based on the research findings.

Three community interviewees commented on how political the city government is. Stated most strongly, this was expressed as, "They don't want to make the administration look bad, so I think that it's hard for them [city agencies] to generate data that reflects on current policies or even generate information that reflects on previous policies." Two researchers and, to a lesser extent, one community interviewee, were concerned that residents participating in the study not be put at risk if they were found, in the course of research, to have violated their lease.

Other ideas that came up were, that the city has 1) a broad responsibility to provide "safe and decent" housing, 2) must give equal access to health services and information, 3) must strive to serve the lowest income households, 4) not enter into the project in order to raise money for itself, and 5) in the words of one researcher, has "a very strong ethical obligation" to share as much data as possible.

Question 8. *What does the term "good science" mean from a community-based research perspective?*
Responses to this question were mostly along two themes. One was that good science is science that provides practical benefits to the community. The other was that good science is defined by adherence to research techniques. Seven interviewees (four from the community, two city agency staff and one consultant) defined good science in terms of what it gives back to the community. One community interviewee said that good science is, "science that the community can benefit from by learning something new about [itself] and use it as a tool to improve [the community]." One of the city agency staff and the consultant seemed to suggest trying to balance the community benefits with academic purpose, but did not get into issues of research technique.

One interviewee from the community simply said that good science was no different when applied to community-based research and did not elaborate further, which may imply support for measuring science primarily by its adherence to traditional methods. All three researchers, however, were unambiguous in their concern about research methods. One considered the main criteria to be whether a study is replicable. Another re-raised the issue of not telling participants what the hypothesis is. The third, saying, "I think that a lot of the rules of good science still apply," pointed to testing a hypothesis as critical.

The third researcher, however, also spoke about how community-based research raises questions, presumably in the minds of other researchers, about the "objectivity" of the work and concluded, "some might say that you don't necessarily have good science, you have standard observation." The second researcher raised a point, perhaps related, in saying that, "this is research [community-based] at its infancy" that still needs to develop new techniques. Perhaps the idea here is to find ways to bridge the gap between community and researcher needs that retain objectivity and validity.

One of the community interviewees related an experience in which researchers not affiliated with the HPHI apparently tested a research method in the community without providing any benefit back to the community. This community member thought that that was "inappropriate" and that it, "caused all sorts of problems". This same person noted that the earlier pilot study by one of the directors of the HPHI was "pretty good". Other important elements also raised by this interviewee were 1) the need to have a reasonably good chance of finding something of value to the community; 2) not deceiving participants (apparently in direct conflict with the researcher who suggested withholding the hypothesis); 3) whether researchers would allow this to be done to themselves; and 4) taking issues of class, race and gender into consideration.

Question 9. *From an ethical standpoint, what defines success in a community-based research study, with respect to study outcomes?*
The most common answer to this question was that the community/residents see improvements as a result of the study. Seven interviewees from all sectors of the project said something to this effect. There was clearly more convergence and overlap on this point than in answering the question on "good science". Five interviewees, again from various sectors, thought that the process of building the partnership and seeing it grow and be able to continue was an important measure of success. Four interviewees (the three researchers and one of the agency staff people) also defined success in terms of data outcomes. Only one of these, a researcher, listed data outcomes as the sole measure of success.

One city agency staff person noted that the earlier pilot studies helped the agency take up the issues that the HPHI is aiming to address, namely housing conditions and health. This person said, "the data was quite alarming and brought a new level of focus to the issue."

Question 10. *Describe how you feel about what defines the appropriate relationship between researchers and participants? What defines the appropriate relationship between researchers and the community?*
Only five interviewees stated the word "respect" or "mutual respect" explicitly, but most of the themes that follow implicitly rest on a foundation of mutual respect. Eight interviewees spoke about relationship building, sometimes using those words and other times being more descriptive. All five community interviewees addressed this theme, the other three were a researcher, a consultant and a city agency staff person.

According to interviewees, some of the ways that relationships could be built included allowing the "other person" to not be perfect, making no assumptions about who participants are, that researchers must remember that they are not part of the community, being aware that "I am in someone else's home," maintaining boundaries, being aware of the "power gap," and getting involved in the community. A city staff person said that, "a researcher [should] not [be] pretending to befriend someone on the street because they are trying to do a survey."

Six interviewees from all sectors also raised honesty, equity and clear communication. Three people (one from the city and two researchers) noted that either the researchers could provide training to the community or that the community had a lot to teach the researchers. One city staff person mentioned "producing" (taken to mean full follow through and implementation) with respect to confidentiality. A consultant wanted to know whether the definition of community is limited to the housing development, the surrounding neighborhood, or all of public housing in Boston.

Question 11. *Thinking about the IRB training you completed, name three amendments you would like to see added to the text, which would educate readers on the ethics of doing community-based research?*
Unlike any of the other questions asked, this question resulted in three interviews without answers, one interviewee who did not have an answer and another who said that the IRB did not have a role in setting ethics guidelines, but rather only in enforcing them. Also, unlike answers to other questions, the remaining answers did not coalesce into clear themes. Instead they are more of a laundry list, with no one mentioned by more than one interviewee.

Possible additions to the IRB training, in no particular order, were: 1) "maybe something about how the information is going to be used at a community level"; 2) how to treat unflattering data; 3) that the IRB is too "after the fact" and too focused on punishment instead of caring; 4) concern and humanity; 5) "its truly the institutions protecting their butt"; 6) to not call participants "subjects" because you are not studying specimens; 7) that the medical model limits the ability to "promote" (taken to mean advocate); 8) that confidentiality is not always applicable; 9) that it takes time to get to know a community; 10) that there were "lots" of researchers seeking to study people in Boston; 11) to make sure you understand the pressures on research participants; 12) to clearly understand the actions that will result from the research; 13) that if you are working with several community partners you will need many meetings for problem solving; and 14) to always maintain a professional manner with participants. One researcher said that the project should do what "is best for the participants and not necessarily what is in the best interests of the project."

Question 12a. *What is the appropriate ethical approach to a situation in which a tenant participating in a research project is found to be engaging in activities considered to be in violation of their contract with the landlords?*
There was broad agreement on this question. Eight interviewees said that the project should ignore tenant violations of their contract with the landlord. None of the remaining four interviewees fully disagreed. One did not answer, one pointed to things the housing authority was not doing, and one thought the project should have a plan. The final person thought people dealing drugs should be evicted.

Question 12b. *What if the researcher witnesses evidence of intentional injury to a child from a participating apartment?*

There was general agreement that this situation was different from that in question 12a and that looking the other way was not an option. Six respondents from all sectors of the project thought that child abuse had to be reported. Three of these people said that they were mandated reporters anyway. Five interviewees thought that something had to be done, but were uncomfortable reporting to authorities. Said, one, "sometimes the system to address it could be worse." These five tended to think that the project should report to an "intermediary" or third party, although their ideas of who that would be were generally vague. The remaining respondent said only that the project should have a plan in place.

Discussion

The methodology was qualitative in form and, consistent with the methods, the goal of the study was to generate ideas. Clearly the task at hand demands more study than what has been done so far, but this is a beginning. The methodology has both strengths and weaknesses. The interviews generated a broad range of interesting ideas with rich detail. It is not easy to summarize such a wide-ranging set of views. In some ways this is positive because it cautions against glib pigeonholing of people into simplistic categories. It is important to note, however, that because of the small sample size (Casken, 1999) the ideas raised should not be uncritically generalized to larger populations.

One thing that stands out about the interviews is that there is more agreement than disagreement despite drawing interviewees from community, university, city and consultant roles. Another general point is that the responses are not always those that might be naively expected. While there may be more commonality between the nonuniversity partners, sometimes community and university interviewees are indistinguishable. At other times they seem to take up concerns naively expected to come from the other, such as when community members worry about how to define the community or when researchers are adamant that the goal is to help the community. The interviewees may be unusual because they have all agreed to work together doing participatory research.

Collaboration of all sorts imposes compromises and distinct responsibilities on the different partners. In the case of HPHI, the researchers must conduct research, the community must protect the interests of the community and the city must act in good faith to change policy in recognition of the findings. All parties must see to it that the work committed to is completed. It is, therefore, not surprising that there is a strong note in the interviews of the need to be flexible to adjust to the other partners and to find common ground.

Interviewees raised numerous ethical issues common to conventional research (e.g., confidentiality). Sometimes these ethical concerns were reported as having a particular form in community collaborations, such as push and pull between the need for confidentiality and the need to organize the community. However, there is also general agreement that there are clearly distinct ethical issues that face projects and individuals who engage in community-based, participatory collaborations. These differences included 1) seeking equality between the partners; 2) the need for the community partner to defend the community; 3) dealing with unflattering data; 4) meeting community expectations; and 5) producing tangible benefits to the community. We doubt this is an exhaustive list given our small sample size, but rather an indication that deeper research is needed into the ethical dimensions of community collaborations in research.

The issue of defining the community bedeviled our interviewees, as it has many before them, raising the critical question, "Who speaks for the community?" We like a particular definition of community that was arrived at through empirical methods, "Community is a group of people with diverse characteristics who are linked by social ties, share common perspectives, and engage in joint action in geographical locations or settings" (MacQueen et al., 2001). We would, however, be the first to admit that there are many other definitions and that none are uniformly accepted at this time. In the HPHI, community organizations are the instrument of community involvement and that was reflected in the interviews.

The use of smaller pilot studies to develop trust was noted by interviewees, as was the importance of establishing relationships based on mutual respect and the need for as much clarity/honesty as possible. For example, there was broad unity of opinion that violations of landlord contractual agreements should not be reportable, and this clearly speaks to the basis for establishing trust. These points have a role in traditional research as well, but the interviewees seemed to be identifying a difference in the form and importance in community collaborations. It should be noted that public housing residents tend to not trust others and place considerable importance on relationships. It may be that this emphasis in the interviews was influenced by the public housing context.

The primary concern raised about presentation of data was the need to consider the impact on the community and to provide an interpretation of the data so that it promoted the policy objectives of the community. Taking a "political stand" as one interviewee put it is anathema to most researchers. Indeed it was the question of what was "good science" that most divided the interviewees. The researchers were firm in the opinion that good science is related to research methods, while the other interviewees were just as certain that good science is science that helped the community solve its problems. The two interpretations are not incompatible with each other and both groups measured success of the project as benefits to the community.

The ethics of how to conduct honest research and still have an interest in the impact of the outcomes could be further developed. One of us (DB) draws the line between data collection and presentation of results (which must be unassailable) and the discussion of results (which is open to relatively broad interpretation). Another way to resolve this dilemma is in the choice of what research one undertakes. By choosing to study housing conditions and health, the HPHI researchers have put themselves in a position where their findings – whatever they are – are more likely to help the community.

The inability of the interviewees, despite their day-to-day involvement in collaborative research, to come up with a set of proposed amendments to traditional IRB training speaks volumes about the need for further thinking and study of community collaborative research ethics. This is an area of thought that is early in its development: at present the interest in ethics of community-based research is driven by studies of molecular genetics (Marshall and Rotimi, 2001), but participatory research such as the HPHI would benefit from more exploration of the ethical issues discussed above.

Acknowledgments

We thank Sabine Jean-Louis and Cat Bui who transcribed the interviews and the HPHI for letting us interview members of the project. We also thank those individuals that we interviewed and Marcia Boumil for helpful comments on the manuscript. The study was funded by a subcontract from NIH grant 1 T15 AI49650 (principal investigator, Dianne Quigley, Syracuse University).

References

Angell, M. (1997), "The Ethics of Clinical Research in the Third World", *New England Journal of Medicine*, **337**, 847–9.

Anonymous (2002), "Fair Benefits for Research in Developing Countries", *Science*, **298**, 2133–4.

Baker, E.A., Homan, S., Schonhoff, R. and Kreuter, M. (1999), "Principles of Practice for Academic/Practice/Community Research Partnerships", *American Journal of Preventive Medicine* **16**(3 Suppl), 86–93.

Bradley, M. (2001), Personal communication, Executive Director, Committee for Boston Public Housing, Boston, MA.

Brown, L.D. (1985), "People-Centered Development and Participatory Research", *Harvard Educational Review*, **55**, 69–75.

Brugge, D., Rice, P., Terry, P., Howard, L. and Best, J. (2001), "Housing conditions and respiratory health in a Boston public housing community", *New Solutions*, **11**, 149–64.

Brugge, D., Vallarino, J., Ascolillo, L., Osgood, N., Steinbach, S. and Spengler, J. (2003), "Comparison of multiple environmental factors for asthmatic children in public housing", *Indoor Air*, **13**, 18–27.

Casken, J. (1999), "Pacific Islander Health and Disease", in Huff, R.M., and Kline, M.V. (eds), *Promotion Health in Multicultural Populations: A Handbook for Practitioners*, Thousand Oaks, CA: Sage Publications, Inc., p. 414.

Christakis, N.A. (1988), "The ethical design of an AIDS vaccine trial in Africa", *Hastings Center Report*, **18**, 31–7.

El-Askari, G., Freestone, J., Irizary, C., Kruat, K.L., Mashiyama, S.T., Morgan, M.A. and Walton, S. (1998), "The Healthy Neighborhoods Project: A Local Health Department's Role in Catalyzing Community Development", *Health Education and Behavior*, **25**, 146–59.

Glesne, C. and Peshkin, A. (1992), *Becoming Qualitative Researchers: An Introduction*, London: Longman.

Hynes, P., Brugge, D., Watts, J. and Lally, J. (2000), "Public health and physical environment in Boston public housing", *Planning, Practice, and Research*, **15**, 31–49.

Inouye, J. (1999), "Chapter 18: Asian American Health and Disease", in Huff, R.M., and Kline, M.V. (eds), *Promotion Health in Multicultural Populations: A Handbook for Practitioners*, Thousand Oaks, CA: Sage Publications, Inc., p. 349.

Israel, B.A., Schulz, A.J. and Parker, E.A. (1998), "Review of Community-Based Research: Assessing Partnership Approaches to Improve Public Health", *Annual Review of Public Health*, **19**, 173–202.

Lehrman, S. (1997), "Jewish leaders seek genetic guidelines", *Nature*, **389**, 322.

Levine, R.J. (1988), *Ethics and Regulation of Clinical Research*, 2nd Ed., New Haven: Yale University Press, p. 13.

MacQueen, K.M., McLellan, E., Metzger, D.S., Strauss, R.P., Scotti, R., Blanchard, L. and Trotter, R.T. (2001), "What is community? An evidence-based definition for participatory public health", *American Journal of Public Health*, **91**, 1928–38.

Marshall, P.A. and Rotimi, C. (2001), "Ethical challenges in community-based research", *American Journal of the Medical Sciences*, **322**, 259–63.

Minkler, M. and Wallerstein, N. (eds) (2003), *Community-Based Participatory Research for Health*, San Francisco: Jossey-Bass.

The National Commission for the Protection of Human Subjects of Biomedical and Behavioral Research (1979), *The Belmont Report: Ethical Principles and Guidelines for the Protection of Human Subjects of Research*, April 18, 1979.

Ryan, L. (2002), *Researching Minority Ethnic Communities: A Note on Ethics*. <http://www.ucc.ie/ucc/units/equality/pubs/Minority/ryan.htm>, accessed June 27, 2002.

Schensul, J.J. (1999), "Organizing Community Research Partnerships in the struggle Against AIDS", *Health Education and Behavior*, **26**, 266–83.

Siedman, I.E. (1991), *Interviewing as Qualitative Research: A Guide for Researchers in Education and the Social Sciences*, New York and London: Teachers College Press.

Suarez, L., and Ramirez, A.G. (1999), "Hispanic/Latino Health and Disease", in Huff, R.M., and Kline, M.V. (eds), *Promotion Health in Multicultural Populations: A Handbook for Practitioners*, Thousand Oaks, CA: Sage Publications, Inc., p. 120.

Sullivan, M., Kone, A., Senturia, K.D., Chrisman, N.J., Ciske, S.J. and Krieger, J.W. (2001), "Researcher and researched-community perspectives: Toward bridging the gap", *Health Education & Behavior*, **28**, 130–49.

United States (2000), *Poverty in the United States 1999*, Washington, D.C.: U.S. Department of Commerce, U.S. Bureau of the Census, Current Population Survey. <http://www.census.gov/prod/2000pubs/p60-210.pdf> accessed June 27, 2002.

United States (2001), *Historical Poverty Tables*, Washington, D.C.: U.S. Bureau of the Census, Current Population Survey, Poverty and Health Statistics Branch/HHES Division, <http://www.census.gov/hhes/poverty/histpov/hstpov4.html> accessed June 27, 2002.

Weijer, C. (1999), "Protecting Communities in Research: Philosophical and Pragmatic Challenges", *Cambridge Quarterly of Healthcare Ethics*, USA: Cambridge University Press, pp. 501–2.

Weijer, C. and Emanuel, E.J. (2000), "Protecting communities in biomedical research", *Science*, **289**, 1142–44.

Chapter 3

The Seattle–King County Healthy Homes Project: Implementation of a Comprehensive Approach to Improving Indoor Environmental Quality for Low-Income Children with Asthma

James Krieger, Tim K. Takaro, Carol Allen, Lin Song,
Marcia Weaver, Sanders Chai and Philip Dickey

Asthma affects 15 million Americans (7% of the population), a third of them under the age of 18 (Mannino et al., 2002). It caused 474,000 hospitalizations, 1.9 million emergency department visits, and 10 million outpatient visits in 1996 (Graves and Kozak, 1998; Schappert, 1996). The national economic burden of asthma was projected to rise to $14.5 billion by the year 2000 (Jack et al., 1999). Asthma especially affects children. It is the most common childhood chronic disease and the leading noninjury cause of hospitalization for children ages 0–15 (Graves and Kozak, 1998). Nationally, asthma prevalence, health service utilization, and mortality (Mannino et al., 2002; Gergen, 1992) have increased among children and young adults since 1980. The self-reported prevalence of childhood asthma in the United States increased by 75% between 1980 and 1994. From 1975 to 1995, the estimated annual number of pediatric office visits for asthma more than doubled, from 4.6 million to 10.4 million. The hospitalization rate has increased among children and mortality rose by 118% between 1978 and 1995.

The causes of the increase in asthma morbidity are not well understood (Crater and Platts-Mills, 1998). However, a large body of evidence suggests that exposures found in indoor environments are major factors in the development and exacerbation of asthma (Institute of Medicine, 2000; Custovic and Woodcock, 2001; Lanphear et al., 2001). Table 3.1 summarizes the major indoor asthma triggers.

Asthma is an environmental justice issue with highly visible health effects. In the United States, low-income people and people of color are disproportionately affected by asthma. Relative to wealthier and White populations, they have higher asthma prevalence (Jack et al., 1999, Aligne et al., 2000; Crain et al., 1994; Litonjua et al., 1999) and experience more severe impacts (Weiss and Gergen, 1992; Wissow et al., 1988; Carr et al., 1992; Marder et al., 1992; Call et al., 1992; Lang and Polansky, 1992; Grant et al., 1999; Eggleson, 1998). In King County in the State of Washington, the asthma hospitalization rate of children living in high-poverty areas is three times that of

Table 3.1   Indoor asthma triggers

Exposure	Source (and contributing factors)
House dust mites	Carpeting, mattresses, bed linens, toys, upholstered furniture (dampness, poor ventilation, unvented cooking, humidifiers)
Animal-derived allergens	Cats, dogs, rodents, birds
Cockroach allergen	Cockroaches (accessible food, food debris, moisture, structural defects, clutter)
Tobacco smoke	Smoking household member (poor ventilation, contact with child)
Mould	Carpeting, walls, windows (leaks, poor ventilation, water damage, dampness)
Nitrogen oxides (NOx)	Space heaters, gas-fueled cooking stove (poor ventilation)
Wood smoke	Wood stoves and fireplaces (poor ventilation, faulty equipment)
Organic compounds	Pesticides, volatile organic compounds, formaldehyde (combustion products, poor ventilation, tobacco smoke, household products)
Viral respiratory infections	Exposures to persons infected (crowding)
Endotoxins	Gram-negative bacteria (soil, moisture, humidifiers)

those living in low-poverty areas (Solet et al., 2000). In addition, being poor or a person of color is associated with increased rates of sensitization to several asthma-associated allergens (Christiansen et al., 1996; Willies-Jacobo et al., 1993; Gelber et al., 1993; Sarpong et al., 1996; Eggleston, 2000; Gergen et al., 1987; Lewis et al., 2001; Strachan, 1996). Sensitization to allergens is one of the main risk factors for developing asthma and its complications (Eggleston and Bush, 2001; Platts-Mills et al., 1995; Sporik et al., 1999). Disparities in asthma morbidity and allergic sensitization may be due, in part, to disproportionate exposure to indoor environmental asthma triggers associated with living in substandard housing (Eggleston, 1998; Huss et al., 1994; Kane et al., 1999; Roberts et al., Johnston et al., 1995; Kitch et al., 2000). Moisture and dampness, poor ventilation, crowding, residence in multiunit dwellings, deteriorated carpeting, and structural deficits can contribute to high levels of indoor asthma triggers. Such conditions are more common in housing inhabited by low-income people and people of color. A strong parallel thus exists between exposure to indoor asthma triggers and the differential exposure of vulnerable populations to hazards in the outdoor environment (e.g., toxic wastes) – a hallmark of environmental racism (Perlin et al., 2001; Macey et al., 2001; Northridge and Shepard, 1997).

The growing understanding of the contribution of indoor environmental exposures to asthma-related health disparities has sparked widespread enthusiasm for interventions to improve the environmental quality of homes of low-income people and people of color. Although the most comprehensive intervention would be assuring access to safe and healthy environments, significant fiscal and political barriers limit the feasibility of this approach, leading advocates to adopt more modest strategies. In recent years, the Healthy Homes approach has gained popularity (Jacobs et al., 1999; Bower, 2001; Healthy Homes for Healthy Kids; Leung et al., 1997). Public health and community-based organizations have offered indoor environmental assessments, advice, resources, and advocacy to assess and improve indoor environmental quality. These programs have been based on current understanding of methods to reduce exposure to indoor asthma triggers (Institute of Medicine, 2000; Wooton and Ashley, 2000). However, information regarding the effectiveness of these methods is incomplete (Institute of Medicine, 2000; Etzel, 1996). While limited evidence regarding the impact of reducing individual exposures exists, even less information is available regarding integrated interventions that address multiple exposures (Institute of Medicine, 2000). To address this gap in knowledge, we designed and implemented the Seattle–King County Healthy Homes (SKCHH) project.

Seattle–King County Healthy Homes Overview

The National Institute of Environmental Health Sciences (NIEHS) Community-Based Prevention/Intervention Research program funded the SKCHH project for 4 years, beginning October 1997. The project was a randomized, controlled trial of an in-home educational intervention to improve asthma-related health status by reducing exposure to allergens, irritants, and toxics. We randomly assigned 274 low-income children 4–12 years of age with asthma to either a high- or a low-intensity group. In the high intensity group, community health workers called Community Home Environmental Specialists (CHES) conducted initial home environmental assessments and provided individualized action plans specifying participant and CHES actions to reduce exposures for each household. The CHES made additional visits to each home over a 12-month period to provide a protocol-defined package of education and social support, encouragement of participant actions, materials to reduce exposures (such as bedding covers and low-emission vacuums), assistance with roach and rodent eradication, and advocacy for improved housing conditions. We also offered free allergy testing. Members of the low-intensity group received the initial assessment, home action plan, limited education during the assessment visit, and bedding covers. One year after joining, low-intensity group participants received the full package of materials and additional advice regarding remaining indoor environmental quality concerns. In this article, we describe the implementation of SKCHH. The evaluation of its effectiveness has been published recently (Krieger et al., 2005). Primary outcomes are asthma-related quality of life (Juniper et al., 1996) and asthma symptoms (days with any symptoms in past two weeks and nights with symptoms), and secondary measures include health service utilization (emergency department, hospital, and unscheduled clinic visits), medication use (days rescue medication used in past two weeks), spirometry (forced expiratory volume in one sec,

FEV1), allergen exposure (dust concentration and floor surface loading of cockroach, mite, cat, and dog antigen and fungal spore counts), and changes in knowledge and actions related to indoor environmental quality. While SKCHH had asthma as its primary focus, the project also addressed other indoor health concerns, including lead, asbestos, pesticides, other toxic household products, and combustion products (CO, NOx) (Wooton and Ashley, 2000; Etzel and Balk, 1999; Schneider and Freeman, 2000). Once a community health worker was in the home, assessing these additional hazards and providing education and referrals to remediate them required little additional effort.

A household was eligible to participate if it included a child 4–12 years of age with health provider–diagnosed asthma of at least mild persistent severity (National Asthma Education and Prevention Program, 1997) and if the child's caretaker spoke English, Spanish, or Vietnamese. All participants had household incomes below 200% of poverty level, and 56% had incomes less than 100% of poverty level. Among caretakers, the most common ethnicities were African American (30%), Vietnamese (24%), Latino (17%), and non-Latino White (16%). The remainder included other Asian groups (7%), Native Americans (2%), and others (5%). Fifty-three percent of caretakers had completed high school, and 8% had completed college. We have reported additional characteristics and baseline findings elsewhere (Krieger et al., 2000).

Project Planning and Organization

The SKCHH project was designed as a community-based participatory research project (Krieger et al., 2002) with overall sponsorship by Seattle Partners for Healthy Communities, an Urban Research Center funded by the U.S. Centers for Disease Control and Prevention. Seattle Partners is a multidisciplinary partnership of community agencies, community activists, public health professionals, academics, and health providers that supports community-based participatory research addressing social determinants of health (Eisinger and Senturia, 2001). The Seattle Partners Board approved the initial proposal to NIEHS, supported project implementation, reviewed project progress, and offered guidance on implementing its principles of community–researcher collaboration (Kone et al., 2000; Sullivan et al., 2001). Development of the proposal to NIEHS, creation of project protocols, and operational oversight of SKCHH were the responsibilities of the steering committee, whose members included the American Lung Association of Washington, the Apartment House Association of Washington, the Center for MultiCultural Health, Engineering Plus, Group Health Cooperative of Puget Sound, the League of Women Voters of Seattle, Public Health – Seattle & King County, the Washington Toxics Coalition, and the University of Washington (Figure 3.1). Both the Seattle Partners Board and the steering committee sought to assure that the project benefited all participants. This led to the staggered intervention design with low- and high-intensity groups. This design assured that low-intensity group participants initially received some immediate benefit [including interventions known to be useful at the time the study was planned, such as bedding encasements; (Arlian and Platts-Mills, 2001)] while ultimately receiving all the benefits accorded the high-intensity group.

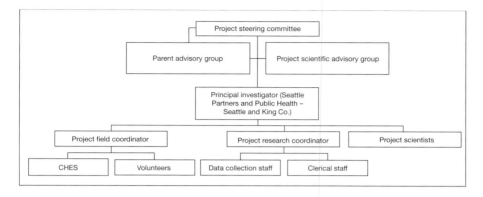

Figure 3.1   Organizational structure of SKCHH project

While this design may have reduced the study's power to demonstrate an effect of the high intensity intervention relative to a "pure" control group receiving no intervention, we felt such a design was not ethical. The Children's Hospital and Regional Medical Center Institutional Review Board approved the protocols.

The health department was responsible for coordination of project operations, project evaluation, and fiscal administration. Other partners developed the project training manual, provided training for project staff, and participated in project evaluation activities. A community agency implemented field activities during the first 18 months, after which the health department assumed responsibility for the remainder of the project with authorization from Seattle Partners. The health department had better capacity to deliver standard intervention protocols and conduct the research and evaluation aspects of the project. Locating activities at a single site improved coordination among project managers, field staff, and evaluators. We recruited project staff from the communities served by SKCHH, and they played important roles in protocol development and project evaluation in addition to their activities as health workers and data collectors. They were invaluable as knowledgeable community advocates.

The Parent Advisory Group consisted of nine participating parents representative of project enrollees. The CHES invited participants to join the group. CHES selected members to assure inclusion of each of the participating ethnic groups. The group met five times over 4 years to review protocols, project implementation, and evaluation findings and to advise on further program development. Its feedback led to development of protocols that were practical and culturally appropriate.

The four members of the scientific advisory group, who are nationally recognized for their expertise in asthma, air pollution, and environmental exposure assessment, contributed additional advice. The principle investigator provided overall leadership and scientific direction to the project while the field and research coordinators managed day-to-day operations.

Implementing SKCHH

The SKCHH project used an integrated approach to reducing exposure to asthma triggers and other indoor environmental risks. We emphasized that a limited number of underlying conditions, such as excessive moisture, dust, carpeting, structural defects, and household cleanliness, were related to exposure to many of the risks. We worked with participants to implement simple, low-cost, and sustainable approaches to addressing these underlying conditions and took more specific measures directed at particular exposures. We assumed that empowering participants with knowledge, tools, and support for taking action, rather than carrying out actions on their behalf, would result in a more sustainable approach. The project focused on education and participant action because the available resources were inadequate to remediate the underlying housing conditions that increase exposure to asthma triggers. We discuss the need for additional interventions at the conclusion of this article.

Because we developed SKCHH *de novo*, implementation was an iterative process. Staff and steering committee developed initial protocols based on existing scientific evidence. The Parent Advisory Group reviewed them and suggested changes. We made further changes after pilot testing in the field. We continued to revise protocols as we gained additional experience during project implementation. This section reviews the strategies and protocols we developed.

Community Health Workers

Our major strategy was the deployment of salaried community health workers (the CHES) to visit the homes of participants, where they conducted environmental assessments and provided education and support for creating a healthier indoor environment. The CHES had characteristics that allowed them to bridge the gap between community members and health agencies and institutions: connection to and understanding of the community; shared ethnic, linguistic, and cultural background with project participants; and recognition as a person who can be respected and trusted (Israel, 1985; Poland et al., 1991; Love et al., 1997; Witmer et al., 1995). Six CHES (including their coordinator) worked for the project over the course of its 4 years, with one or two full-time workers and their coordinator providing services at any one time. The CHES were of diverse ethnic backgrounds (four African Americans, one Latin American, and one Vietnamese). Five were female, and all lived in the targeted geographic area. Four were either personally affected by asthma or had a child who was, and the remaining two had close family members with asthma. We used several methods for recruiting CHES, including word of mouth, networking with community-based organizations, advertising in city and community newspapers, and posting in the county personnel system. The first two approaches were most effective and have been used by other community health worker programs (Jackson and Parks, 1997).

The CHES completed a 40-hr SKCHH training program that included didactic sessions, in-class exercises, role-playing, and field practice. We developed a training manual adapted from one prepared by the Master Home Environmentalist (MHE) program of the American Lung Association of Washington (Dickey, 1998) (see below). CHES also participated in 10–20 hr of continuing education per year. They met with the principal investigator every two weeks and the steering committee every two to three months to review protocols and discuss challenging cases. We also prepared a protocol manual for use in the field [a list of training topics and the training manual are available at the project's website (www.metrokc.gov/health/asthma/healthyhomes/)] The CHES supervisors found frequent review and reinforcement of protocols and field observation valuable for assuring quality of services.

During the early years of the project, CHES visited participants nine times over the course of a year, according to a defined visit protocol. The interval between the first four visits was two weeks, after which subsequent visits occurred every two months. We expected CHES to complete specific tasks at each visit as well as work in a more open-ended manner to meet participants' unique needs. As we accumulated feedback from participants and CHES, we reduced the number of visits per client to five to seven total visits. We now follow a structured six-visit schedule (Table 3.2), with supplemental visits as needed.

Table 3.2   CHES visit schedule
X indicates the activities that all homes receive; (X) additional activities per protocol that homes with specific issues receive.

Activity	Visit 1	Visit 2	Visit 3	Visit 4	Visit 5	Visit 6
Time (months)	0.0	0.5	1.0	4.5	7.5	10.5
General activities						
Project overview	X	X				
Set home priorities and make plan	X	X				
Revisit household priorities		X	X	X	X	X
Assessments						
Home environmental assessment	X					
Screen for urgent issues[a]	X				X	
Dust sampling (allergens)	X					
Deep dust assessment[b]		X	X	X	X	X
Dust mite control reassessment		X[c]	X	X	X	
Roach assessment: traps	X	X		(X)[d]		(X)[d]

Tobacco reassessment			X	(X)	(X)	(X)
Pet reassessment				X	(X)	(X)
Rodent reassessment			X	(X)	(X)	(X)
Moisture reassessment			X	X		X
Vacuuming and cleaning technique reassessment			X^e	X	X	X
Toxins reassessment				X		
Education and action						
Asthma basics	X			X		
Dust mites	X	X	X		X	
Discuss household action plan items		X	X	X	X	X
Household cleaning			X	X	X	(X)
Household toxins			X	(X)	X	(X)
Moisture control		X^f	X^g	$(X)^h$	(X)	(X)
Pets			X	$(X)^i$		(X)
Tobacco		X^j	$(X)^k$	(X)	(X)	(X)
Roaches	X	X		X	(X)	
Rodents			X		(X)	
Outdoor air			X			
Referrals Skin testing		X^l	$(X)^l$			
Tobacco cessation		X^m	X	(X)	(X)	(X)

a Pesticide (canceled/suspended), car exhaust (attached garage and idle >15 sec), flammable products near heat/fire, hazardous products within reach of children, hazardous products in rusting, leaking or open container, use of wood stove, use cooking source to heat house, unvented gas/kerosene heater, smell heating fuel (gas or oil), wet carpet present, roaches present, rodents present.

b Three-spot vacuuming test.

c Check if allergy-control covers are installed.
d Households with "severe" roach problem may need additional assessments.
e Review frequency and check technique.
f Brief introduction, how to use relative humidity meter.
g Overview (sources, general control measures).
h Only for high moisture homes.
i Only for homes with pets.
j General information for all households with/without tobacco problem.
k Brief reminder for homes with tobacco problem.
l Arrange if not yet completed (appointment for skin testing will have been made at intake interview).
m If issue and caretaker or smoker desires to quit and participate in a smoking cessation class.

Participants often had unpredictable schedules that initially made it challenging to set appointments. Ultimately, CHES developed a process in which they fixed the next visit date before leaving the home and confirmed the next visit by telephone the day before. The most effective method for assuring participant presence at the appointed time was giving them a calendar to post in the kitchen and circling the visit date. While participants occasionally were not home for a scheduled visit, this was not a major problem and overbooking the CHES schedules was not necessary. The Vietnamese CHES and his clients were comfortable with unscheduled drop-in visits, but this was not acceptable to other participants.

We developed a computer-based system for tracking home visits, assessment findings, client contact activities, and action plan implementation. The CHES supervisor used the system extensively to prepare visit schedules and develop weekly work plans for each CHES, but the CHES did not regularly use this system because data entry was too time consuming. We are redesigning the system with input from the CHES and will enlist clerical staff to enter encounter data collected by CHES after each visit.

Each full-time equivalent CHES had a caseload of 40–80 clients at any point in time. Carrying a caseload at the high end of this range required considerable overtime. A reasonable load is approximately 50 clients. During an average week, each full-time equivalent CHES scheduled 12 visits and completed 10. The initial assessment visit averaged 50 min (range, 30–90 min), and follow-up visits averaged 45 min (range, 20–120 min). CHES needed additional time for other operational tasks such as travel, assessing client eligibility, scheduling appointments, attending team meetings, training, and picking up supplies. The CHES completed 970 visits over the course of two years.

It was important that the CHES performed their work with cultural competence (Kleinman et al., 1978; Manson, 1988). When possible, we matched the ethnicities of CHES and participants (54% of participants shared ethnicity with their CHES). CHES communicated in the primary language of nearly all of their clients. All staff participated in 6 hr of cultural competency training, which emphasized effective communication with diverse clients. CHES would have liked further training to understand the specific values, beliefs, and concerns of each of the ethnic groups with which they worked. The basic educational materials used by the CHES were available in Spanish, Vietnamese, and English. Adequate materials, especially in Vietnamese, were not available when we began our work. We translated some resources, but culturally appropriate, low-literacy, visually oriented materials are needed.

Another important CHES activity was provision of instrumental, informational and emotional support. Social support can be a powerful motivator and reinforcer of behavioral change (Heaney and Israel, 1997; Berkman and Glass, 2000). CHES had a caring, empathetic attitude and genuine interest in the well being of their participants. They helped clients initiate cleaning and make minor repairs. They referred caretakers to the Asthma and Allergy Foundation's dedicated help line for additional advice and to local asthma support groups. CHES served as role models for clients, demonstrating the skills for making a healthier home. Many participants had issues that took precedence over asthma, such as inadequate income, risk of eviction, unemployment, child behavior problems, teen suicide, drug addiction, and inability to pay utility bills. The CHES and their coordinator identified appropriate community resources [using the local "Where to Turn" manual (The Crisis Clinic, 2001) and a network of contacts] and linked participants with them. Other assistance included finding free furniture (some homes had no beds), collecting funds to assist clients in the purchase of asthma medication, enrollment in a program to receive Christmas gifts, and weatherization program assistance. The need for these support activities could become overwhelming, and it was important to provide CHES with support and counseling in setting boundaries on the roles they played in participants' lives. At times, sustained assistance and case management beyond the scope of CHES skills was necessary.

The stresses of setting boundaries with clients and being confronted with their difficult life circumstances were only some of the challenges faced by the CHES. Another challenge was changes in roles and responsibilities because we modified protocols based on field experience. A third was that some of the CHES felt too constrained when following project protocols that allowed limited flexibility in working with their clients. A fourth was the daily logistical hassles such as spending much time traveling heavily trafficked roads, carrying cumbersome vacuums and other equipment, working evenings and weekends, and arriving for home visits only to find the client not in. Finally, family issues such as difficulties in arranging childcare when working evenings and weekends played a role. These issues contributed to high staff turnover during the first two years of the project. However, once the project matured during the third year, staff stabilized and we completed the project with CHES who were skilled at their work and committed to SKCHH. The difficulties faced by the CHES underscore the need for debriefing them when experiences become overwhelming, providing emotional support, offering incentives such as attendance at conferences, and assuring periods of less intensive activity.

Community Volunteers

We originally intended to use community volunteers from the MHE program to implement the low-intensity intervention. The MHE program provides trained volunteers who visit homes to educate residents about improving indoor environmental quality. Volunteers receive a 40-hr training covering indoor pollution, communication and community outreach skills, and cultural diversity. They use the Home Environmental Assessment List (HEAL) (Leung et al., 1997) to identify pollutants and develop an action plan that prioritizes problems and low-cost or no-cost solutions that reduce exposures. The initial visit is followed up with a telephone call to assess progress.

A special recruitment and training prepared 20 volunteers for participation in SKCHH. We focused recruitment efforts on reaching people who lived in the communities to be served or who had worked with low-income community members.

The volunteer component faced a number of challenges and ultimately was ineffective. This result was surprising because the MHE program routinely employs volunteers successfully. Multiple factors may have contributed to this outcome. First, an 8-month delay occurred between completion of the training and commencement of interventions. In this time, volunteers had limited contact with the program. When home visits by volunteers did begin, project staff supported volunteers consistent with past MHE practice, but this was insufficient for the specific needs of the SKCHH project volunteers. A new project coordinator assumed this responsibility and devoted considerable time to calling active volunteers every 7–14 days to answer questions, providing support, and requesting submission of visit reports. Second, despite the recruiting efforts, volunteers were generally not from the participants' communities. This led to reluctance of volunteers to work in inner-city neighborhoods and limitations on the cultural competence of the volunteers. Third, scheduling home visits was difficult for the volunteers, who often were not available at the times preferred by participants and had limited ability to adjust their schedules. Fourth, volunteers had difficulty in adhering to protocols, fully completing home assessments, keeping to timelines, and returning visit reports. Because of these difficulties, the CHES assumed responsibility for providing services to the low-intensity group.

Participant Recruitment and Retention

To obtain participants, we collected lists of potential participants from community and public health clinics, hospitals, and emergency departments; publicized the project through local media and at community events; and received referrals from public schools, government and community agencies, public housing, churches, sororities, and other community organizations. The most efficient approach was identifying potential participants through their sources of medical care. All these sources yielded 1,111 potentially eligible children, whose asthma diagnosis we verified through chart review. We reached 709 (64%) of their caretakers and were unable to contact the remaining 402 households because of disconnected or incorrect phone numbers, or no response after six phone calls and one mailing. Of the households we reached, 355 (50%) were eligible; the remainder either refused the eligibility interview (90) or were not eligible (258). Of the eligible households, we randomly assigned 138 (39%) to the high-intensity group and 136 (38%) to the low-intensity group; 67 (19%) declined participation, and 14 (4%) did not enroll because of logistical difficulties.

Of the original participants, 226 (82%) completed the 1-year program. The difficulties in maintaining contact with participants in health-related outreach and research projects have been well described (Senturia, 1998). The most common reason for dropping out of our project was being too busy. A small number of participants (12) seemed motivated to join in order to obtain the supplies and dropped out after receiving the vacuum. CHES followed a protocol to maximize retention, which included up to seven phone calls, a postcard, a letter, two home visits, three attempts to reach an alternate personal contact, contacting workplace and source of medical care, and consulting residence directories. Recruitment and retention may have been facilitated by offering cash incentives ($45 for completion of baseline data collection and $65 for completing the project), as well as providing resources such as the vacuum and bedding encasements.

Conducting Home Environmental Assessments

The CHES conducted a comprehensive home environmental assessment at their first visit. They repeated portions of this assessment at subsequent visits to assess progress in resolving problems or development of new concerns. If households moved (3% of SKCHH participants did so), the CHES performed a complete assessment of the new home. To conduct the assessment, the CHES administered a questionnaire, joined participants in conducting a visual inspection of the home, and made environmental measurements. Dharmage et al. (1999) have shown that interview and inspection provide valid measures of home environmental conditions. We collected data using the Healthy Homes Baseline Questionnaire and the Home Environmental Assessment List – II (HEALII), both of which are available on the SKCHH website. We adapted the latter from the HEAL developed by the MHE program. Areas covered in the assessment included:

● knowledge of asthma triggers and prior asthma education
● assessment of asthma severity and medications used
● access to medical care for asthma
● tobacco smoke exposure
● exposure to allergen sources (mites, cockroaches, rodents, dust, pets)
● dust control behaviors (track-in, vacuuming/cleaning, use of allergen-control bedding encasements)
● mould and moisture problems and contributing structural factors (condensation, water infiltration and damage, sources of leaks, ventilation [windows and fans, appliances], weatherization, heating, insulation, vapor barriers)
● structural conditions (carpeting, building age, condition of paint, structural deficits, recent remodeling)
● additional factors contributing to exposure (food debris and storage, trash, clutter, heating system filters and ducts, heating and cooking sources, location of garage)
● use and storage of hazardous and toxic products
● additional indoor air contaminants (asbestos, combustion products)
● tap and washing machine water temperature
● exposure to take-home hazards from work

We encouraged participants to obtain free skin-prick allergy testing to determine the specific exposures most relevant for their children. Ten allergens (dust mite [Der p1 and Der f1], regional mould mix, cat, dog, cockroach [American and German], alder, birch, grass mix) and histamine and saline controls were applied intradermally with bifurcated needles using standard procedures (Nelson, 1995). We made arrangements with three clinical sites in the target area to provide this service on weekday afternoons and Saturday mornings. We also held an allergy testing fair that included food, games, door prizes, and a raffle. Despite these efforts, only 23% of children received the test. Lack of easy transportation and competing demands were the major obstacles. Having the child's health provider order the test and increasing client appreciation of its benefits may have increased testing. Future efforts may require taxi vouchers or collecting blood samples for radioallergosorbent allergy testing during a regular clinic visit rather than relying on skin prick tests.

We collected additional environmental exposure data as part of our research and evaluation protocol. Briefly, CHES collected floor dust from the child's bedroom that was sieved and weighed prior to analysis for cat, dog, cockroach, and dust mite antigen and viable mould counts (Tokaro et al., 2004).

The Action Plan

The CHES developed a Home Action Plan with each client. A computerized system generated a draft action plan by linking each assessment finding with protocol-derived action steps for the residents and CHES. The following section summarizes these protocols. Because the protocols specified a wide range of actions and because clients' interests varied, the CHES and client together prioritized the action steps to prepare a final individualized action plan. A standard form logged actions taken by the CHES and clients after each visit for entry into the data system, which then generated an updated action plan for the next visit. As actions were accomplished, the CHES and participants moved on to address other items.

A key component of our intervention, therefore, was promoting participant actions to improve control of asthma. Social cognitive theory (Bandura, 1977; Bandura, 1986; Baranowski et al., 1997) and the transtheoretical stages of change model (Prochaska and DiClemente, 1983; Prochaska et al., 1994; Prochaska et al., 1997) suggest the value of an individualized, stage-specific approach that sets manageable priorities, of providing clients with feedback on their implementation of action plans, and of CHES serving as role models who demonstrate actions to reduce exposures (e.g., vacuuming and cleaning mould). CHES used several techniques to encourage participant actions: simplification to adapt to the participant's lifestyle; monitoring and reinforcement; individualizing, reviewing, and adjusting plans as needed; encouraging family involvement; being attentive to client concerns and fears; and giving participants simple, brief, written materials that reinforced the actions recommended and skills taught (Roter et al., 1998; Willey, 1999; Clark et al., 1995; Haynes et al., 1979; Evans, 1993; Meichenbaum and Turk, 1987).

Table 3.3 Exposure reduction protocols used in Seattle–King County Healthy Homes project

Exposure	Action	
	Resident	CHES
Asthma triggers		
Moisture and mould (Bush and Portnoy, 2001)	Use ventilation properly (kitchen, bath, crawl space), avoid fish tanks, clean with 5% bleach/detergent solution, heat all rooms and closets, open windows often, repair leaks, maintain humidity below 50%, reduce household plants if present in large quantity (Burge et al., 1982), remove carpeting, place vapor barrier between concrete floors and carpet, remove mould damaged carpet, furniture and other items	Educate on moisture sources/barriers, provide cleaning materials, replace moldy shower curtain, inspect and clean ventilation fans, plug holes between crawl space and home with steel wool and foam
Dust	Vacuuming and dusting (Munir et al., 1993; Adilah et al., 1997; Lioy et al., 1998; Murray and Ferguson, 1983), use double-layer vacuum bags and/or low-emission vacuum (Vaughan et al., 1999), use high-quality door mats and remove shoes (Roberts et al., 1991)	Educate and provide with low-emission vacuum with dirt finder, double-layer microfiltration vacuum bags, clean green cleaning kit (vinegar, baking soda, oil soap, etc.), mop and bucket, gloves, door mat, furnace filters, lint-free dusting rags
Mites (Arlian and Platts-Mills, 2001)	Vacuuming, cleaning and dusting, wash bedding weekly in ≥130°F water (pillows monthly), remove or wash stuffed animals, replace (or vacuum) upholstered furniture, carpet and drape removal, maintain humidity below 50% (Ehnert et al., 1992; Cabera et al., 1995; Arlian et al., 2001; Shapiro, 1999)	Educate, provide and install allergy-control bedding encasements on pillows and mattresses (Ehnert et al., 1992; Shapiro, 1999; Owen et al., 1990; ven der Heide et al., 1997; Vaughan et al., 1999; Hill et al., 1997)
Roaches (Reid and Bennett, 1989) (O'Connor and Gold, 1999)	Food clean up and storage, clean up clutter, remove garbage from home daily, cleaning, eliminate sources of standing water (e.g., leaks, refrigerator drip pans), cleaning before and after eradication	Educate, integrated pest management methods (provide food storage containers, caulk or steel wool and foam to seal small defects; Abamectin gel bait[a] (Reid and Bennett, 1989); vacuuming and intensive cleaning post-eradication)
Rodents	As per roaches and clean up outdoor rodent hiding places and attractants	Seal small defects, screens on exhaust vents, glue boards and snap traps

Tobacco smoke	Quit smoking or smoke outside using smoking jacket, launder clothes exposed to smoke, avoid smoking in the car	Assess stage of change (Prochaska et al., 1983), brief non-confrontational counseling (Wahlgren et al., 1997), refer to the Free and Clear smoking cessation program[b] (telephone counseling and nicotine replacement)
Wood smoke	Use alternative heat source or maintain stove and flue	Educate and refer to weatherization program for replacement with natural gas
Pets (Chapman and Wood, 2001)	Remove from home or keep outside bedroom, vacuuming, carpet removal, bedding covers (De Blay et al., 1991)	Educate
NOx	Ventilate kitchen, assure furnace properly vented	Educate on combustion sources
Toxics		
Toxic or hazardous chemicals	Store safely, dispose of properly and switch to less toxic alternative	Educate about safer use, storage, and disposal and encourage use of alternatives, provide safer cleaning alternatives in "clean green" cleaning kit
Pesticides	Use integrated pest management alternatives	Educate about integrated pest management alternatives
CO	Identify combustion sources vented to living area	Educate[c]
Lead	Vacuuming and cleaning (Lioy et al., 1998; Mielke et al., 1992), and reducing track-in of exterior dust	If lead risk present, refer child to primary medical provider for lead testing
Asbestos		Identify materials potentially containing asbestos; refer to certified remediation team (U.S. EPA, 1998)

a   Whitmire Micro-Gen Research Laboratories, St. Louis, MO.
b   Group Health Cooperative of Puget Sound, Seattle, WA.
c   For households with combustion appliances/furnaces.

Reducing Specific Exposures

Table 3.3 summarizes the protocols used by the CHES, and details are available at our website. Recent reviews summarize the justification for including these interventions (Institute of Medicine, 2000; Wooton and Ashley, 2000; Bierman, 1996; Eggleston and Bush, 2001; Gold, 2000; Tovey and Marks, 1999; Platts-Mills et al., 2000), and Table 3 cites additional supporting literature.

The experience of implementing SKCHH and new findings in the research literature has shown us ways to improve our protocols. A major lesson learned was that the "best practices" as described in the literature and guidelines may not be feasible to implement in low-income households similar to those that participated in our project. A project that emphasizes actions that are easy to adopt, that use simple protocols, and that encourages participants to take on a limited number of actions may increase chances of success. We summarize what we have learned in the following paragraphs.

Mites. Providing allergy-control bedding covers was not sufficient; participants often needed assistance in placing them on the mattress. Less expensive vinyl covers ripped easily, and we recommend the more durable woven fabric type. We measured the temperature of hot water in homes and found that it was below the 130°F needed for killing mites in 74%. We considered adding eucalyptus oil to cooler wash water (Tovey and McDonald, 1997), but it is expensive and leaves a residual odor.

Drying bedding at 130°F for at least 20 min also kills mites and is an alternative (Miller and Miller, 1996; Mason et al., 1999). Many (82%) children had stuffed toys, but few participants (26%) washed them regularly. Freezing toys and small items for at least 24 hr kills mites and may be easier than washing. We elected not to use acaricides because evidence of their effectiveness is inconclusive (Arlian and Platts-Mills, 2001) and not to use tannic acid because of its unacceptability to participants (it may stain fabrics).

Mould. Not all homes with visible mould were able to eliminate it through cleaning with bleach solution, yet replacement of contaminated building material was beyond the scope of this project. Although we recommended the use of a high-efficiency particulate air (HEPA) filter if a child was sensitized to moulds and ongoing exposure was present, most participants could not afford one (Bush and Portnoy, 2001; American Lung Association, 1997). We will include provision of air filters for such situations in future work.

Tobacco smoke. Despite making available free telephonic smoking cessation counseling and nicotine replacement patches, only 20% of smoking caretakers quit. We found that motivating smoking household members to smoke outside the home was useful: among smokers who did not go outside to smoke prior to intervention, a quarter did so after education by the CHES. We also recommended use of a HEPA filter (although we were unable to offer one) if tobacco smoke was present in the house (American Lung Association, 1997), and we will provide HEPA filters in future work.

Cockroaches. Education regarding cockroaches and asthma emerged as an especially important topic. Participants frequently were unaware of the relationship of roaches to asthma (Krieger et al., 2000) and did not often realize that they could be present without being visible. In fact, some participants who reported no roaches were offended when the CHES placed roach traps in the participants' homes. We would modify some aspects of our eradication protocol. Authorities recommend a repeated application of gel bait 1–2 weeks after the initial application, and we will revise our protocol accordingly (Eggleston and Arruda, 2001). One challenge we faced was that some homes required an intensive amount of work to eliminate clutter and food sources before eradication and to clean comprehensively after eradication for removal of remaining allergen. Assistance for participants from professional house cleaners for some homes would have been beneficial. Other issues were the limited effectiveness of eliminating roaches in homes contained in multiunit structures without treating the entire building and difficulties in addressing some of the underlying structural conditions that allowed entry of roaches. Solutions to these issues require additional resources and cooperation from landlords.

Pets. Because removal of pets from the home is difficult, we have considered other alternatives. Cat and dog allergens accumulate in clothing and fabric, and washing them may be of some benefit (Patchett et al., 1997). Although some studies have suggested that washing cats twice weekly may reduce exposure to allergen (Avner et al., 1997), we rejected pet washing because experts (Wood, 1997; Chapman and Wood, 2001) and our participants felt that this was not an effective, practical approach. The role of HEPA filters remains controversial (Institute of Medicine, 2000; van der Heide et al., 1999; Wood et al., 1998).

Hazardous household chemicals. Given our focus on reducing asthma morbidity, the intervention for household chemical products was directed primarily at respiratory irritants.

However, we took advantage of the opportunity to educate household members about other product hazards that could affect children. We identified products of concern by category (e.g., pesticides), by federally mandated label warnings (U.S. EPA, 2001; U.S. Consumer Product Safety Administration, 2001) (e.g., corrosive products), or by the presence of certain ingredients (e.g., chlorine bleach, solvents) and placed them on one of two priority lists. High-priority products included canceled or suspended pesticides, pesticides in U.S. Environmental Protection Agency hazard category I or II, pesticide dusts, products containing chlorine bleach or ammonia, and solvent-based products used once per week or more. CHES helped participants eliminate these products from homes to minimize exposure. Lower-priority items included corrosive products, other pesticides, solvent products used less than once per week, other volatile organic compounds, and other potential asthma triggers such as air fresheners and fragrances. For these products, CHES suggested alternatives where possible. For all products, CHES looked for unsafe storage, suggested proper disposal, and recommended safer alternatives.

Combustion products. Most (70%) homes relied upon electricity for heat and cooking; exposure to NO_2 and CO was therefore not an issue for most participants. In the homes with hydrocarbon energy sources, CHES counseled participants on maintaining adequate ventilation while cooking and on the value of regular furnace maintenance. We plan to add assessment of CO levels in such homes.

Addressing Underlying Conditions

Exposure is affected by underlying housing conditions. For example, excessive indoor moisture increases exposure to mites and moulds, whereas poor ventilation can exacerbate exposure to tobacco smoke, combustion products, irritants, and moisture. Structural deficits allow entry of pests and water. As shown in Table 3.3, our protocols spoke to these conditions to varying degrees, and we now describe lessons learned as we addressed them.

Moisture. Moisture problems were present in 77% of homes. We collected evidence of excessive moisture by asking questions about humidifier use, fog on glass surfaces, presence of vapor barriers and vents in crawl spaces, and by direct inspection for mould, leaks, wet carpeting, and water damage. We also attempted to assess relative humidity by asking participants to record daily maximum and minimum relative humidity over two-week periods in a diary using a digital hygrometer, but the very low completion rate (36%) invalidated the diary as a useful tool. We partially addressed excessive moisture by the protocols described in Table 3.3. However, we did not usually accomplish some of these interventions (e.g., installation of ventilation fans, installation of vapor barriers and ventilation of moist crawl spaces), given the resource constraints of this project. Controlling indoor relative humidity to less than 50% is effective in reducing mite and possibly mould exposure (Bush and Portnoy, 2001; Cabera et al., 1995), but doing so by simple ventilation may not be practical in Seattle and other coastal areas where high relative humidity is common year-round (in Seattle, seasonal humidity ranges from 49–53% in the summer to 74–78% in the winter) (National Weather Service). More expensive options such as dehumidifiers may be efficacious (Warner et al., 2000), but their feasibility and effectiveness have been questioned (Fletcher et al., 1996). Our project was limited in its ability to correct structural deficits permitting water intrusion, which we noted in over 20% of the homes. Remediation of mould-contaminated wallboard or carpet was also beyond project resources, and participants did not have the means to do so independently. Healthy Homes demonstration and education projects funded by the Department of Housing and Urban Development are currently assessing the benefits of more aggressive structural remediation interventions. We have recently received such a grant to conduct remediation of 35 homes at an average cost of $4,400.

Dust and housecleaning. CHES found that conveying basic information about housecleaning and its benefits for a child with asthma was valuable, and most participants became more effective cleaners (the proportion vacuuming at least weekly increased from 62% to 78% in the high intensity group). It was important to help participants distinguish between aspects of household appearance relevant to asthma control (e.g., clutter, dust, mould) and those of a more cosmetic nature (e.g., stains). Providing simple tips such as cleaning on a schedule, giving oneself a reward for cleaning, and doing a little bit each day seemed helpful, as did provision of vacuums and cleaning supplies.

Household clutter was a significant problem in 42% of homes, and participants had widely varying tolerances for its extent. They had limited understanding of how clutter contributed to increasing levels of allergens by impeding implementation of other cleaning strategies, such as vacuuming, dusting, and removal of food debris. CHES had to work alongside a limited number of participants to help them attain a reasonable level of cleanliness in their home so that they could implement action plan items related to cleaning. Providing professional housecleaning services for participants with large cleaning needs or those whose homes harbor roaches may be useful. Visual information such as a video of housecleaning or before-and-after pictures demonstrating successfully cleaned homes may also be helpful.

Carpets are an important reservoir of dust and allergens (Vaughan and Platts-Mills, 2000). While most (85%) homes had carpets, few (7%) participants were able to remove them because they were renters or could not afford to install alternative flooring. As a partial solution, vacuuming may be moderately effective in reducing dust and allergen exposure (Munir et al., 1993; Adilah et al., 1997; Lioy et al., 1998). We enhanced the effectiveness of vacuuming by providing participants with low-emission, power-head vacuums equipped with a dirt detector and gave them feedback regarding effectiveness of vacuuming through the "three-spot" vacuum test (Roberts et al., 2001). The test uses a vacuum with a dirt detection system that allows the deep carpet dust to be estimated. The detector used in this project has a red light that changes to green when nearly all the dust is out. The three-spot test measures the time in seconds to get green lights on three spots three feet apart. Ten seconds or less is considered a clean carpet (<10 g/m^2 of deep dust). The three-spot test appears to be useful in assessing the effectiveness of efforts to reduce dust levels in carpets and may reinforce good cleaning habits by demonstrating progress in removing dust from carpets. Details of the test are available at our website. About 10% of vacuums we provided required repairs after use. Many of the repairs were related to motors jammed with vacuumed material. In the future, we will use a vacuum in which vacuumed material is deposited directly into the bag, rather than passing through the motor.

Removing shoes and leaving them at the door was difficult for many households, as homes lacked space for shoe storage. We are exploring the provision of shoe storage bags or shelving and inexpensive house slippers.

Ventilation. We assessed ventilation by observing the presence and use of exhaust fans and operable windows in kitchen and bath, and testing the function of the fan by observing whether it generated sufficient suction to hold a piece of two-ply tissue paper against the grille. While those participants who had working fans used them, project resources did not permit installation of fans in homes without them or repair of nonworking units. We are currently working with subsidized weatherization programs for help in repairing and installing ventilation fans. While we recommended opening windows to increase ventilation, participants felt unsafe with open windows and did not follow this advice. We will begin to provide window locks.

Landlord–tenant relations. Remediation of underlying conditions sometimes required involvement of a landlord because 86% of participants were renters. In some cases, tenants were afraid to approach the landlord because of fear of retaliation in the context of a very tight housing market. In other cases, CHES assisted tenants approach their landlords by helping draft letters and speaking directly to the landlords as needed. In the few cases in which the landlord was not responsive, we referred participants to the Seattle Tenants Union for additional assistance.

Because many participants lived in public housing or were on the waiting list, we worked closely with the Seattle Housing Authority (SHA). Participants on the waiting list were moved to the top and offered housing that met Healthy Homes criteria. For participants already living in SHA units, SHA immediately repaired unhealthy conditions upon contact by the project coordinator and gave priority to eradication of roaches in participants' homes. If the only solution was a move to a different unit, SHA moved the client.

Participant Feedback

We collected data from participants regarding their perceptions of the program as part of an exit interview conducted one year after enrollment by an interviewer with no prior contact with the participant. Questions included close-ended items covering the usefulness of the information provided, supplies received, and the action plan on a 4-point response scale (extremely useful, very useful, somewhat useful, not useful) and satisfaction with CHES worker (excellent, very good, good, fair, poor). Additional questions asked the participant how much of the action plan they carried out (all, most, some, none) and the reasons why participants had not completed parts of the plan (the questions included six specific items such as "not enough time or being too busy," "cost too much," "didn't think the actions would be helpful," as well as an open-ended probe asking about "other things that got in your way"). A set of open ended questions asked the respondent to describe the most important actions he or she took as a result of the project, things most liked about the project, things to improve the project, things liked best about the CHES worker, and things the CHES could do to improve the service received.

Caretakers in the high-intensity group generally gave positive feedback: 93% said that the information they received was extremely useful or very useful. Most considered the supplies provided to be extremely useful or very useful (97% for the vacuum cleaner, 96% for the mattress cover, 93% for the door mat, and 89% for the cleaning kit). Of those who remembered receiving an action plan (78% of caretakers), 88% thought it was extremely useful or very useful, and 77% were able to carry out all or most of the action plan. Among those who did not carry out all of the action plan items, the main barriers were "not enough time or being too busy" (55%) and "cost too much money to do" (44%).

The actions the caretakers described as most important for controlling their child's asthma were cleaning, dusting, and vacuuming more often and more thoroughly; covering bedding with allergy control encasements; washing or changing bedding more regularly; cleaning mould; keeping the child away from tobacco smoke; and getting rid of stuffed animals.

The aspects of the project the caretakers liked most included the information and education provided, supplies (especially the vacuum cleaner and allergy-control encasements), home visits, and help from CHES. Most (84%) of the caretakers described their experience working with the CHES workers as excellent or very good. When asked about things that could improve the project, the most frequent response was reducing the length or repetitiveness of the evaluation questionnaires. Some caretakers would have preferred fewer visits, but a few others would have liked more. A few would have liked the project to have the school involved.

Conclusions

We have described the organization and implementation of the SKCHH project. It is a promising approach to address the disparities in exposures to indoor asthma triggers and in asthma morbidity seen among low-income households. The SKCHH project members worked with 274 low-income families to identify and take actions to control indoor health hazards. We developed protocols to address major indoor environmental quality problems associated with asthma that low-income and ethnically diverse caretakers of children with asthma can implement with assistance from community health workers. Project participants were enthusiastic about SKCHH, felt they derived important benefits and would like to see the project made available more widely. Before doing so, we need evidence of the effectiveness of this and other Healthy Homes projects (e.g., Boston and Cambridge, Massachusetts; Detroit, Michigan; Cleveland, Ohio; Philadelphia, Pennsylvania; and San Diego and San Francisco, California) that have employed similar approaches to improving indoor environmental quality. Our evaluation of SKCHH found that it reduced asthma symptoms and urgent health service use and increased asthma-related quality of life (Krieger et al., 2005). Other Healthy Homes projects will also be reporting on their evaluations in coming years. Until these evaluations are complete, it seems reasonable to use existing evidence to guide education and actions to improve home environmental quality, as summarized in Table 3.3 and elsewhere (Institute of Medicine, 2000; Wooton and Asthley, 2000; Bierman, 1996; Etzel, 1996; Etzel and Balk, 1999; Schneider and Freeman, 2000; National Asthma Education and Prevention Program, 1997; Tovey and Marks, 1999; Platts-Mills et al., 2000).

We limited our protocols to asthma triggers, dust control, and elimination of hazardous chemical products and did not address other indoor hazards. We plan to add additional protocols to address injury hazards. Lead and radon are not major issues in the Seattle area, so we did not emphasize them. However, dust control is an important tool for prevention of lead and pesticide exposure (Davies et al., 1990), and our current protocols would be expected to reduce these exposures if present in house dust. We are planning to add more explicit linkages with health care providers, who have expressed an interest in receiving information about the homes of their patients and the changes they are making as a result of SKCHH, and would like assistance with improving medication use and self-management of asthma. Participants indicated a desire for more education regarding asthma medications and help in communicating with medical providers. Community health workers are well suited to meet these needs. While the SKCHH project members worked with children with asthma and their caretakers, our protocols should be useful for adults with asthma as well. We expect that the SKCHH approach could also be used among higher-income homes, where many of the barriers to implementing action plans would be absent.

The SKCHH project was designed as a culturally competent approach for addressing indoor environmental conditions in low-income, ethnically diverse homes. Our work illustrates the gaps between literature-based recommended practices and what is practical in these homes. Many recommended resources (e.g., allergy-control bedding encasements or HEPA filters) are not affordable. Some recommended behavioral changes are impractical (e.g., pet washing, washing in hot water), and others are difficult to sustain given other pressing demands (e.g., regular vacuuming). Continued support from community health workers, health care providers, and others may help. Continuously collecting feedback from caretakers and field staff on how well protocols are working is essential. Protocols should be viewed as guidelines that can be adapted to fit the values, beliefs, and resources of diverse communities.

Strategies for improving indoor environmental quality must go beyond asking household members to take individual actions. Structural changes are needed to reduce exposure sources, yet are often not completed given the cost to the households or lack of landlord interest (e.g., installation of ventilation systems, removal of water-damaged carpet or wallboard, or replacement of windows). Our local public housing authority, although able to make improvements in the units it manages, lacks resources to do so in the homes of Section 8 tenants. Financially strapped, small-scale landlords may need assistance in making remediations to assure that their units are code compliant and healthy. Updating and enforcement of housing codes are needed, as are policies that assure access to housing units that meet basic guidelines for healthy living conditions. Project staff successfully worked with the local public housing agency to increase its awareness of the impact of housing conditions on asthma and to arrange for tenants with asthma to move to more suitable units (e.g., second-floor units with less dampness). However, a single research project could not achieve the goal of addressing the impact of housing quality on asthma. The complexity of this issue suggests that further progress will depend on organizing effective advocacy efforts and increasing funding for programs such as the above-mentioned Housing and Urban Development Healthy Homes initiative.

Policy changes to assure health insurance coverage of durable medical equipment (e.g., bedding encasements) and home visitation services are needed in order to make progress, and we are beginning advocacy efforts to address them. If evaluations of our and other Healthy Homes projects demonstrate potential for cost savings through decreased health services utilization, insurers may be more likely to cover these services and the costs of remediation.

The community health workers were critical to the implementation of SKCHH. Using full-time, salaried CHES enabled us to develop a knowledgeable cadre of workers who understood and followed project protocols and were able to work well with their clients. The CHES also faced many challenges as they implemented the project. It is important that prospective community health workers have a clear understanding of the nature of the type of work before accepting the position. We observed several characteristics that contributed to CHES success (Nguyen et al.). They included being outgoing and skilled at establishing rapport with diverse participants, being nonjudgmental in their relationships with their clients, having an ability to adapt to changing job requirements, being able to set priorities independently in the context of a carefully defined weekly work plan, having flexibility to work evenings and weekends, being able to learn new skills and information and transmit them to their clients, understanding and being comfortable with their clients and communities, being good communicators, being caring and respectful, connecting well with clients in their cultural context, knowing their communities and being involved in them as volunteers and members of social networks, having good organizational skills and paying attention to details (e.g., reporting and documentation, scheduling), being motivated to help others, being reliable with good follow-through and self management, and having lots of energy, enthusiasm, patience and perseverance. These attributes of successful community health workers are similar to those described by other projects (Poland et al., 1991; Love et al., 1997; Collier et al., 2000).

Providing a supportive work environment is critical for ensuring their success. Their supervisor must be able to observe their work closely, review challenging clients, offer advice and resources, provide a detailed weekly work plan, arrange a consistent work schedule, assure that the pace of work is reasonable, allow for administrative and "catch-up" time, and provide emotional support. Emotional support can also come from peer support groups and networks. Providing opportunities for enhancing skills and sharing knowledge through peer networks and more formal conferences is valuable. Involving CHES in program design and evaluation not only increases their morale and skill but also yields a better program. Adequate training and ongoing opportunities for feedback and continuing education add to job satisfaction.

We considered alternatives to using community health workers, and tried some of them. We were not successful in using volunteers; this approach may have required more resources for volunteer recruitment and support than were available to this project. An uncontrolled post-participation evaluation of 36 MHE program clients showed that self-reported knowledge of indoor environmental issues increased and that most participants made at least one behavior change (Leung et al., 1997). A "natural helper" or peer educator model (Israel, 1985) based upon volunteers from the participants' communities is another possible alternative. Additional, more rigorous evaluation of these programs, and comparison with staff-model programs, would be helpful. We considered using group classes and support groups, but community partners indicated attendance would be low, the format would not permit attention to the specific issues of each participant, and the approach would not allow direct observation of the home. One promising approach that we did not test was training other home visitors (e.g., public health nurses, social workers, environmental health inspectors) in Healthy Homes protocols so that they could integrate these protocols into their work.

The SKCHH project was designed and implemented with the participation of parents of children with asthma, community-based organizations, community health workers, public health staff, and university faculty. Guided by principles of community– researcher collaboration, they worked together and developed a project that was more suited to community desires, more effective, and more likely to be sustained than if traditional approaches to research had been employed. An important goal of community-based participatory research is to provide tangible benefits to community members. Participants valued the knowledge, support, and resources received from the project. Project staff hired from the community gained jobs along with specialized skills and knowledge. We have shared the knowledge resulting from the project with the participants and the broader community. We sent a summary of project findings to all participants and discussed them in more detail with the Parent Advisory Group. Our experience has informed the activities of the King County Asthma Forum, the local asthma coalition, and the asthma-related activities of the King County Health Action Plan, a local partnership of health care institutions, insurers, foundations, public health, and consumer organizations. Both the Forum and Action Plan have provided support to sustain SKCHH activities.

In conclusion, we have presented one of the first descriptions of the implementation of a Healthy Homes project. We hope that the lessons we have learned will be of use to others who are developing similar projects in their communities. The cumulative potential of all these efforts is great for addressing the growing burden of asthma, especially among low-income and ethnically diverse communities.

References

Adilah, N., Fitzharris, P., Crane, J., Siebers, R.W. (1997), "The effect of frequent vacuum cleaning on the house dust mite allergen, Der p 1 in carpets: a pilot study", *NZ Med J*, **110**, 438–9.

Aligne, C.A., Auinger, P., Byrd, R.S., Weitzman, M. (2000), "Risk factors for pediatric asthma: contributions of poverty, race, and urban residence", *Am J Respir Crit Care Med*, **162**, 873–7.

American Lung Association (1997), *Residential Air Cleaning Devices: Types, Effectiveness, and Health Impact*, Washington, DC: American Lung Association.

Arlian, L.G., Neal, J.S., Morgan, M.S., Vyszenski-Moher, D.L., Rapp, C.M., Alexander, A.K. (2001), "Reducing relative humidity is a practical way to control dust mites and their allergens in homes in temperate climates", *J Allergy Clin Immunol*, **107**, 99–104.

Arlian, L.G., Platts-Mills, T.A. (2001), "The biology of dust mites and the remediation of mite allergens in allergic disease", *J Allergy Clin Immunol*, **107(suppl)**, S406–S413.

Avner, D.B., Perzanowski, M.S., Platts-Mills, T.A., Woodfolk, J.A. (1997), "Evaluation of different techniques for washing cats: quantitation of allergen removed from the cat and the effect on airborne Fel d 1", *J Allergy Clin Immunol*, **100**, 307–12.

Bandura, A. (1977), *Social Learning Theory. Englewood Cliffs*, New Jersey: Prentice-Hall.

Bandura, A. (1986), *Social Foundations of Thought and Action: A Social Cognitive Theory. Englewood Cliffs*, NJ: Prentice Hall.

Baranowski, T., Perry, C.L., Parcel, G.S. (1997), "How individuals, environments and health behavior interact: social cognitive theory", in Glanz, K., Lewis, F.M., Rimer, B.K., eds, *Health Behavior and Health Education*, 2nd ed., San Francisco: Jossey-Bass, pp. 153–78.

Berkman, L.F. (2000), "Glass T. Social integration, social networks, social support, and health", in Berkman, L.F. and Kawachi, I., eds, *Social Epidemiology*, New York: Oxford University Press, pp. 137–73.

Bierman, C.W. (1996), "Environmental control of asthma", *Immunol Allergy Clin North Am*, **16**, 753–65.

Bower, J. (2001), *The Healthy House: How to Buy One, How to Build One, How to Cure a Sick One*, 4th ed., Bloomington, IN: Healthy House Institute.

Burge, H.A., Solomon, W.R. and Muilenberg, M.L. (1982), "Evaluation of indoor plantings as allergen exposure sources", *J Allergy Clin Immunol*, **70**, 101–8.

Bush, R.K., Portnoy, J.M. (2001), "The role and abatement of fungal allergens in allergic diseases", *J Allergy Clin Immunol*, **107(suppl)**, S430–S440.

Cabera, P., Julia-Serda, G., Rodriquez de Castro, F., Caminero, J., Barder, D. and Carillo, T. (1995), "Reduction of house dust mite allergens after dehumidifier use", *J Allergy Clin Immunol*, **95**, 635–6.

Call, R.S., Smith, T.F., Morris, E., Chapman, M.D. and Platts-Mills, T.A.E. (1992), "Risk factors for asthma in inner city children", *J Pediatr*, **121**, 862–6.

Carr, W., Zeitel, L. and Weiss, K. (1992), "Asthma hospitalization and mortality in New York City", *Am J Public Health*, **82**, 59–65.

Chapman, M.D., Wood, R.A. (2001), "The role and remediation of animal allergens in allergic diseases", *J Allergy Clin Immunol*, **107(suppl)**, S414–S421.

Christiansen, S.C., Martin, S.B., Schleicher, N.C., Koziol, J.A., Hamilton, R.G. and Zuraw, B.L. (1996), "Exposure and sensitization to environmental allergen of predominantly Hispanic children with asthma in San Diego's inner city", *J Allergy Clin Immunol*, **98**, 288–94.

Clark, N.M., Nothwehr, F., Gong, M., Evans, D., Maiman, L.A., Hurwitz, M.E., Roloff, D. and Mellins, R.B. (1995), "Physician-patient partnership in managing chronic illness", *Acad Med*, **70**, 957–9.

Collier, C., Krieger, J.W., Song, L., Wright-Thompson, D., Grimes, S., Hubbard, C., Linear, D., Townsend, M. and Trinidad, D. (2000), Unpublished data.

Crain, E.F., Weiss, K.B., Bijur, P.E., Hersh, M., Westbrook, L. and Stein, R.E.K. (1994), "An estimate of the prevalence of asthma and wheezing among inner-city children", *Pediatrics*, **94**, 356–62.

Crater, S.E. and Platts-Mills, T.A. (1998), "Searching for the cause of the increase in asthma", *Curr Opin Pediatr*, **10**, 594–9.

Custovic, A. and Woodcock, A. (2001), "On allergens and asthma (again): does exposure to allergens in homes exacerbate asthma?", *Clin Exp Allergy*, **31**, 670–73.

Davies, D.J., Thornton, I., Watt, J.M., Culbard, E.B., Harvey, P.G., Delves, H.T., Sherlock, J.C., Smart, G.A., Thomas, J.F. and Quinn, M.J. (1990), "Lead intake and blood lead in two-year-old U.K. urban children", *Sci Total Environ*, **90**, 13–29.

De Blay, F., Chapman, M.D. and Platts-Mills, T.A. (1991), "Airborne cat allergen (Fel d I): Environmental control with the cat in situ", *Am Rev Respir Dis*, **143**, 1334–9.

Dharmage, S., Bailey, M., Raven, J., Mitakakis, T., Guest, D., Cheng, A., Rolland, J., Thien, F., Abramson, M. and Walters, E.H. (1999), "A reliable and valid home visit report for studies of asthma in young adults", *Indoor Air*, **9**, 188–92.

Dickey, P. (ed.) (1998), *Master Home Environmentalist Training Manual*, American Lung Association of Washington, Washington, DC.

Eggleston, P.A. (1998), "Urban children and asthma", *Immunol Allergy Clin North Am*, **18**, 75–84.

Eggleston, P.A. (2000), "Environmental causes of asthma in inner city children", The National Cooperative Inner City Asthma Study, *Clin Rev Allergy Immunol*, **18**, 311–24.

Eggleston, P.A. and Arruda, L.K. (2001), "Ecology and elimination of cockroaches and allergens in the home", *J Allergy Clin Immunol*, **107 (suppl)**, S422–S429.

Eggleston, P.A. and Bush, R.K. (2001), "Environmental allergen avoidance: an overview", *J Allergy Clin Immunol*, **107 (suppl)**, S403–S405.

Ehnert, B., Lau-Schadendorf, S., Weber, A., Buettner, P., Schou, C. and Wahn, U. (1992), "Reducing domestic exposure to dust mite allergen reduces bronchial hyperreactivity in sensitive children with asthma", *J Allergy Clin Immunol*, **1**, 135–8.

Eisinger, A. and Senturia, K. (2001), "Doing community-driven research: a description of Seattle Partners for Healthy Communities", *J Urban Health*, **78**, 519–34.

Etzel, R. (1996), "Indoor air pollution and childhood asthma: effective environmental interventions", *Environ Health Perspect*, **103 (suppl 6)**, 55–8.

Etzel, R.A. and Balk, S.J. (1999), *Handbook of Pediatric Environmental Health. Elk Grove Village*, American Academy of Pediatrics, IL.

Evans, D. (1993), "To help patients control asthma the clinician must be a good listener and teacher" [Editorial]. *Thorax*, **48**, 685–7.

Fletcher, A.M., Pickering, C.A., Custovic, A., Simpson, J., Kennaugh J, Woodcock A (1996), "Reduction in humidity as a method of controlling mites and mite allergens: the use of mechanical ventilation in British domestic dwellings", *Clin Exp Allergy*, **26**, 1051–56.

Gelber, L.E, Seltzer, L.H., Bouzoukis, J.K., Pollart, S.M., Chapman, M.D. and Platts-Mills, T.A. (1993), "Sensitization and exposure to indoor allergens as risk factors for asthma among patients presenting to hospital". *Am Rev Respir Dis*, **147**, 573–8.

Gergen, P.J. (1992), "The increasing problem of asthma in the United States", *Am Rev Respir Dis*, **146, 823**–4.

Gergen, P.J., Turkeltaub, P.C. and Kovar, M.G. (1987), "The prevalence of allergic skin test reactivity to eigth common aeroallergens in the US population", *J Allergy Clin Immunol*, **80**, 669–79.

Grant, E.N., Alp, H. and Weiss, K.B. (1999), "The challenge of inner-city asthma", *Curr Opin Pulm Med*, **5**, 27–34.

Graves, E.J., Kozak, L.J. (1998), "Detailed diagnoses and procedures, National Hospital Discharge Survey, 1996", *Vital Health Stat*, **13**, 1–151.

Gold, D.R. (2000), "Environmental tobacco smoke, indoor allergens, and childhood asthma", *Environ Health Perspect*, **108 (suppl 4)**, 643–51.

Haynes, R.B., Taylor, D.W. and Sackett, D.L. (eds), (1979), *Compliance in Health Care. Baltimore*, Johns Hopkins University Press, MD.

Healthy Homes for Healthy Kids, Available: http://www.hcfama.org/hcfa_contents. php3?fldID=92 [accessed 23 July 2001].

Heaney, C.A. and Israel, B.A. (1997), "Social networks and social support", in Glanz, K., Lewis, F.M. and Rimer, B.K. (eds), *Health Behavior and Health Education*, 2nd ed., Jossey-Bass, San Francisco, 179–205.

Hill. D.J., Thompson, P.J., Stewart, G.A., Carlin, J.B., Nolan, T.M., Kemp, A.S. and Hosking, C.S. (1997), "The Melbourne House Dust Mite Study: eliminating house dust mites in the domestic environment", *J Allergy Clin Immunol*, **99**, 323–9.

Huss, K., Rand, C.S., Butz, A.M., Eggleston, P.A., Murigande, C., Thompson, L.C., Schneider, S., Weeks, K. and Malveaux, F.J. (1994), "Home environmental risk factors in urban minority asthmatic children", *Ann Allergy*, **72**, 173–7.

Institute of Medicine (2000), *Clearing the Air: Asthma and Indoor Air Exposures*, Washington, DC: National Academy Press.

Israel, B. (1985), "Social networks and social support: implications for natural helper and community level interventions", *Health Educ Q*, **12**, 65–80.

Jack, E., Boss, L. and Millington, W. (1999), *Asthma: A Speakers Kit for Public Health Professionals,*Centers for Disease Control and Prevention, Atlanta, GA.

Jackson, E.J. and Parks, C.P. (1997), "Recruitment and training issues from selected lay health advisor programs among African Americans: a 20-year perspective", *Health Educ Behav*, **24**, 418–31.

Jacobs, D.E., Friedman, W., Ashley, P. and McNairy, M. (1999), *The Healthy Homes Initiative: A Preliminary Plan,* U.S. Department of Housing and Urban Development, Washington, DC.

Johnston, S.L., Pattemore, P.K., Sanderson, G., Smith, S., Lampe, F., Josephs, L., Symington, P., O'Toole, S., Myint, S.H., Tyrrell, D.A. and Holgate, S.T. (1995), "Community study of role of viral infections in exacerbations of asthma in 9–11 year old children", *Br Med J*, **310**, 1225–9.

Juniper, E.F., Guyatt, G.H., Feeny, D.H., Ferrie, P.J., Griffith, L.E. and Townsend, M. (1996), "Measuring quality of life in children with asthma", *Qual Life Res*, **5**, 35–46.

Kane, M.P., Jaen, C.R., Tumiel, L.M., Bearman, G.M. and O'Shea, R.M. (1999), "Unlimited opportunities for environmental interventions with inner-city asthmatics", *J Asthma*, **36**, 371–9.

Kitch, B.T., Chew, G., Burge, H.A., Muilenberg, M.L., Weiss, S.T., Platts-Mills, T.A., O'Connor, G. and Gold, D.R. (2000), "Socioeconomic predictors of high allergen levels in homes in the greater Boston area", *Environ Health Perspect*, **108**, 301–7.

Kleinman, A., Eisenberg, L. and Good, B. (1978), "Culture, illness, and care: clinical lessons from anthropologic and cross-cultural research", *Ann Intern Med*, **88**, 251–8.

Kone, A., Sullivan, M., Senturia, K., Chrisman, N., Ciske, S. and Krieger, J. (2000), "Improving collaboration between researchers and communities", *Public Health Rep*, **115**, 243–8.

Krieger, J.W., Song, L., Takaro, T.K. and Stout, J. (2000), "Asthma and the home environment of low-income urban children: preliminary findings from the Seattle-King County healthy homes project", *J Urban Health*, **77**, 50–67.

Krieger, J.W., Takaro, T.K., Song, L., Weaver, M. (2005), "The Seattle–King County Healthy Homes Project: A randomized, controlled trial of a community health worker intervention to decrease exposure to indoor asthma triggers", *Am J Pub Health*, **95**, in press.

Krieger, J.W., Allen, C., Cheadle, A., Ciske, S., Schier, J.K., Senturia, K. and Sullivan, M. (2002), "Using community-based participatory research to address social determinants of health: lessons learned from Seattle Partners for Healthy Communities", *Health Education & Behavior*, **29**, 361–82.

Lang, D.M. and Polansky, M. (1992), "Patterns of asthma mortality in Philadelphia from 1969 to 1991", *N Engl J Med*, **331**, 1542–6.

Lanphear, B.P., Aligne, C.A., Auinger, P., Weitzman, M. and Byrd, R.S. (2001), "Residential exposures associated with asthma in US children", *Pediatrics*, **107**, 505–11.

Lewis, S.A., Weiss, S.T., Platts-Mills, T.A.E., Syring, M. and Gold, D.R. (2001), "Association of specific allergen sensitization with socioeconomic factors and allergic disease in a population of Boston women", *J Allergy Clin Immunol*, **107**, 615–22.

Leung, R., Koenig, J.Q., Simcox, N., van Belle, G., Fenske, R. and Gilbert, S.G. (1997), "Behavioral changes following participation in a home health promotional program in King County, Washington", *Environ Health Perspect*, **105**, 1132–5.

Lioy, P.J., Yiin, L.M., Adgate, J., Weisel, C. and Rhoads, G.G. (1998), "The effectiveness of a home cleaning intervention strategy in reducing potential dust and lead exposures", *J Expos Anal Environ Epidemiol*, **8**, 17–35.

Litonjua, A.A., Carey, V.J., Weiss, S.T. and Gold, D.R. (1999), "Race, socioeconomic factors, and area of residence are associated with asthma prevalence", *Pediatr Pulmonol*, **28**, 394–401.

Love, M.B., Gardner, K. and Legion, V. (1997), "Community health workers: who they are and what they do", *Health Educ Behav*, **24**, 510–22.

Macey, G.P., Her, X., Reibling, E.T. and Ericson, J. (2001), "An investigation of environmental racism claims: testing environmental management approaches with a geographic information system", *Environ Manage*, **27**, 893–907.

Mannino, D.M., Homa, D.M., Akinbami, W., Moorman, J.E., Gwynn, C., Redd, S.C. (2002), "Surveillance for Asthma–United States, 1980–1999", *Morb Mortal Wkly Rep Surveil Summ*, **51**, 1–13.

Mannino, D.M., Homa, D.M., Pertowski, C.A., Ashizawa, A., Mixon, L.L., Johnson, C.A., Ball, L.B., Jack, E. and Kang, D.S. (1998), "Surveillance for asthma – United States, 1960–1995", *Morb Mortal Wkly Rep*, **47**, 1–27.

Manson, A. (1988), "Language concordance as a determinant of patient compliance and emergency room use in patients with asthma", *Med Care*, **26**, 1119–1128.

Marder, D., Targonsky, P., Orris, O., Persky, V. and Addington, W. (1992), "Effect of racial and socioeconomic factors on asthma mortality in Chicago", *Chest*, **101**, 427S–430S.

Mason, K., Riley, G., Siebers, R., Crane, J. and Fitzharris, P. (1999), "Hot tumble drying and mite survival in duvets", *J Allergy Clin Immunol*, **104**, 499–500.

Meichenbaum, D. and Turk, D. (1987), *Facilitating Treatment Adherence: A Practitioners Guidebook*, New York: Plenum Press.

Mielke, H.W., Adams, J.E., Huff, B., Pepersack, J., Reagan, P.L., Stoppel, D. and Mielke, P.W. Jr (1992), "Dust control as a means of reducing inner-city childhood Pb exposure", in Hemphill, D.L. and Beck, B. (eds), *Trace Substances in Environmental Health*, University of Missouri, Columbia, MO, 121–8.

Miller, J.D. and Miller, A. (1996), "Ten minutes in a dryer kills all mites in blankets", *J Allergy Clin Immunol*, **97**, 423.

Munir, A.K., Einarsson, R. and Dreborg, S.K. (1993), "Vacuum cleaning decreases the levels of mite allergens in house dust", *Pediatr Allergy Immunol*, **4**, 136–43.

Murray, A.B. and Ferguson, A.C. (1983), "Dust-free bedrooms in the treatment of asthmatic children with house dust or house dust mite allergy: a controlled trial", *Pediatrics*, **71**, 418–22.

National Asthma Education and Prevention Program (1997), *Expert Panel Report 2: Guidelines for the Diagnosis and Management of Asthma*, National Health, Lung, and Blood Insitute, Bethesda, MD.

National Weather Service. Available: http://www.nws.mbay.net/rh.html [accessed 6 December 2001].

Nelson, H. (1995), "Clinical application of immediate skin testing", in Spector, S.L., (ed.), *Provocative Testing in Clinical Practice*, New York: Marcel Dekker, pp. 754–66.

Nguyen, M., Allen, C. and Krieger, J.W. Unpublished data.

Northridge, M.E. and Shepard, P.M. (1997), "Environmental racism and public health", *Am J Public Health*, **87**, 730–32.

O'Connor, G.T. and Gold, D.R. (1999), "Cockroach allergy and asthma in a 30-year-old man", *Environ Health Perspect*, **107**, 243–7.

Owen, S., Morganstern, M., Hepworth, J. and Woodcock, A. (1990), "Control of house dust mite antigen in bedding", *Lancet*, **335**, 396–7.

Patchett, K., Lewis, S., Crane, J. and Fitzharris, P. (1997), "Cat allergen (Fel d 1) levels on school children's clothing and in primary school classrooms in Wellington, New Zealand", *J Allergy Clin Immunol*, **100**, 755–9.

Perlin, S.A., Wong, D. and Sexton, K. (2001), "Residential proximity to industrial sources of air pollution: interrelationships among race, poverty, and age", *J Air Waste Manage Assoc*, **51**, 406–21.

Platts-Mills, T.A., Sporik, R.B., Wheatley, L.M. and Heymann, P.W. (1995), "Is there a dose-response relationship between exposure to indoor allergens and symptoms of asthma?" *J Allergy Clin Immunol*, **96**, 435–40.

Platts-Mills, T.A., Vaughan, J.W., Carter, M.C. and Woodfolk, J.A. (2000), "The role of intervention in established allergy: avoidance of indoor allergens in the treatment of chronic allergic disease", *J Allergy Clin Immunol*, **106**, 787–804.

Poland, M.L., Giblin, P.T., Waller, J.B. Jr and Bayer, I.S. (1991), "Development of a paraprofessional home visiting program for low-income mothers and infants", *Am J Prev Med*, **7**, 204–7.

Prochaska, J.O. and DiClemente, C.C. (1983), "Stages of and processes of self-change of smoking: towards an integrative model of change", *J Counseling Clin Psychol*, **51**, 390–95.

Prochaska, J.O., Norcross, J.C. and DiClemente, C.C. (1994), *Changing for Good*, New York: Morrow.

Prochaska, J.O., Redding, C.O. and Evers, K.E. (1997), "The transtheoretical model and stages of change", in Glanz, K., Lewis, F.M. and Rimer, B.K. (eds), *Health Behavior and Health Education*, 2nd ed, San Francisco: Jossey-Bass, pp. 60–84.

Public Health: Seattle and King County. *Seattle Healthy Homes Project: Environmental Interventions to Improve Chilren's Health,* available: http://www.metrokc.gov/health/pnhr/eapd/healthyhomes.html [accessed 15 August 2001].

Reid, B.L. and Bennett, G.W. (1989), "Apartments: field trials of abamectin bait formulations", *Insecticide Acaracide Tests*, **14**, 4.

Roberts, J.W., Bidd, W.T., Ruby, M.G., Camann, D.E., Fortmann, R.C., Lewis, R.G., Wallace, L.A. and Spittler, T.M. (1992), "Human exposure to pollutants in the floor dust of homes and offices", *J Expos Anal Environ Epidemiol*, **1 (suppl)**, 127–46.

Roberts, J.W., Camann, D.E. and Spittler, T.M. (1991), "Reducing lead exposure from remodeling and soil track-in older homes", in Proceedings of the annual meeting of the Air and Waste Management Association, 1991, Vancouver, BC. Pittsburgh, PA: Air and Waste Management Association, **15**, 134.2.

Roberts, J.W., Glass, G., Krieger, J. and Song, L. Unpublished data, 2001.

Roter, D.L., Hall, J.A., Merisca, R., Nordstrom, B., Cretin, D. and Svarstad, B. (1998), "Effectiveness of interventions to improve patient compliance: a meta-analysis", *Med Care*, **36**, 1138–61.

Sarpong, S.B., Hamilton, R.G., Eggleston, P.A. and Adkinson, N.F. (1996), "Socioeconomic status and race as risk factors for cockroach allergen exposure and sensitization in children with asthma", *J Allergy Clin Immunol*, **97**, 1393–1401.

Schappert, S.M, (1998), "Ambulatory care visits to physician offices, hospital outpatient departments, and emergency departments: United States, 1996", *Vital Health Stat*, **13**, 1–37.

Schneider, D. and Freeman, N. (2000), *Children's Environmental Health: Reducing Risk in a Dangerous World*, Washington, DC: American Public Health Association.

Senturia, Y.D., McNiff, Mortimer K., Baker, D., Gergen, P., Mitchell, H., Joseph, C. and Wedner, H.J. (1998), "Successful techniques for retention of study participants in an inner-city population", *Control Clin Trials*, **19**, 544–54.

Shapiro, G.G., Wighton, T.G., Chinn, T., Zuckrman, J., Eliassen, A.H., Picciano, J.F. and Platts-Mills, T.A. (1999), "House dust mite avoidance for children with asthma in homes of low-income families", *J Allergy Clin Immunol*, **103**, 1069–74.

Solet, D., Krieger, J.W., Stout, J. and Lui, L. (2000), "Childhood asthma hospitalizations – King County, Washington, 1987–1998", *Morb Mortal Wkly Rep*, **49**, 929–32.

Sporik, R., Squillace, S.P., Ingram, J.M., Rakes, G., Honsinger, R.W. and Platts-Mills, T.A. (1999), "Mite, cat, and cockroach exposure, allergen sensitisation, and asthma in children: a casecontrol study of three schools", *Thorax*, **54**, 675–80.

Strachan, D. (1996), "Socioeconomic factors and the development of allergy", *Toxicol Lett*, **86**, 199–203.

Sullivan, M., Kone, A., Senturia, K.D., Chrisman, N.J., Ciske, S.J. and Krieger, J.W. (2001), "Researcher and researched-community perspectives: toward bridging the gap", *Health Educ Behav*, **28**, 130–49.

Takaro, T.K., Krieger, J.W., Song, L. (2004), "Effect of environmental intervention to reduce exposure to asthma triggers in homes of low-income children in Seattle", *J Expos Anal Environ Epidemiol*, **14 Suppl 1**, S133–43.

Tovey, E. and Marks, G. (1999), "Methods and effectiveness of environmental control", *J Allergy Clin Immunol*, **103**, 179–91.

Tovey, E.R., McDonald, L.G. (1997), "A simple washing procedure with eucalyptus oil for controlling house dust mites and their allergens in clothing and bedding", *J Allergy Clin Immunol*, **100**, 464–6.

The Crisis Clinic (2001), *Where to Turn: Health and Human Services in King County,* Seattle.

U.S. EPA. *Asbestos in Your Home*. Washington, DC: US Environmental Protection Agency, 1998. Available: *http://www.epa.gov/iaq/pubs/asbestos* [accessed 7 December 2001].

U.S. EPA (rev 2001), Code Fed Reg 40(pt 156.10). **20**: 54–62.

U.S. Consumer Products Safety Commission (rev 2001), Code Fed Reg 16(pt 1500.3). **2**: 404–412.

van der Heide, S., van Aalderen, W.M., Kauffman, H.F., Dubois, A.E. and de Monchy, J.G. (1999), "Clinical effects of air cleaners in homes of asthmatic children sensitized to pet allergens", *J Allergy Clin Immunol*, **104**, 447–51.

van der Heide, S., Kauffman, H.F., Dubois, A.E. and de Monchy, J.G. (1997), "Allergen reduction measures in houses of allergic asthmatic patients: effects of air-cleaners and allergenimpermeable mattress covers", *Eur Respir J*, **10**, 1217–23.

Vaughan, J.W., McLaughlin, T.E., Perzanowski, M.S. and Platts-Mills, T.A. (1999), "Evaluation of materials used for bedding encasement: effect of pore size in blocking cat and dust mite allergen", *J Allergy Clin Immunol*, **103**, 227–31.

Vaughan, J.W. and Platts-Mills, T.A. (2000), "New approaches to environmental control", *Clin Rev Allergy Immunol*, **18**, 325–39.

Vaughan, J.W., Woodfolk, J.A. and Platts-Mills, T.A. (1999), "Assessment of vacuum cleaners and vacuum cleaner bags recommended for allergic subjects", *J Allergy Clin Immunol*, **104**, 1079–83.

Wahlgren, D.R., Hovell, M.F., Meltzer, S.B., Hofstetter, C.R. and Zakarian, J.M. (1997), "Reduction of environmental tobacco smoke exposure in asthmatic children: a 2-year followup", *Chest*, **111**, 81–88.

Warner, J.A., Frederick, J.M., Bryant, T.N., Weich, C., Raw, G.J., Hunter, C., Stephen, F.R., McIntyre, D.A. and Warner, J.O. (2000), "Mechanical ventilation and high-efficiency vacuum cleaning: a combined strategy of mite and mite allergen reduction in the control of mite-sensitive asthma", *J Allergy Clin Immunol*, **105**, 75–82.

Weiss, K.B. and Gergen, P.J. (1992), "Inner-city asthma: the epidemiology of an emerging US public health concern", *Chest*, **101 (suppl)**, 362S–367S.

Willey, C. (1999), "Behavior-changing methods for improving adherence to medication", *Curr Hypertens Rep*, **1**, 477–81.

Willies-Jacobo, L.J., Denson-Lino, J.M., Rosas, A., O'Connor, R.D. and Wilson, N.W. (1993), "Socioeconomic status and allergy in children with asthma", *J Allergy Clin Immunol,* **92**, 630–32.

Wissow, L.S., Gittelsohn, A.M., Szklo, M., Starfield, B., Mussman, M. (1988), "Poverty, race and hospitalization for childhood asthma", *Am J Public Health*, **78**, 777–82.

Witmer, A., Seifer, S.D., Finocchio, L., Leslie, J. and O'Neil, E.H. (1995), "Community health workers: integral members of the health care work force", *Am J Public Health*, **85**, 1055–8.

Wood, R.A. (1997), "Indoor allergens: thrill of victory or agony of defeat?", *J Allergy Clin Immunol*, **100**, 290–92.

Wood, R.A., Johnson, E.F., Van Natta, M.L., Chen, P.H. and Eggleston, P.A. (1998), "A placebo-controlled trial of a HEPA air cleaner in the treatment of cat allergy", *Am J Respir Crit Care Med*, **158**, 115–20.

Wooton, M. and Ashley, P. (2000), *Residential Hazards: Asthma. Healthy Homes Initiative Background Information*, Washington, DC: U.S. Department Housing and Urban Development.

SECTION B:
OPEN SPACE

Chapter 4

Environmental Justice Across the Mystic: Bridging Agendas in a Watershed

Julian Agyeman and Dale Bryan

Introduction

For years, activists and researchers in environmental justice (EJ) have discussed issues such as what is the most appropriate scale of action and study and what should be the spatial units of analysis (Harner et al., 2002). This developed out of debates in the 1980s and 90s regarding the utility of zip codes (based on the volume of mail) and census tracts, blocks and block groups (based on sociological characteristics) in identifying and taking action in communities at risk. Whatever the answers are, and there may be no "one size fits all" solution, here we[1] describe and analyze a participatory community research effort of which we were part that promoted an EJ agenda in the Mystic River watershed, part of the Boston metro area in Massachusetts.

Environmental Justice Across the Mystic (EJAM) was a project of the Mystic Watershed Collaborative (MWC), the Massachusetts Executive Office of Environmental Affairs' (EOEA) Environmental Justice Program and its now defunct Massachusetts Watershed Initiative, the United States Environmental Protection Agency New England's Urban Environmental Initiative, and the Urban Ecology Institute. The MWC is a long-term partnership between the Mystic River Watershed Association (MyRWA) and Tufts University. The MyRWA submitted a grant proposal to the EPA Small Grants Program in February 2002 and EJAM began in September 2002.

The purpose of EJAM was to bring a participatory, critical dialogue approach to the issues of disproportionate adverse environmental exposure or lack of access to desirable environmental resources and to begin shifting the thinking of watershed residents, activists, regulatory workers and other stakeholders. Our objectives were to work with communities in the watershed to promote an understanding of EJ issues, identify specific problems affecting the watershed, and plan a course of action to correct existing environmental injustices and prevent them from arising in the future. This "combination of collaborative inquiry, critical analysis, and social action" is fundamental to many community-based research practices which attempt to build a knowledge and "information base from which community and agencies can plan and act" in order to meet community-identified needs (Strand et al., 2003).

We also aimed to build local and regional capacity to address EJ issues while pursuing urban watershed restoration. To facilitate communication and information exchange, we developed a multi-tiered approach and offered different levels of community engagement in order to stimulate involvement and generate the investment of a broad audience, with emphasis on community-based organizations and individuals. The long-term goal of this approach is the development of more sustainable communities in which "economic vitality, ecological integrity, civic democracy, and social well-being are linked in complementary fashion, thereby fostering a high quality of life and a strong sense of reciprocal obligation among its members" (Hempel, 1999).

Early on we held an EJ training workshop in Chelsea, a city in the lower watershed, designed in large part to help community members and public officials better understand and implement the Commonwealth's new EJ policy. Subsequently we held three public forums in Medford, East Boston and Woburn, each of which included presentations on water quality, watershed restoration and EJ issues and solutions, panel responses, and open discussion about the various perspectives on these issues in the Mystic watershed. These were "listening sessions" for us, and were followed by another EJ training session held in Arlington. This brought forward the issues and strategic concerns discussed in the previous training and community forums.

The culmination of this "issue cascade" project was an EJ Summit, held at Tufts University in November 2003, at which participants reviewed and added to lists of *issues* identified at previous trainings and public forums, and identified specific *actions* to address these issues. The action plan is to be represented in a final document, *The Mystic Environmental Justice Accord*.

In this chapter we want to look briefly at some demographic and some community issues in the Mystic River Watershed; at EJ issues in the watershed; at community research and our approach to it; and at combining what we perceived to be two (competing) agendas, or "frames": the *"science and management based"* watershed agenda and the more *'human and ethic-centered'* EJ agenda. We will conclude with a reflection on the watershed as a unit of action and analysis.

Mystic River Watershed

The Mystic River Watershed has an area of approximately 76 square miles, encompassing 21 municipalities (in whole or in part) north and west of Boston (Map 1). The headwaters of the system begin in Reading and form the Aberjona River, which flows into the Upper Mystic Lake in Winchester. The Mystic River flows from the Lower Mystic Lake through Arlington, Medford, Somerville, Everett, Charlestown, Chelsea, and East Boston before emptying into the Boston Harbor. Main tributaries to the Mystic River include Mill Brook, Alewife Brook, Malden River, and Chelsea Creek (also known as the Chelsea River). The watershed contains 44 lakes and ponds, the largest of which is Spot Pond in the Middlesex Fells, with an area of 307 acres.

Home to about 8% of Massachusetts' population (nearly half a million people) in less than 1% of its land area, the Mystic River watershed is one of the most densely populated and urban watersheds in the state. The watershed includes relatively wealthy "economically developed suburbs" such as Winchester and Stoneham, as

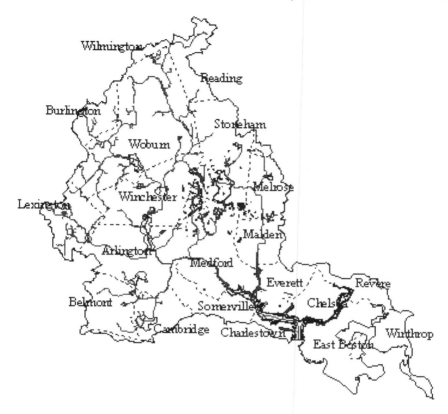

Figure 4.1   The Mystic River watershed
         (http://www.mysticriver.org/images/maps/WshedOhead.gif).

well as low-income "urbanized center" communities such as Somerville and
Chelsea (Figure 4.1). The 1999 per capita income in these communities varied from
$14,628 in Chelsea and $19,845 in Everett, to $50,514 in Winchester and $46,119 in
Lexington. According to the MA Dept of Revenue(http://www.dls.state.ma.us/
MDMSTUF/Socioeconomic/Wealth.xls http://www.dls.state.ma.us/MDMSTUF/
Socioeconomic/ComparisonReport.xls), the range of median family income was
between $32,130 in Chelsea and $49,876 in Everett, to $111,899 in Lexington and
$110,226 in Winchester. As of September 2003, unemployment rates across Mystic
communities indicate similar disparities. Not surprisingly, Chelsea and Everett
residents endure a steeper rate of joblessness, 8.8% and 7.1%, respectively, while
Lexington and Winchester citizens fair relatively better in securing the means to a
livelihood: 3.7% and 4.2%, respectively.

   True to sprawling metropolitan development patterns most everywhere,
population density varies across the watershed, thinning out as one moves away from
the Boston metro core. In its urbanized center communities, for example,

approximately 35,080 Chelsea residents inhabit 2.19 square miles (land area), or 16,038 people per square mile, and in Somerville roughly 50,454 people reside in 2.67 square miles of land in the watershed (which is about 65% of the city's land mass), or 18,897 people per square mile. For the relatively well-off suburb of Stoneham, approximately 21,159 residents occupy 5.86 square miles (3,611/sq. mi.), whereas in Lexington 1,900 people live in each square mile (6,100 people on 3.21 sq. mi). Significantly, communities in the lower watershed (e.g., Chelsea, East Boston and Somerville) are notably more ethnically diverse and have significant numbers of recent immigrants.

Development in the watershed began in the 1600s and has included extensive industrial and manufacturing facilities across the area's 76 square miles. This has resulted in the release of hazardous chemicals to soils, groundwater, and surface waters. At present there are two Superfund sites and several hundred state-identified hazardous waste disposal sites in the watershed. The lower half of the watershed contains Combined Sewer Overflows (CSOs) that degrade overall water quality by discharging untreated sewage into the Mystic River and the Alewife Brook during storm events (Perez et al., 2002). Remaining illicit connections of sanitary waste pipes into storm water drains contribute to dry weather inputs of sewage. Excessive application of nutrients from urban and industrial landscaping practices, perhaps chief among the non-point source pollution factors[2] (Kirshen et al., 2000), affect water quality from runoff of storm water across impervious surfaces. In the Mystic watershed, only 17% is designated as open space, and in Somerville, 85% of the land is impermeable, making urban runoff a substantial problem. The large amount of organic matter in the river leads to generally low dissolved oxygen levels, high turbidity and high quantities of pathogenic bacteria. Industry in the lower watershed threatens both water and air quality standards. While the towns of Everett and Chelsea are both significantly bounded by the Mystic and its tributaries the Malden and Chelsea Rivers, respectively, neither have appreciable public access to the waterfronts. Since 1978 Chelsea's waterfront has been rezoned a designated port area (DPA) as part of the Boston Harbor, whereby development for industrial use is prioritized (Hynes, 2003). Everett's waterfront to the Mystic is also a DPA (though not it's waterfront to the Malden River, a Mystic tributary); the Mystic along both East Boston and Charlestown was part of the 1978 designation. As a result of industry and regional energy distribution facilities and Logan International Airport cargo terminals, heavy commercial and industrial truck traffic impact residential neighborhoods throughout the lower watershed communities.

State Level EJ Policy

Partially in response to injustices in watersheds such as the Mystic, some individual states have developed environmental justice policies, for example, Massachusetts, which set up the Massachusetts Environmental Justice Advisory Committee (MEJAC), in 2000 and launched its policy in October 2002 (Eady, 2003). One of the authors (Agyeman) was on the Committee. The Commonwealth of Massachusetts uses the following definition in its Environmental Justice Policy:

Environmental justice is based on the principle that all people have a right to be protected from environmental pollution and to live in and enjoy a clean and healthful environment. Environmental justice is the equal protection and meaningful involvement of all people with respect to the development, implementation, and enforcement of environmental laws, regulations, and policies and the equitable distribution of environmental benefits.

(Commonwealth of Massachusetts 2002)

Three weeks after the Commonwealth of Massachusetts released its environmental justice policy in a public comment draft (December 2000), Faber and Krieg (2002) unveiled their long anticipated report, *Unequal Protection: Ecological Injustices in the Commonwealth of Massachusetts*.[3] In a revealing look at Environmental Justice Communities[4] in Massachusetts, they undertook an in depth analysis of the socio-geographic distribution of hazards across 368 communities in the Commonwealth. They looked at both income based and racially based biases in the distribution of 17 types of hazardous sites and industrial facilities. Using enforcement and other public data from Massachusetts' own regulatory agencies, they developed a point system for measuring and ranking cumulative exposure to these 17 types of sites and facilities which showed (Table 4.1) that "hazardous sites and facilities are disproportionately located and concentrated in communities of color and working-class communities" (Faber and Krieg, 2002; p. 277).

Table 4.1   Most intensively overburdened communities in Massachusetts (total points per square mile from Faber and Krieg, 2002)

Rank	Town name	Points per square	Class status of town	Racial status of town
1	Downtown Boston[a]	224.8	Low income ($29,468)	High minority (31.9%)
2	Charlestown	134.3	Medium-low ($35,706)	Moderate-low (5.1%)
3	Chelsea	127.4	Low income ($24,144)	High minority (30.3%)
4	South Boston	126.2	Low income ($25,539)	Low minority (4.2%)
5	East Boston	123.3	Low income ($22,925)	Moderate-high (23.6%)
6	Cambridge	115.0	Medium-low ($33,140)	Moderate-high (24.9%)
7	Somerville	104.7	Medium-low ($32,455)	Moderate-low (11.3%)
8	Roxbury	101.3	Low income ($20,518)	High minority (94.0%)
9	Allston/Brighton	100.0	Low income ($25,262)	High minority (26.9%)
10	Watertown	98.6	Medium-high ($43,490)	Low minority (3.8%)
11	Everett	98.1	Medium-low ($30,786)	Moderate-low (6.0%)
12	Boston (all)	84.0	Low income ($29,180)	High minority (37.0%)
13	Dorchester	81.3	Low income ($29,468)	High minority (50.7%)
14	Lawrence	59.3	Low income ($22,183)	Moderate-low (34.9%)
15	Malden	57.8	Medium-low ($34,244)	Moderate-low (10.1%)
Totals	15 towns		14 of the 15 most intensively overburdened towns are of lower-income status (less than $40,000)	9 of the 15 most intensively overburdened towns are of higher minority status (15% or more people of color)

[a] Downtown Boston encompasses Central Boston and Chinatown, Back Bay and Beacon Hill, the South End, and the Fenway/Kenmore neighborhoods.

To the surprise of many, largely depending on where they lived or worked, the report revealed that (Table 1) eight out of the 15 most overburdened communities in Massachusetts are in the Mystic River Watershed (Charlestown, Chelsea, East Boston, Everett, Malden and portions of Cambridge, Somerville and Watertown). As we imply above, residents and activists from the Mystic's "EJ communities," or those with significant percentages of people of color and/or low-income populations,[5] were already well aware of the poor environmental conditions and numerous burdensome facilities throughout their neighborhoods. More so than the majority of residents across the Mystic, environmental management and regulatory professionals and watershed restoration activists were not altogether surprised by the findings in many of the specific locales. They were, though, in important respects taken aback by the overall extent and disproportion of the environmental burdens their Mystic neighbors endured in daily life. For the recently formed MWC and its *stated* priority of advancing EJ in the watershed, the report was received with critical interest and as an important new resource. At MyRWA's next annual meeting, Faber was the keynote speaker.

Community Research

The EJAM concept was developed by the steering committee of the MWC, the long-term partnership between Tufts University and the MyRWA. The MWC itself represents an emerging and largely promising organizational form among community research practices, where institutions of higher education and community-based organizations (and sometimes including both private enterprise and public institutions) combine resources around mutual interests in attempts to address community needs and local matters of social policy, social betterment, and social justice. These "civic engagement" partnerships and their innovative efforts have become the premiere intellectual and programmatic concern for scholars, administrators and many students recently involved in "community service learning" projects in their surrounding host communities. (Strand et al., 2003; Sirianni and Friedland, 2001; Bringle and Hatcher, 2002; Morton, 1995) EJAM's collaborative and community-dependent design attempted, in part, to discover and disseminate useful knowledge which ultimately could "make some contribution to changing the social arrangements that create and sustain inequality and injustice" in the Mystic watershed (Strand et al., 2003). For it is significant disparities of wealth and power that undermine environmental quality and general quality of life (Boyce et al., 2003) and compromise restoration efforts. Indeed, Agyeman, Bullard and Evans (2003) argue that, "the issue of environmental quality is inextricably linked to that of human equality" and Pastor argues persuasively, that "a more equitable distribution of social goods and services can help the environment" (2003).

In the spring of 2000 then Tufts President John DiBiaggio and MyRWA leadership held a press conference with state and federal officials to announce their active commitment to "solve" local watershed problems. Perhaps dramatically, they jointly claimed their intention to make fishing and swimming in the Mystic River possible by 2010. Now after almost four years and a variety of activities, a more tempered understanding of the scale of some of the causes and solutions has led to a less ambitious time frame in restoring the river itself to more healthful and useful conditions. Moreover and importantly, many of the key MWC players have come to the realization that "watershed restoration work is really community restoration" (Ferguson, 2003).

From the outset the MWC has given priority to issues that are anchored in concerns raised by watershed citizens, with a particular emphasis on problems and actions that are likely to benefit from cooperation between the university and citizen groups. MWC objectives include: raising awareness of the environmental problems of the bioregion and how human actions create or ameliorate them; augmenting the resources available to MyRWA in its efforts; engaging students and faculty in specific watershed management problems that require professional expertise; training citizens to deal with ongoing problems and translate scientific knowledge into information usable by concerned citizens; educating Tufts students in the skills of active citizenship; and enabling Tufts University to improve its own watershed management practices and deepen relationships of mutual trust and benefit with local municipal, governmental and community-based organizations.

The MyRWA was founded thirty years ago as an incorporated 501(c)(3) organization, with a mission to restore clean water in the Mystic River watershed, protect water and related natural resources, and establish relevant public information and education programs. For much of its history, MyRWA was a volunteer-run organization, mobilizing activists on a project-by-project basis. In 1999, MyRWA merged with the Mystic River Watershed Coalition, a coalition of groups that had been created to address the needs of the many smaller localized citizens' groups in the watershed. As part of this merger, MyRWA expanded its membership and board format to include organizational members. The result of the merger is a stronger organization that can better represent and advocate on behalf of watershed community needs. MyRWA's organizational capacity has grown significantly in the past few years. Its website (www.tufts.edu/mystic) highlights both history and recent accomplishments such as establishment of volunteer water monitoring, research on watershed open space protection, and increased public access.

MyRWA currently has approximately 250 organizational and individual members, 125 volunteers, and three full-time staff. A Board of Directors is elected annually and meets on a bi-monthly basis. Committees focus on outreach and stewardship, policy, water quality, and development/fundraising. Current organizational members represented on the board include the Alewife/Mystic River Advocates, Belmont Citizens Forum, Coalition for Alewife, East Arlington Good Neighbor Committee, Friends of the Upper Mystic Lake, Mystic View Task Force and Woburn Residents' Environmental Network. MyRWA collaborates with volunteers, local groups, municipalities, state and federal agencies, businesses and universities to accomplish its mission.

MWC priorities are determined by a Steering Committee which also works to set and implement its plans. The committee is made up of representatives from the MyRWA and its member organizations that are able to speak for diverse citizen concerns in different sections of the watershed. In addition, Tufts faculty, staff and student members represent the academic units closely involved in the MWC: the WaterSHED Center, the Department of Civil and Environmental Engineering, Tufts Institute of the Environment, the Center for Interdisciplinary Studies, the Department of Urban and Environmental Policy and Planning, and the University College of Citizenship and Public Service. In order to maintain clear communication and ensure that the MWC reflects current concerns among watershed citizens, priorities and planning are communicated by Steering Committee members to their constituents for comment and input. This committee meets on a monthly basis.

To date MWC accomplishments include two substantial grants, one to coordinate and archive research on the Mystic, and the other a successful EPA EMPACT[6] proposal to develop "real time" water quality monitoring and modeling for equitable recreation on the Mystic River. The MWC has also been able to offer seed grants for community-based projects, supporting research, clean-ups and celebrations. Otherwise, a growing number of academic offerings at Tufts address content related to watershed efforts, with student research and service learning increasingly dedicated to Mystic efforts. Longest running among these was the River Institute (RI), a summer project that placed students in internships combined with twice-weekly half-day seminars for reflection and deeper exposure to concerns of sustainable community change and issues of leadership for the future. The curriculum addressed six priority areas first determined in MyRWA's "Future Search"[7] conference of residents from across the Mystic at Tufts in 2000: watershed awareness and identity, water quality and quantity, habitat restoration, new governance and partnerships, increased public access, and EJ. Each topic served as a foundation for exploring the issues of watershed restoration in the context of environmental movement strategies and leadership. Three internships for the RI in 2003 were to begin integrating strategic actions identified in the Summit for building new partnerships and capacities for addressing EJ and watershed issues. As it happened, the Summit was postponed from its original schedule in Spring 2003 to late Fall that year. The RI internships were thus based on initial results from the training and public forums, as well as the EJ objectives held by local organizations. The internship organizations were the Toxics Action Center, Groundwork Somerville, and the Chelsea Creek Restoration Project.

As we mentioned, EJAM was made possible by a U.S. EPA grant from the EJ Small Grants Program managed by the New England office. Coincidently, another EPA facilitated effort, the EJ Training Collaborative (EJTC), served as a contributing resource for EJAM. One of the authors (Bryan) was among the initial cohorts to complete a "train the trainers" curriculum program, which was to be applied nationwide in outreach efforts. The "EJ Fundamentals" Course thus became a pillar of the EJAM trainings.

The target audience for EJAM was the Mystic River watershed and its residents. Based on the premise that all residents share the same watershed address, and on the reality that rivers have tended to harbor a disproportionate level of environmental problems, all constituencies have a stake in the wide range of work to be accomplished. Thus, a focus on facilitating communication and information exchange, with an emphasis on partnership and capacity building, would begin building a foundation for future watershed health.

We envisioned the outcomes of EJAM as being fourfold. First, we wanted to "reframe" EJ in the eyes of local communities. We aimed to move away from it being seen as dealing only with *problems*, towards a more *solutions-oriented* approach to local sustainability. In effect, we wanted EJ to become a framework for action.

Second, we wanted to show how EJ is integral to the development of sustainable communities, and a sustainable watershed. We interpret sustainability in its broadest sense, as "ensuring a better quality of life for all, now, and into the future; in a just and equitable manner; while living within the limits of supporting ecosystems" (Agyeman, Bullard and Evans, 2003). The social and policy learning from this project will inform development of strategic objectives addressing EJ and sustainability issues in the watershed. Third, we viewed the project as a pilot for integrating EJ objectives into watershed management. And fourth, mindful that calls for greater EJ are coming in from around the world, another outcome of the dialogue and training sequence would be to link actions at the local level to their more global consequences.

As of yet, there is no comprehensive framework for researching, teaching and learning EJ that is universally agreed upon by scholars, activists or regulators. Competing definitions and theoretical interpretations are in dynamic flux and "contest" as practitioners and academics attempt to engage issues for understanding, assessment, prediction and prescription. Accepting this context as one of challenge and promise, an EJAM objective via the trainings and forums was to cultivate residents, activists, regulators and municipal officials' creative *thinking about* and *agency for* EJ. "The Four Domains" curriculum tool for analysis developed by the EJTC provided trainers and trainees with a means for discussing both problems and solutions.[8] The various conditions these categories aim to reveal include, though are not limited to: vulnerable or susceptible populations, lack of capacity to meaningfully participate in decision making processes, adverse health or environmental impacts, disproportionate or cumulative impacts, or unique exposures or benefits to communities or localities.[9]

From Issues to Action

An outcome of our forums and trainings was a fairly comprehensive set of *"issues"* which the EJAM team loosely grouped into four categories: *land use and transportation; exposures and public health; water quality and improvements; and communication and participation*. These categories became the themes of the small group sessions at the Summit. Table 4.2 reflects the four categories of *"issues"*, and Table 4.3, the *"actions"* suggested in the small group sessions at the Summit to support resolution of those issues.

At this final public stage of our collaborative inquiry our objective was to facilitate a process which enabled all participants a voice in the decision-making process as to which issues would be most useful to prioritize on behalf of the community. To deepen our understanding of the diverse issues and interests expressed throughout EJAM, two questions guided the Summit's deliberations: "What do we know?" and "What do we need to know?" Our primary purpose, to determine action items, was addressed in a two-step discussion that moved from prioritizing issues to identifying potential and priority activities.

Here we address only the *Exposures and Public Health* category and some of the "findings" which emerged. Perhaps not surprisingly, scientific knowledge and socioeconomic data embodied in academic reports, agency or community

Table 4.2   The four categories of "*issues*"

1) Land Use and Transportation	2) Exposures and Public Health
Public access	Fish consumption
Open space	Swimming
Recreational opportunities	Boating
Growth and development	Flooding
Sprawl	Housing
Waterfront use	Public notice of bacterial levels
Fences	Air exposures
Housing	Fencing
Transit oriented development	Ingesting pollutants
Regional equity and sustainability (incl. social	Baseline public health data – what are the health
equity, environmental health & economics)	problems?
Regional planning – need better metrics	Open space and recreational opportunities
Transit-oriented development	Noise
Mixed waterfront use – incl. transportation	Access to health care
Better bike/pedestrian access	Non-point source pollution
Municipal infrastructure	
Agricultural use	
Air pollution – impact on public health	
Outreach to immigrant communities	
3) Water Quality and Improvements	**4) Communication and Participation**
Water Quality	Coalition building
Sediments	Education
Regulations and enforcement	Youth opportunities for involvement
Testing and monitoring	Activist fatigue
Flooding	Empowering communities
Understanding pollution sources – cause and	NIMBY
effect	Social-cultural awareness
CSOs	Activating "early retirees"
Salt pile	Cooperation across boundaries
Boating as a pollution source	Focus on the positive
Trash, illegal dumping	Conflicting state laws & regional coordination
Oil tanks on Chelsea Creek (recent oil spill)	Non-human communities
Used oil disposal	Age issues
Catch basins, sewage and storm drains	Decision-making
Illegal connections	Reporting back to communities
Animal waste – dogs	Increased translation services/opportunities
Landfill in Woburn	Lack of local advocacy groups
Island End coal tar plant	Building government capacity to outreach and to
Too much asphalt	address issues
	YIMBY – Yes in My Back Yard; willingness to
	accept burdens and responsibilities
	On-going structure of EJAM post-grant period
	Increase communications capacity among existing
	advocacy groups

Table 4.3   The "*actions*" suggested in the small group sessions at the Summit to support resolution of those issues

Priority Issues for Action Planning: Land Use and Transportation	**Priority Issues for Action Planning: Exposures and Public Health**
Understanding the linkages: land use/transportation/public health/water quality Networking systems Preserving natural spaces	How to figure out what's important? Communication – synchronizing the information that exists, and simplifying so that community can use
Potential Actions: Role of regional organizations (MAPC, MyRWA, Boston MPO) (MPO not responsive to EJ issues – need systemic change, increase community representation) Have state EJ policy apply to non-EOEA agencies – e.g., transportation and housing agencies People in communities should have a say about how agencies work with the communities. Standardize and improve the 37 land-use categories – include square footages, impervious surface Identify, correlate and improve data sets: e.g., need data on vehicle miles traveled Help citizens use the data Broaden MEPA review – consider regional impacts, use more metrics (vehicle miles added, total jobs added, total household units) Training of municipal officials and community members Balancing of quantitative and qualitative data – case studies needed Funding for community groups and municipalities for technical assistance Promulgate regulations to implement EJ policy More accountability on projects – clear explanation of EJ outreach on all projects, how implemented and audited Review criteria for transportation system expansion.	**Potential Actions:** **Defining Priorities:** Public health NGO/clearinghouse Community mapping – overlay health + pollutants + EJ; discover gaps & set priorities Pilot program with Fed $$ Outreach to empower people, communities Health center survey – survey public health infrastructure & organizations Exposure & emissions research Small grant-based local actions & participation => awareness & engagement (mini-RFPs) Door-to-door concurrent survey & engagement Use what we already know (e.g., EMPACT, Faber) **Communication:** Distribute literature door-to-door Web-site links Communicate on 2 levels – technical and lay person (churches, city centers, day care, cable TV) Political base
Priority Issues for Action Planning: Water Quality Characterizing pollution levels Identifying pollution sources Making monitoring information available to the public Educating towns/decision makers about what has to happen to improve Addressing CSOs Shared expertise	**Priority Issues for Action Planning: Communication and Participation** Empowering communities Education about issues and health impacts facing the 8:15 EJ watershed communities Increased coalition building Cooperation across boundaries
Potential Actions: **Pollution and Pollution Sources:** Measure pollution – coordination needed to measure all types Use community observations – e.g., Riverkeepers in NYC Continued and expanded water quality monitoring Identify an organization to play a communications role **CSOs:** Different parts of watershed have different polluters and levels of pollution Focus advocacy on CSOs to get federal, state and local government action Work on low-impact development Storm drain stenciling. **Highest Priorities:** Continued & expanded monitoring Advocacy for government action on CSOs: lobbying, op eds, publicity around the Mystic River movie	**Priority Actions:** Public education campaign about 8:15 EJ communities in watershed Construct a post-EJAM structure Speakers bureau to promote social-culture awareness and meaningful involvement of all watershed residents

organizational monitoring data was the foundation of what is "known." For example, Toxic Release Inventory, EMPACT, the Faber report, and municipal and regulatory and municipal data on CSOs were sources familiar to many of the participants. The knowledge from hands-on experience and grounded in social location, however, also "knew" that such professional expertise often omitted input from different population groups and that risks from exposure are not readily and easily translated at the "street" level. Thus, in what needs to be learned the community members especially addressed grassroots ways to both better and more meaningfully involve residents and diverse groups in getting information from and to them. Outreach and inquiry via numerous languages and in diverse settings, e.g., community health centers, cultural centers, houses of faith, youth groups, and web-based and local mapping projects were all discussed.

This group's deliberations revealed how difficult and complex the process of moving from *knowing issues* to *taking actions* is. Strengthening and deepening information and facilitating communication were key concerns and challenges. Strategic planning for action requires this knowledge in determining steps to be taken and in moving diverse people into active participation.

As we reviewed the video taping of the event, the various note sheets crafted during the Summit, and the categories for Tables 4.2 and 4.3, two other matters stand out. First, the issues raised were mostly not "*EJ issues*" in the traditional sense, such as toxics and facilities, but were either very specific concerns such as water quality, sedimentation, CSOs or air exposures, or they were broader sustainability issues (interrelated social – economic – environment issues) such as regional planning, coalition building, outreach to immigrant communities or access to health care. In short, the "*science and management based*" watershed agenda issues can be seen as having a "*narrow focus*" civic environmentalism, and the "*human and ethic-centered*" EJ agenda issues are examples of a "*broad focus*" civic environmentalism[10] (Agyeman and Angus 2003).

As Agyeman and Angus (2003) argue, "'narrow focus' civic environmentalism looks at 'the interconnected nature of environmental problems' themselves, whereas the 'broad focus' is on the connections between environmental problems and economic and social issues such as urban disinvestment, racial segregation, unemployment, and civic disengagement". Second, we noticed during the public forums, Summit and trainings that whether people were coming from an established "watershed perspective" (narrow focus, largely science and management based), or an "environmental justice perspective" (broad focus, more human and ethic-centered) affected how they framed these issues, and the nature of their prescribed actions. Framing is "the process by which individuals and groups identify, interpret, and express social and political grievances" (Taylor, 2000, see also Entman, 1993). It is therefore a useful analytical device in community research, upon which we rely more in our final discussion.

Bridging Agendas via Movement Frames and Social Capital

Though it unfolded over the course of fifteen months, EJAM was a snapshot in an on-going encounter of competing social movement (SM) narratives in an urban watershed. The storyline we have been describing is one which reveals the confluence of two movements, namely *watershed restoration* with a (narrow) focus on resource protection and pollution prevention, and *EJ* with a (broader) focus on race and class (Moyer, 2001; Sirianni and Friedland, 2001:102). This confluence follows Taylor's (2000) delineation of the *"New Environmental Paradigm"* (NEP) of scientific environmentalism and the *"Environmental Justice Paradigm"* (EJP) focused on linking "environment and race, class, gender and social justice concerns in an explicit framework" (Taylor, 2000). The storyline also marks the intersections of their joint mobilization of adherents and stakeholders in each, individuals and organizations alike, across and on behalf of an urban watershed setting.

These SMs have separate but complementary frames for describing problems, attributing cause or blame for particular and general conditions, and proposing alternative realities or prescribing possible solutions (Snow and Benford, 1992; Taylor, 2000). The participants in these meaning-making and place-making activities of collective agency are in a dynamic process of negotiating forms of collaboration and coexistence based on trust, norms, and different stocks of cultural images, creating and/or engaging different forms of social capital in their shared bioregional context, a densely populated and environmentally overburdened urban watershed (Sirianni and Friedland, 2001; Pastor, 2003; Lepofsky and Fraser, 2002).

Whatever the concerns of a particular SM, they need to be described and defined, given meaning such that supporters, opponents, and possibly most crucially, bystanders come to a better understanding of them as a "causal story"; a narrative of cause and effect. This is a strategic challenge for any SM because it needs to interpret a social problem or complex issues in such a way that participants and bystanders are motivated to action on behalf of some claim (Best, 1987), solution or alternative (social or cultural), and that bystanders and the broader public accept the legitimacy of both (ideally) the claims and the claims-makers of the collective action. And for the movement's opponents and the political context(s) in which it occurs, framing is crucial to the extent it can shape a conflict or set the agenda of public discourse, even if it falls short of attaching blame or complicity on the part of particular groups, institutions, or enterprises. Importantly, the interpretive frame is as much an indispensable aspect of getting citizens to engage and/or organize their social capital forms on behalf of an SM, as it is to get them to first pay attention to a movement's claims.

What we witnessed, we believe, are two fundamental and related developments. First, we initially noticed at the "listening sessions" and then more so at the Summit that a process of "frame alignment" was occurring (Taylor, 2000). In effect, as EJ meanings and interpretations were clarified and linked to watershed issues (Table 4.2), the actions deliberated and prioritized by the strategic stakeholders' groups (Table 4.3) made EJ perspectives and concerns more directly relevant to watershed residents' livelihoods, if not their daily lives. This amplification and extension of the EJ frame to watershed activists and residents who largely were not from EJ communities, constituencies or groups holds promise for future dialogue and collaboration among the different movement groups.

In part, this alignment was facilitated by the political opportunity (Eisinger, 1973) created by the Faber and Krieg Report (2002) into environmental injustices in Massachusetts, the development and passage of the Commonwealth of

Massachusetts Environmental Justice Policy, and current efforts by State Senator Jarrett T. Barrios' to sponsor an EJ bill, S.190, "The Clean and Healthy Communities Act". Senator Barrios is joined by Representative David Sullivan, who has introduced to the House H. 2112, an Act to Promote Environmental Justice in the Commonwealth. The bills would require "the state to develop statewide regulations that give communities greater protections from even more pollution, and would establish a procedure under which additional communities that do not fall under direct demographic definition of an EJ Population may petition for such status" (from promotion literature).

Second, we also observed the beginnings of the bridging of social capital between the representatives of the two SMs, an essential element if further community development and watershed restoration collaborations are to take place. The formal groups and informal networks found in every community, as well as the norms and trust found in a place, are the reservoir of social capital from which community members draw when addressing contentious issues or revitalizing their community (Pastor, 2003; Sirianni and Friedland, 2001). This same stock of social capital is engaged or manipulated when groups or community members attempt to advance their own favorable claims and meanings for a place (Lepofsky and Fraser, 2003). Thus, the formation and mobilization of social capital is also a strategic concern of SMs.

While social capital can be put to use or assembled for all manner of policy or cultural objectives (Sirianni and Friedland, 2001), the basic forms are *bonding* and *bridging* types. Pastor describes the former as involving building or utilizing connections within a community and the latter as the cultivation of allies or connections across different communities. In the context of the EJM, "bonding social capital among those suffering most environmental negatives and bridging social capital [that] reaches out for support from other communities" is facilitated by grassroots community organizing, coalition-building among SM organizations, and new alliances with different community groups and constituencies (2003). Further below we will add the watershed context to this conceptual outline.

To most students of SM, the EJM frame is characterized by its aspirations and appeals to transformative and paradigmatic change (Agyeman et al., 2003; Cole and Foster, 2000; Taylor, 2000). Noted for its collective voice and agency of marginalized minorities and low-income populations, the EJM both advocates cooperation and agitates with confrontation when deemed necessary for realizing social justice in daily lived experience (Bryant, 1995). Fundamentally, EJ makes claims about the right to clean water, air, and surroundings for everyone, which has helped to redefine and broaden the meaning of environment beyond wilderness or natural resources to include "built" settings "where people live, work, play and pray." The EJM combines its demands for "equitable access to a healthy environment" with similar claims for "the distribution of other social resources, such as schools, housing, open space, and employment" (Pastor, 2003). This framing stands squarely on "rights" claims established in earlier Civil Rights struggles (Taylor 2000), as well as on the quality of life claims embodied in the nonviolent aspirations for a "beloved community," where no one would suffer the selective victimizations largely but not totally concealed by structural and cultural violence, where everyone would be free from fear and domination (King, 1963; Johnston, 1994; Muro, 1999; Thiele, 1993).

In comparison to the *transformative* EJM, the watershed movement frame is arguably more *reformative* in its quest for resource protection, restoration, and management. We believe this is the fundamental nature of watershed restoration even when claims of "watershed democracy" are promoted within the watershed movement or made by scholars celebrating its contributions to civic innovation (Sirianni and Friedland, 2001). The primary change objective is for the direct benefit to natural resources, albeit typically simultaneously for the recreational, productive or aesthetic use for people (to the chagrin of radical environmentalists like Deep Ecologists). Policy proposals and political objectives are crafted and pursued with this primary motivation. Where social and cultural relations are matters of change, a redistribution of power or the status quo for shaping the political landscape and forming social policy would be, of course, considered strategically relevant. But in the eyes of "narrow focus" civic environmentalism, this is a "controversial" matter mainly for the procedural injustices faced by some population groups. This is a far cry from the liberatory EJ analysis that understands empowerment, agency, and participatory democracy through critiques of domination and oppression (Kreisberg, 1992), and that intentional moral engagement is the foundation for effective civic action (Kaza, 2002).

It is through these different and sometimes competing lenses and narratives that EJAM's proceedings and its action outcomes can be best understood. In every public forum and training session, the watershed and EJ frames competed for exposure and domination of the discourse.[11] There is not the space here to illustrate this differential framing in the case of each issue in each of our four categories (Table 4.2), however. A couple of examples should help make the point.

While discussing the issue of "Transit Oriented Development" (TOD) in the *Land Use and Transportation Group* at the Summit, it was clear that TOD was looked at primarily as an environmental issue by those using the watershed frame, and as primarily an issue of equity by those using the EJ frame. Of course, TOD is both an environmental and equity issue, but the differential framing prioritizes one over the other. Similarly, the issue of the infamous Chelsea salt pile – a 100,000 ton mountain of toxin-treated salt used for roadway de-icing purposes, which went uncovered (though it sits across the street from a residential neighborhood and is on the river front) until activism pressure eventually met with success (though it is still in violation of environmental regulations) – was addressed at a public forum held in East Boston and was discussed by the *Water Quality and Improvements* group at the Summit. The "narrow focus" or watershed frame saw this more in terms of its detrimental effects on the biota of the watershed ecosystem, whereas the "broad focus" or EJ frame was much more concerned with the human health implications and the inequity of siting road salt for the Commonwealth in one of its most environmentally overburdened communities. In the *Exposures and Public Health* group at the Summit, housing issues were discussed. This is a perennial thorn for many "narrow focus" environmentalists, who are generally middle class and do not face severe housing issues (Brulle 2000; Kempton et al., 1996) whereas the "broad focus" saw housing as a much more fundamental issue. In the *Communication and Participation* group at the Summit, a discussion around Youth opportunities for involvement yielded a division between seeing Youth as volunteers in cleaning up the watershed ("narrow focus") and Youth as agents in political activism ("broad focus").

Conclusion

Roseland (1998) writes that "social capital is the shared knowledge, understandings, and patterns of interactions that a group of people brings to any productive activity. The term refers to the organizations, structures, and social relations that people build themselves, independently of the state or larger corporations. It contributes to stronger community fabric, and, often as a by-product of other activities, builds bonds of information, trust, and inter-personal solidarity." The sharing of knowledge, especially across the "narrow" and "broad" foci during the EJAM process, we believe, will contribute to a better understanding of the watershed and EJ frames and, potentially, a realization that both frames are legitimate and not mutually exclusive.

During closing remarks at the Summit, which effectively concluded EJAM's public proceedings, Fred Paulsen, President of MyRWA's Board of Directors, said: "if there is no formal structure going forward, then it does become important for MyRWA and its Board and committees to make sure that EJAM is part of that on-going work of MyRWA." In this, Paulsen is signaling that MyRWA understands the importance of the EJ frame. More importantly, since then MyRWA has been directed by the Board of Directors to begin an internal assessment of how it can best integrate EJ analysis across all its committees. To that end a member of the Board, who happens to be a lawyer at a prominent Boston-based advocacy organization, Alternatives for Community and Environment, and a key volunteer are having part of their time redirected to carry this out. In this MyRWA has taken an important step in further aligning its watershed frame with that of EJ.

Moreover, it is also beginning to construct a form of bridging capital between the two movements. MyRWA, though facing financial challenges familiar to most community-based organizations, can offer to extend hard to come by resources to EJ groups in the watershed. Namely, in the form of its well-publicized partnership with a major private research institution (Tufts) and the recognition accorded it by the Massachusetts Watershed Initiative and the EOEA as the primary watershed-wide environmental organization working on behalf of the Mystic River, MyRWA brings a degree of weighted legitimacy as a stakeholder in place-making restoration activities and claims-making about land use and community development. Used strategically, a partnership with MyRWA could be a useful asset to EJ groups in the lower watershed's urbanized centers.

For example, during an EJAM forum Chelsea Creek Restoration Project activists outlined part of their plan for integrating local waterfront restoration with EJ objectives meeting residents' recreational and green space needs. Steps by MyRWA and the MWC to take action on behalf of locally defined needs embodied in the plan would strengthen the social capital bridge between them.

Yet, this same step would also facilitate bonding social capital. From a watershed perspective, increasing ties among groups, neighborhoods and communities across the entire watershed is an essential task toward effective restoration. Building capacity and utilizing connections within the Mystic watershed as a unit of analysis and action is among the necessary though not sufficient conditions for cultivating a watershed identity and increasing awareness of both MyRWA and MWC objectives.

Indeed, we argue that understanding both SM frames and creating both forms of social capital will result in greater and stronger social capital, a more powerful movement towards sustainable communities, and, ultimately, a more sustainable watershed. As Pastor and others argue persuasively, "a more equitable distribution of social goods and services can help the environment. Recent research by Boyce et al. (1999) and Morello-Frosch (1997) demonstrates that lower levels of social inequality are associated with higher levels of environmental protection, presumably because the fairer distribution of power makes it difficult to place hazards in someone's backyard and thus enhances incentives to engage in source reduction and cleanup at the regional and state levels" (2003). EJAM's participatory community dialogue appears to have taken modestly effective steps toward such movement and restoration objectives.

Although the information in this document has been funded wholly or in part by the United States Environmental Protection Agency under assistance agreement (EQ98170901) to the Mystic River Watershed Association, it has not been submitted to the Agency's publication's review process and therefore, may not reflect the view of the Agency and no official endorsement should be inferred.

Notes

1   The other EJAM team members were Nancy Hammett and Grace Perez, MyRWA, Lisa Brukilacchio and Veronica Eady, Tufts University, Kwabena Kyei-Aboagye and Joan Robes, EOEA, Elisabeth Miley Krautscheid, MA Dept. of Housing and Community Development, Aaron Toffler, Urban Ecology Institute, Kristi Rae, EPA New England, and Susan Loucks, NOAH. The authors of this paper must make clear that the ideas contained in this paper are ours, and do not necessarily reflect those of all EJAM team members.

2   Non-point source pollutants do not come from a specific, easily-identifiable source, such as a pipe or smokestack.

3   Faber and Krieg's initial report was embargoed until January 9th 2001. Our later citation (2002) is their preferred citation in Environmental Health Perspectives.

4   They were called EJ "Populations" in the Commonwealth's final policy document. See note 5.

5   EJ Populations are those segments of the population that EOEA has determined to be most at risk of being unaware of or unable to participate in environmental decision-making or to gain access to state environmental resources. They are defined as neighborhoods (U.S. Census Bureau census block groups) that meet *one or more* of the following criteria:

   ● The median annual household income is at or below 65 percent of the statewide median income for Massachusetts; *or*
   ● 25 percent of the residents are minority; *or*
   ● 25 percent of the residents are foreign born, *or*
   ● 25 percent of the residents are lacking English language proficiency".

   (Commonwealth of Massachusetts 2002)

6   EMPACT (Environmental Monitoring for Public Access and Community Tracking) had the goal of helping communities bring people up-to-date local environmental information they can understand and use in making daily decisions about protecting their health and environment.

7   "Future search brings people from all walks of life into the same conversation - those with resources, expertise, formal authority and need. People tell stories about their past, present and desired future. Through dialogue they discover their common ground. Only then do they make concrete action plans." http://www.futuresearch.net/method/whatis/index.cfm.

8   For some, the EJTC model appears to start from a regulator's point of view, thereby privileging their knowledge or sets of concerns. The community is not centered, it is a variable to be treated as object and manipulated.

9   EPA EJ Assessment Tool http://www.epa.gov/enviro/ej.

10   Over the past 10 years, civic environmentalism has emerged as the dominant US discourse on sub-national environmental policy making. DeWitt John, formerly of the US National Academy of Public Administration, was the first person to articulate and name "civic environmentalism" as an emergent policy framework that recognized the limits of top-down environmental regulation, during the "regulatory reinvention" initiative of the Clinton-Gore years. The approach stems from an increasing awareness in the EPA and elsewhere, that centrally imposed, media specific environmental policy found in legislation like the Clean Air Act or Clean Water Act is not sufficient for dealing with contemporary environmental problems and that more flexible and collaborative solutions should be found.

11   This was also true within EJAM team deliberations, as it is on the MWC steering committee.

References

Agyeman J., Bullard, R. and Evans, B. (eds) (2003), *"Just sustainabilities: Development in an unequal world"*, London: Earthscan Publications/MIT Press.

Agyeman, J. and Angus, B. (2003), "The role of civic environmentalism in the pursuit of sustainable communities", *Journal of Environmental Planning and Management*, **46**, 345–63.

Anthony, C. (1998), "Foreword", in Faber, D. (ed) (1998), *The Struggle for Ecological Democracy: Environmental Justice Movements in the United States*, New York and London: The Guilford Press.

Best, J. (1987), "Rhetoric in claims making", *Social Problems*, **34**, 101–21.

Boyce, J.K., Klemer, A.R., Templet, P.H. and Willis, C.E. (1999), "Power distribution, the environment, and public health: a state level analysis", *Ecological Economics*, **29**, 127–40.

Boyce, J.K. and Shelley, B.G. (eds) (2003), *Natural assets: Democratizing environmental ownership*, Washington: Island Press.

Bringle, R.G. and Hatcher, J.A. (2002), "Campus-community partnerships: The terms of engagement", *Journal of Social Issues*, **58**, 503–16.

Brulle, R. (2000), *Agency, democracy, and nature: The U.S. environmental movement from a critical theory perspective*, Cambridge: MIT Press.

Bryant, B. (ed.) (1995), Environmental justice: Issues, policies, and solutions, Washington, D.C.: Island Press.

Cole, L. and Foster, S. (2001), *From the ground up. Environmental racism and the rise of the environmental justice movement*, New York: NYU Press.

Commonwealth of Massachusetts (2002) *Environmental Justice Policy*. Boston: State House.

Eady, V. (2003), "Environmental justice in state policy decisions", in Agyeman, J. Bullard R. and Evans, B. (eds) (2003), *Just sustainabilities: Development in an unequal world*, London. Earthscan: MIT Press.

Eisinger, P. (1973), "The conditions of protest behavior in American cities", *American Political Science Review*, **67**, 11–28.

Entman, R. (1993), "Framing: Toward clarification of a fractured paradigm", *Journal of Communication*, **43**, 51–8.

Faber, D. (ed.) (1998), *The struggle for ecological democracy: Environmental justice movements in the United States*, New York and London: The Guilford Press.

Faber, D. and Krieg, E. (2002), "Unequal exposure to ecological hazards: Environmental injustices in the Commonwealth of Massachusetts", *Environmental Health Perspectives, Supplements*, **110**, 277–88.

Ferguson, L. (2003), "Hands across the Mystic", *Tufts Magazine*, Winter, pp. 34–42.

General Accounting Office (1983), *Siting of hazardous waste landfills and their correlation with racial and economic status of surrounding communities*, Washington D.C.: GPO.

Goldman, B. (1993), *Not just prosperity. Achieving sustainability with environmental justice*, Washington D.C.: National Wildlife Federation.

Harner, J., Warner, K., Pierce, J. and Huber, T. (2002), "Urban Environmental Justice Indices", *Professional Geographer*, **54**, 318–31.

Hempel, L.C. (1999), "Conceptual and analytical challenges in building sustainable communities", in Mazmanian, D.A. and Kraft, M.E. (eds), *Towards Sustainable Communities: Transition and Transformations in Environmental Policy*, Cambridge: MIT Press.

Hynes, H.P. (2003), "The Chelsea River: Democratizing access to nature in a world of cities", in Boyce, J.K. and Shelley, B.G. (eds), *Natural assets: Democratizing environmental ownership*. Washington D.C.: Island Press.

Johnston, B.R. (ed.) (1994), *Who pays the price: The socio cultural context of environmental crisis*. Washington D.C.: Island Press.

Kaza, S. (2002), "Teaching ethics through environmental justice", *Canadian Journal of Environmental Education*, **7**, 99–109.

Kempton, W., Boster, J. and Hartley, J. (1996), *Environmental values in American culture*, Cambridge, MA: MIT Press.

King, M.L. Jr. (1963), *Strength to Love*, New York: Harper Row.

Kirshen, P., Durant, J. and Perez, G. (2000), "Water resource management in the Mystic River II: University and community collaboration through service learning and active citizenship", Watershed Management 2000, American Society of Civil Engineers, 21–3 June 2000.

Kreisberg, S. (1992), *Transforming power: Domination, empowerment, and education*, Albany, NY: SUNY Press.

Lavelle, M. and Coyle, M. (eds) (1992), The racial divide in environmental law: Unequal protection (Special Supplement), *National Law Journal*, September 21.

Lepofsky, J. and Fraser, J.C. (2002), "Building community citizens: Claiming the right to place-making in the city", *Urban Studies*, **40**, 127–42.

Morton, K. (1995), "The irony of service: Charity, project, and social change in service-learning", *Michigan Journal of Community Service Learning*, **2**, 19–32.

Morello-Frosch, R. (1997), *Environmental justice and California's "Riskscape". The distribution of air toxics and associated cancer and non cancer risks among diverse communities*. Unpublished dissertation, Department of Health Sciences, University of California, Berkeley.

Moyer, B., with MacAllister, J., Finley, M.L. and Soifer, S. (2001), *Doing democracy: The MAP Model for organizing social movements*, Gabriola Island, BC: New Society Publishers.

Muro, A.M. (1999), *Toward the Beloved Community: The Fellowship of Reconciliation's Statement on Racial and Economic Justice*, FOR, Nyack, NY.

Pastor, M. (2003), "Building social capital to protect natural capital: The quest for environmental justice", in Boyce, J.K. and Shelley, B.G. (eds) *Natural assets: Democratizing environmental ownership.* Washington DC: Island Press.

Perez, G., Durant, J. and Senn, D. (2002), "Don't flush when it rains?" *Cambridge Chronicle*, 30 April 2.

Roseland, M. (1998), *Toward sustainable communities: Resources for citizens and their governments*, Gabriola Island, BC: New Society Publishers.

Sirianni, C. and Friedland, L. (2001), *Civic innovation in America: Community empowerment, public policy, and the movement for civic renewal*, Berkeley, Los Angeles, London: University of California Press.

Snow, D.A. and Benford, R.D. (1992), "Master frames and cycles of protest", in Morris, A.D. and Mueller, C.M. (eds), *Frontiers in social movement theory*, New Haven, CT: Yale University Press.

Strand, K., Marullo, S., Cutforth, N., Stoecker, R. and Donohue, P. (2003), "Principles of best practice for community-based research", *Michigan Journal of Community Service-Learning*, **9**, 5–15.

Taylor, D. (2000), "The rise of the environmental justice paradigm", *American Behavioural Scientist*, **43**, 508–80.

Thiele, L.P. (1993), "Making democracy safe for the world: Social movements and global politics", *Alternatives*, **18**, 273–305.

Chapter 5

A Program to Improve Urban Neighborhood Health Through Lead-Safe Yard Interventions

Jill S. Litt, H. Patricia Hynes, Paul Carroll, Robert Maxfield,
Pat McLaine and Carol Kawecki

Introduction

Childhood lead poisoning is one example of a contemporary environmental health problem that has been treated and managed through a panoply of environmental and biomedical interventions and prevention strategies. It is an issue that has been imbedded in public health for decades and has been addressed quite successfully from a national perspective. By eliminating two major sources of exposures – leaded gasoline and leaded paint – blood lead levels for the majority of Americans have dropped dramatically over the past two decades.

Unfortunately, for those who live in poorly maintained housing in older urban neighborhoods, environmental lead continues to pose health threats, particularly for those under the age of six (Centers for Disease Control and Prevention, 1997). The threats of lead poisoning are most prevalent in poor, minority, and immigrant communities and are compounded by additional environmental hazards including indoor air contaminants (e.g., allergens, combustion by-products, volatile organic compounds, pesticides) and neighborhood factors such as deteriorating infrastructure, housing demolition, abandoned housing, congested roadways, violence, industrial land uses, and vacant land. These environmental hazards are signals of compromised neighborhoods and are linked to declines in community health (Fullilove et al., 2000).

The complexities of inner-city lead poisoning and the significance of this issue to millions of affected children and their families continue to motivate tens of thousands of public officials, medical providers, environmental scientists, engineers, lawyers, and policy makers in managing lead exposures and preventing adverse health effects. One new focus of national and local lead poisoning prevention efforts is the residential yard in older urban neighborhoods. From 1998 to 2001, a collaboration of government, university and community partners conducted a 3-phase lead safe yard intervention pilot project in Boston. The Boston Lead-Safe Yard Project was funded by the U.S. Environmental Protection Agency's (US EPA) Environmental Monitoring for Public Access and Community Tracking (EMPACT) program. Its goal was to generate real-time data on lead in urban soil that would enable us to design and implement a community-based program to reduce exposure to soil lead in residential yards of two Boston neighborhoods, Roxbury and Dorchester. The project components included: outreach and education to homeowners and residents; soil analysis to establish baseline lead levels in soil; development and application of cost-effective landscape measures to reduce exposure to high lead soil; communication with homeowners about design decisions and long-term maintenance; and dissemination of the project methods to community agencies, local government, and cities in other regions for replication.

A previous publication presents the initial project planning, yard selection criteria, the risk-reducing landscape techniques used in the intervention; and lead soil data from the first two phases of this three-phase project (including 43 of the 102 yards sampled in entire project) (Hynes et al., 2001). In addition, a project handbook was developed, as the project was concluding its final phase, to provide detailed instructions for community and public agencies on how to organize and implement a Lead-Safe Yard program. The project handbook contains sample consent forms; sample yard plans color-coded by lead levels and yard uses; construction details and specifications for landscape measures; and cost estimates of materials and labor (U.S. Envrionment Protection Agency, 2001a).

This chapter has two interrelated purposes. First, it will contextualize the Lead-Safe Yard project within the current arena of environmental health policy. Second, it will present the descriptive soil lead data from all three phases of the project in order to: 1) establish a baseline profile of soil lead for Boston inner-city yards, and 2) compare the baseline and average levels found in yards with current regulatory levels for lead in residential soil. Throughout the pilot project, we employed principles of community-based research, and we report within this chapter on the results and impact of the community-university-government partnership.

Part I defines environmental health in its fullest sense, describes the changing boundaries of environmental health, recent developments in community-based environmental health, and the changing face of public sector agencies in their support of localized environmental health research and practice. Part II provides background information on lead poisoning trends and policy guidelines. Part III describes and discusses the methods and results from the soil lead analysis and intervention in residential yards. The concluding section includes a summary of the project evaluation process as well as possible next steps with phytoremediation.

Part I: The Urban Setting and Environmental Health

Understanding, harmonizing, and sustaining the relationships between environment and public health requires a broadening of 'environment health' as a concept and its respective theoretical underpinnings, research protocols, and practice strategies. While the current environmental health paradigm, which reflects the continuum from source of contaminant to environmentally-related health outcome, is useful in looking at the relationships between individual substances, individual pathways of exposure, and individual health risks, it falls short of providing a useful framework to consider other non-chemical environmental factors and the interaction of multiple environmental factors in shaping population health status. Such factors include among others, physical and biological hazards, severely diminished natural resources, deteriorating infrastructure and blight, and housing and school quality. For the purposes of this paper, we have adopted the following definition of environmental health to provide a broader context when considering lead poisoning in urban communities and environmental interventions, such as the EMPACT Lead-SafeYard project:

> Environmental health includes "those aspects of human health, including quality of life, that are determined by interactions with physical, chemical, biological, and social factors in the environment. It also refers to the theory and practices of assessing, correcting, controlling, and preventing those factors in the environment that may adversely affect the health of present and future generations"
>
> (Goldman et al., 1999)

Changing Times

The toxics movement of the late 1980s, the environmental and social justice movements of the 1980s and 1990s, and regulatory reform efforts of the 1990s have been instrumental in identifying the shortcomings of existing regulations, expanding the scope of environmental health, and forcing innovations in related research, policy making, and practice. As this sea change has liberated some institutional, financial, and political resources, scientists and policy makers have been able to pursue and investigate the multifaceted aspects of environmental health by developing and employing more systematic approaches that capture cumulative environmental risk, the complicated nature of the built environment and its role in community health, and community priorities and concerns. Importantly, such approaches advocate and require, in some cases, that research and implementation strategies address "pollution" together with "poverty" to ultimately improve and sustain community health and well-being.

Paradigmatic shifts in environmental health have been embraced by community researchers, practitioners, and affected communities, who recognize the need for more holistic, bottom-up approaches to community development, local environmental management and public health protection. One approach that befits this new direction in environmental health is "assets-based community development (ABCD)"; an approach that is assets-oriented rather than deficiency-oriented and needs driven. "ABCD" spotlights community strengths by focusing on what is present in the community, including local resources, bolstering ties among residents, associations, and institutions – in essence, building from the ground up (Kretzman and McKnight, 1993). Moreover, an assets-based approach recognizes the fundamental building blocks of a community – social capital (e.g., neighborhood cohesion), human capital (e.g., competencies and skills), physical capital (e.g., infrastructure), and natural capital (e.g., natural resources and living systems), as critical to improving health and well-being in communities (Ambler, 2001; Boyce and Paster, 2001).

Within public health, community-based approaches premised on community assets have emerged in response to calls for more comprehensive and integrated approaches to research and practice solutions that affect change at the neighborhood level (Chaskin, 2001; Institute of Medicine, 2001; Israel et al., 1998). The "Healthy Cities" and "Healthy People" initiatives throughout the United States and abroad are two efforts that have renewed recognition of the local authority as the front line defense in public health and argue for the return of public health decision-making to the local and community level (International Healthy Cities Foundation, 2001; van Oers, 1993).

From Theory to Action The call for locally based environmental health action has been met with a surge of interest in and allocation of resources to support community-based research and activities. Various government committees and commissions, non-profit organizations, and religious organizations have endorsed or argued for such considerations including the Institute of Medicine, U.S. Department of Health and Human Services, the United States Environmental Protection Agency (EPA), the Presidential/Congressional Commission on Risk Assessment and Risk Management, the United Nations Development Program (Ambler, 2001; Institute of Medicine, 1999; Institute of Medicine, 1988; U.S. Department of Health and Human Services, 2000; National Research Council, 1996; Presidential/Congressional Commission on Risk Assessment and Risk Management, 1997a and 1997b).

The EPA EMPACT Program The US Environmental Protection Agency's Environmental Monitoring for Public Access and Community Tracking (EMPACT) program, which was designed to work with communities to collect, manage, and present environmental information to the public (U.S. Environmental Protection Agency, 2001b), is one example of a federally-funded initiative that is community-based and assets-oriented. The EMPACT program, which organizationally resides in EPA's Office of Environmental Information, aims to transfer timely environmental information and technological innovations to communities in order to inform local environmental decision-making (U.S. Environmental Protection Agency, 2001a). Moreover, such a program offers financial resources to build capacity at the community level to tackle and respond to vexing issues such as air pollution, hazardous waste management, water quality, and community exposures to toxic substances.[1]

Thus far, a national network of 84 EMPACT-related projects has been created. Not only are resources being transferred across communities throughout the United States but also, for the first time, a national picture of local needs is being defined, which will help close the gap between national priorities and regional and local environmental health needs. Ultimately this will meet the goals of environmental protection – to protect and improve population health and well-being. The EMPACT funded Lead-Safe Yard Project in Boston focused on lead in soil as an important contributor to the lead story in urban America, and thus moved beyond traditional lead poisoning prevention strategies that have addressed housing, nutrition and clinical interventions.

Part II: Lead in Soil as an Urban Environmental Hazard

Lead as a human toxicant is widely recognized to cause deleterious effects in children and adults, including developmental delays, learning disabilities, behavioral disorders, and depression. Technological improvements and advancements in epidemiologic methods continue to elucidate the clinical and sub-clinical effects of lead poisoning (Lanphear et al., 2000). Lead's persistence in the environment, its widespread use in industry, its presence in older homes, and its remnants in soil from leaded gasoline and deteriorating exterior paint on aging homes make it a public health threat in aging urban neighborhoods (Mielke et al., 1983; Mielke and Reagan, 1998).

From a national perspective, federal policies and regulations that recommended or mandated the removal of lead from food cans and gasoline, respectively, have contributed to reductions in baseline blood lead levels, from 77.8 % of the population with blood lead levels (BLLs) greater than or equal to 10 µg/dl in late 1970s to 4.4 % in the early nineties (Anonymous, 1997; Mahaffey et al., 1982).[2] Additionally, national standards have been set to guide states and localities in their efforts to stabilize interior and exterior lead levels in the home setting. The implementation of local programs to achieve these standards and eliminate or prevent lead exposures varies depending on the local "lead-scape". Low-income and minority families, those living in older housing, those living in older urban areas, and those living near point sources (e.g., lead smelters) and major roadways still suffer from excess exposures to lead in the environment. Specifically, nearly one million children are estimated to have blood lead levels (BLLs) greater than 10µg/dl (Anonymous, 1997) and millions more are estimated to have BLLs in the range of 2.5 to 10 µg/dl (Pirkle et al., 1994).

The intervention strategy for reducing and preventing lead exposure should reflect risk factors specific to the affected community. Historically, risk factors have included lead paint, lead pipes and interior dust. Specialized interventions to control and prevent lead poisoning include clinical interventions such as oral chelating agents for moderately lead poisoned children, nutritional guidance, and environmental interventions including abatement of house dust and lead-based paint, and restoration or replacement of aging housing infrastructures (e.g., windows). Urban soil, on the other hand, is a significant sink of bio-available lead (lead that can be absorbed by the body) that has not, until recently, been regulated or included in a comprehensive prevention strategy. In December 2000, the US EPA promulgated standards for residential lead-contaminated bare soil that took effect in March 2001. In addition to revising hazard standards for lead in house dust and paint (interior environment), it established two hazard standards for lead in soil – 400 parts per million (ppm) for bare soil in play areas and 1200 ppm average for bare soil in the rest of the yard (Federal Register, 2001).

In 1993, the EPA published the Integrated Report of the Urban Soil Lead Abatement Demonstration Project, which synthesized the findings from scientific studies carried out in three cities: Boston, Baltimore, and Cincinnati. The aims of the studies were to determine whether lead in soil was an important pathway of exposure for children and whether soil abatement was an effective measure in reducing blood lead levels. Based on these studies, the EPA concluded that when soil is a significant source of lead in the child's environment, the abatement of that soil will result in a reduced exposure and consequently a reduction in blood lead levels (U.S. Environmental Protection Agency, 1993; U.S. Environmental Protection Agency, 2001a). From these studies, the EPA identified four major factors that would mediate the effectiveness of a soil-based intervention: 1) past history of childhood exposure to lead; 2) a direct exposure pathway between soil and the child; 3) magnitude of other sources of lead exposure; and 4) magnitude of reduction in soil-lead concentrations.

In the Boston pilot study, investigators found that lead in soil was a significant pathway for population exposures (Aschengrau et al., 1994; Weitzman et al., 1993). The large inventory of older wood-framed housing (generally sided with wooden clapboard), which is likely to have exterior lead-based paint, was found to be a major source of lead in soil. Heavily traveled roadways also were recognized as potential contributors to high lead concentrations in soil from historic uses of leaded gasoline. Figure 5.1 illustrates the major pathways of soil-lead exposures. This figure was adapted from the EPA and modified to reflect our focus on lead in soil in Boston, Massachusetts (EPA 747-R-97-006).

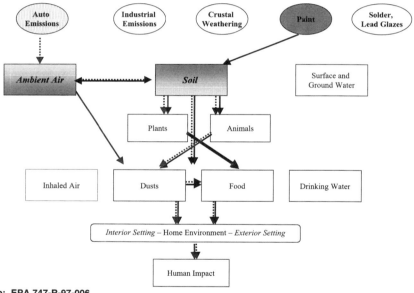

Source: EPA 747-R-97-006

Figure 5.1   The major pathways of soil-lead exposures

In studying the impact of exterior and interior lead abatement on children's blood lead levels, the Boston research team found that a soil lead reduction of 2060 ppm was associated with a 2.25 to 2.70 µg/dL decline in blood lead levels (Aschengrau et al., 1994). These results are supported by other research that has estimated that interior house dust is comprised of anywhere from 30 to 50% of soil dust (Calabrese and Stanek, 1992; Fergusson et al., 1986). Lanphear and others found that blood lead concentrations at levels down to 5 μg/dl are associated with deficits in children's cognitive skills (Lanphear et al., 2000). More recently, Canfield and others found that for children with blood lead levels below 10 μg/dl, IQ (composite score on the Stanford-Binet Intelligence Score) declined by 7.4 points as lifetime average blood lead concentrations increased from 1 to 10 mg/dl (Canfield et al., 2003). Finally, Bellinger and Needleman reported that, in a reanalysis of data from their prospective cohort study, IQ was inversely and significantly associated with blood lead concentrations and that this finding persisted at blood lead levels below 5 mg/dl (Bellinger, 2003). Given these recent findings, a soil lead hazard reduction program could prove to be very important for young children at risk for lead exposure.

Part III: Boston Lead Safe Yard Initiative

The Lead-Safe Yard Project in Boston, Massachusetts, which was funded by the EMPACT program for three phases from 1998 through 2001, was developed to quantify lead levels in residential soil, reduce exposure to lead-contaminated areas through low-cost landscaping interventions, and develop educational and instructional materials for reducing exposure to soil-lead in at-risk urban neighborhoods (Hynes et al., 2001). Moreover, the study aimed to answer the following questions:

1   What are average lead concentrations for residential yards in an urban area like Boston that result from multiple sources of contamination, in particular leaded gasoline and exterior lead-based paint?
2   Is there a relationship between the distance from a building structure and soil lead concentrations in residential yards?

The intervention project was designed in response to the findings from EPA's Urban Soil Lead Abatement Demonstration project in Boston, Massachusetts (as discussed above) that found associations between soil treatment to reduce exposures in residential yards and reductions in blood lead levels in children.

The project involved a range of partners including local community organizations, the residents of affected communities, local businesses, a university, and federal and city environmental protection, public health and housing agencies. The primary partners included the US EPA New England Regional Laboratory, the Boston University School of Public Health, the Bowdoin Street Community Health Center, the Dudley Street Neighborhood Initiative, and local landscape contractors. The project widened the partnership to include Boston's Childhood Lead Poisoning Prevention Program, Lead-Safe Boston, and the National Center for Healthy Housing (NCHH) in its last phase. This partnership enabled the Lead-Safe Yard project to move the project from a pilot program to the possibility of an institutionalized program within municipal health and housing agencies; to improve the specifications and protocols, and to participate in an evaluation of the lead-safe yard intervention directed by the NCHH.

The Lead Safe Yard Project offers an example of the translation of scientific results to sound public health practice. Additionally, it is a model that can: 1) serve as a catalyst for other neighborhood interventions and citywide initiatives; 2) restore neighborhood assets; and 3) return pride to disenfranchised communities – all essential ingredients to improving community health. The methods and results of this intervention to control lead exposures in the residential setting are described in the following section.

Methods

Community-Based Methods

We have employed community-based methods in many aspects of the intervention project. The principles of community-based research include receptivity toward the knowledge of community partners; sharing of skills and knowledge with community partners; fair compensation to community members for work done on the project; data gathering for the purpose of education, action and social change; and sharing of results with community participants (Israel et al., 1998).

Neighborhood Selection Criteria

In the past three years, the EMPACT Lead Safe Yard Project included two neighborhoods – Bowdoin Street (North Dorchester) and Dudley Street (Roxbury). The Bowdoin Street neighborhood was selected based on the following criteria (Hynes et al., 2001):

1   Prevalence of lead poisoning;
2   Concentration of pre-1978 painted housing (generally wooden clapboard siding);
3   Low-income/immigrant population;
4   Contiguous yards (to improve potential for neighborhood-wide impact);
5   Presence of health organization focused on community environmental health issues; and
6   Established neighborhood environmental activities upon which the EMPACT project could build.

In the Dudley Street area, we added the criterion that eligible homes had to be certified as de-leaded in order to promote a holistic model of lead-safe homes that includes the house and yard. Phase III of the EMPACT project was extended to include properties from two "spin-off" lead safe yard programs initiated by the Lead-Safe Boston program within the Boston Department of Neighborhood Development (BDND) and the Boston Public Health Commission's Office of Environmental Health (OEH), which were based on the EMPACT prototype. These latter programs worked closely with the EPA initiative to ensure consistency in research methods, intervention approaches, and documentation and are included in the project evaluation by National Center for Healthy Housing.

Outreach and Education

Outreach and education were essential components of the EMPACT project. During the first phase of outreach and education, outreach staff from community organization partners provided homeowners with information about the hazards of lead in soil and invited them to participate in the project. Outreach strategies to reach homeowners included mailings, phone calls, door-to-door solicitation, and distribution of lead-safe yard literature at community events. Education materials initially included multicultural printed handouts; later we added a video produced by the Boston Childhood Lead Poisoning Prevention Program and a quiz that tested parents' knowledge about lead poisoning. Once participants agreed to enroll in the project, outreach staff conducted the education session and coordinated the soil analysis with other members of the team. Homeowners were briefed throughout the process about the findings from the on-site soil analysis in their yard, the development of a treatment plan, and long-term maintenance of the yard intervention.

Sampling Technology and Data Collection

Soil samples were analyzed in situ with a Niton model 702 field portable X-ray fluorescence (FPXRF) analyzer according to procedures outlined in EPA Method 6200 (U.S. Environmental Protection Agency, 1997). The depth of in-situ measurements was approximately two to three millimeters and sample results were obtained within 30–60 seconds. Clark et al. have demonstrated that the FPXRF is an effective method to gather "real-time" data on lead and other metals in soil environments (Clark et al., 1999). Quality assurance and quality control (QA/QC) for the FPXRF analysis included calibration checks, replicate sample analyses and confirmation sampling (U.S. Environmental Protection Agency, 1998).[3]

We evaluated four types of areas of interest in each yard during the on-site soil analysis: (1) the house drip line area (3-foot wide perimeter of a house); (2) areas of unique use, such as children's play areas and picnic and gardening areas; (3) areas of bare soil and high foot traffic; and (4) 'other' areas noted by the sampling team that could present a source of lead contamination to the subject property other than the house. Examples of 'other' areas include soil near painted perimeter fences, painted tool sheds and other non-residential buildings, auto repair sites, and so on.

The number of samples and sampling plan depended on the size and shape of the yard areas of interest. A line pattern was used for linear sampling sites (e.g. house drip line). Soil measurements were taken at approximately 5-foot intervals along the line. A large X was transcribed over other areas of concern, such as children's play areas. Soil measurements were taken at regular intervals along each line of the X unless the field technician determined that additional resolution was needed because of anomalous readings or suspected sources of lead contamination other than residential house paint.

FPXRF readings and descriptive information about each site, including distance of sample site from house structure, housing characteristics, and weather, were recorded on a site sheet. Each data point collected during on-site sampling was considered a sub-sample and averaged with others in the area of interest (e.g., west drip line) to determine the mean value for that area. Composite results of the soil analysis were transcribed onto a color-coded plot plan of the property for use in the exposure-reduction landscape design. Color codes were used on the property map to indicate the nature and extent of lead contamination in each area sampled and to delineate particular yard uses of concern, such as play and gardening areas.

Exposure-Reduction Measures

Once baseline data for each yard were collected and mapped onto the plot plans, landscaping teams were contracted to carry out the residential yard treatment. A coordinator for each landscaping team first met with the homeowner(s) to review the pattern of lead in soil with the homeowner, to discuss yard treatment strategies with the homeowner and to design a treatment plan. Engaging the homeowner in understanding the pattern of lead soil contamination and in choosing the components of the lead-safe yard landscape options was central to the project's goal of informing residents about their residential environment and including them as decision-makers in the environmental improvements to their home environment.

The project developed a suite of yard treatment options that reduced the risk of human exposure, that were affordable and replicable by community organizations, and that could be maintained by homeowners. The yard treatments included wood-framed drip-line boxes, newly planted grass and shrubs, stone walkways and modifications to the resident's yard use patterns (for example, relocating and constructing a child's play area or a vegetable garden in a safer part of the yard). By year three of the project, the construction specifications were fully standardized and priced, thus improving the reliability and durability of the exposure-reduction work. When the yard treatments were completed, the property owner was given a maintenance manual with instruction on maintaining the treatments. Table 5.1 describes the lead safe yard treatment measures (see Hynes et al., 2001 and U.S. Environmental Protection Agency, 2001a) for samples of yard plans and specifications, materials used, costs, and maintenance manuals and contracts).

Data Analysis

Lead sample data were analyzed using SAS 8.0®. The "yard" rather than the individual soil sample is the primary unit of analysis. Aggregating data at the yard level reduces the variability introduced into the sub-yard results because of over-sampling in areas, such as nearby wooden garages and fences that warranted further investigation.

The concentration of soil-lead in the yard is plotted at regular intervals (0–3 feet, 3–8 feet, 8–12 feet, 12 to 16 feet, and > 16 feet) in order to illustrate the distribution of soil lead with distance from the house. Results are reported by geometric mean, arithmetic mean, and range. The geometric mean, like the median, is an appropriate metric since it is less sensitive to outliers and thus provides a better statistical profile of lead in soil trends in an urbanized area. On the other hand, outliers, that may be a result of common urban sources such as paint chips, waste burning, or auto repair, are important because they represent "hot spots" of potential residential exposure. Thus, we also report lead levels using the arithmetic mean and range (Asante-Duah, 1996).

Urban Geochemical Baseline

To estimate the urban geochemical baseline for lead in soil in our study (hereinafter referred to as 'urban baseline'), we included all soil samples averaged in all yards, including those with average levels less than 400 ppm where we did not do any

Table 5.1   The lead safe yard treatment measures

Soil-Lead Level (parts per million)	EMPACT LSYP Treatment Measures
> 5,000 (very high)	If soil removal or permanent barriers are not possible: ● Install semi-permanent barrier, such as a wood-framed dripbox filled with gravel or mulch ● Relocate gardens – unsafe for all types of gardening
2,000-5,000 (high)*	● Relocate gardens – unsafe for all types of gardening ● Relocate children's play area, pet area and picnic area, if possible. If not, install wood platform or wood-framed raised play and picnic area filled with woodchips. ● Install path of walking stones for high-traffic areas ● Seed and fertilize grassy areas, or cover with mulch or woodchips if not suitable for grass
400-2,000 (moderately high)*	● Install raised-bed garden and supplement with clean topsoil. ● Install wood-framed raised play and picnic area filled with woodchips. ● Install path of walking stones for high-traffic areas. ● Seed and fertilize grassy areas or cover with mulch or woodchips if not suitable for grass.
<400 (EPA Action Level)	● No treatment necessary.

* The lower limit of this range was based on the existing EPA standards at the time of the study. As of January 5, 2001, lead is considered a hazard in soil if there are greater than 400 parts per million of lead in bare soil in children's play areas and 1,200 parts per million of lead in soil in the rest of the yard. Our data analysis reflects these revised standards (40 CFR Part 745, January 5, 2001).

exposure-reduction measures. The urban baseline was determined by examining the relationship between the mean and geometric mean lead levels with distance from housing structure by fitting exponential curves to the data and evaluating the curves for their convergence (n= 2920).

Results

Community-Based Activities

We relied upon and incorporated our community partners' knowledge of their neighborhoods and residents in the selection of sites for the lead-safe yard project and in the design of improved community outreach and education. As a result, the project moved from passive education methods, such as distributing educational pamphlets, to more active and interactive communication with a video, quiz, and discussion about lead hazards and the importance of lead-safe yards. A small number of businesses approached by one of the community partners to donate materials and tools to the project did so, local businesses more so than the large chain stores. The project offered employment opportunities for residents from the community to do the outreach, education, and landscaping work. Initially, we trained and employed youth; next we contracted with a local non-profit organization that builds community gardens and parks. In the last year of the project (Phase 3), we employed a pool of landscaping companies that work in the city of Boston with the intention of building their capacity to continue creating lead-safe yards as a component of their business and also to make the cost as competitive as possible. A focus group discussion with the landscapers, held midway through the last phase, yielded many interesting ideas and recommendations about materials and techniques used for future lead-safe yard projects.

Residents who agreed to participate in the Lead-Safe Yard project were educated about lead and its health effects by the outreach worker and kept informed of the soil sample results by the field team and the landscaper and were given a maintenance manual at the culmination of the project. Finally, we disseminated the model of community-institution partnership as well as information about the technology used, sampling plan, and construction techniques in three ways: 1) making presentations to community organizations in many local forums, using local media, and being featured in a documentary film about selected EMPACT projects; 2) creating a comprehensive handbook for community and public sector agencies interested in replicating the project (U.S. Environmental Protection Agency, 2001a); and 3) conducting an EPA-funded technology transfer workshop for city and state agencies from other EPA regions. All community, government, private sector and university project partners participated in the various aspects of project dissemination.

Profile of Study Yards and Intervention Costs

From the summer of 1998 through the fall of 2001, the EPA-funded Lead Safe Yard Project completed 61 lead-safe yards. By 2001, the Lead Safe Boston program completed 22 lead-safe yards, and the Office of Environmental Health completed six. Since some sampled yards were not eligible for the program because of low soil lead values and, in other cases, homeowners did not participate, more yards were sampled than were completed as lead-safe yards. All sample results from 102 yards, including replicate samples, are included in this analysis.[4]

The Bowdoin Street neighborhood in Dorchester and the Dudley Street neighborhood in Roxbury consist mostly of older wood-framed homes with painted exteriors and unpaved yards where soil is present and soil lead is bio-available. In this area, the median year housing structures were built in 1939. Additionally, 95% of homes were built prior to 1980, based on 1990 US Census data (compared to the citywide average of 91%). Based on data from the 2000 census, children aged five years or younger constituted 7.9% of the population, compared to a citywide average of 5.5%. In general, these inner-city neighborhoods are densely populated with a higher percentage of children and an older housing stock than the city overall. The average cost of interim measures per yard in Phases I and II was approximately $3000, with a breakdown of $2,100 average per yard for materials and construction costs and $900 per yard for project management and indirect costs. We were able to reduce costs in these phases by obtaining some materials at no cost, including gravel from a local company and wood chips and compost. The average cost of Phase III projects was $2800. These figures were not broken down by direct and indirect costs. Because many of the houses in Dorchester and Roxbury are two-and three-family dwellings, we were able to benefit multiple families for the cost of one lead-safe yard.

Construction time per yard ranged from one day to eight weeks, and the average time per yard was under one week. Factors that delayed or preempted yard treatment included inclement weather, availability of contractor and/or homeowner, and insufficient removal of large debris from yards (e.g. trash, appliances, and cars).

Profile of Soil Lead in Yards

For each yard, approximately 30 samples were collected yielding a total of 2920 sample results across 102 yards. The arithmetic mean for lead in soil at the yard level was 1456 ppm (range: 65 ppm–12875 ppm) and the standard deviation was 318 ppm. The geometric mean for lead in soil at the yard level was 1064 ppm (range: 580 ppm–1631 ppm). Figure 5.2 describes the percent distribution of yards by lead concentration. Approximately 87% of yards had average lead concentrations exceeding 400 ppm and approximately half of the yards had average lead concentrations between 400 and 1200 ppm. Figure 5.3 provides percentage distributions within each distance category to show how the concentration levels varied within each group. For example, 96% of all yard averages in the first distance category (0-3 feet) exceeded 400 ppm. More specifically, 32% were between 400 and 1200 ppm, 56% within the range of 1200 to 5000 ppm and 8% exceeded 5000 ppm.

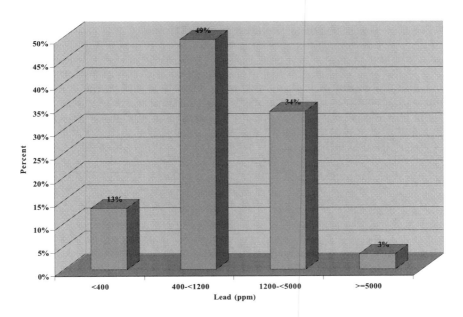

Figure 5.2   The percent distribution of yards by lead concentration

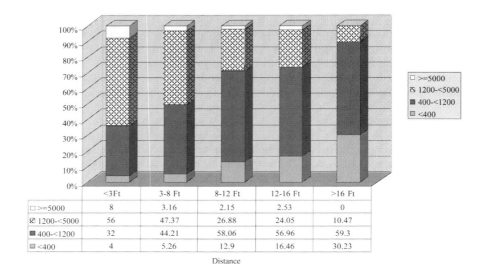

	<3Ft	3-8 Ft	8-12 Ft	12-16 Ft	>16 Ft
□ >=5000	8	3.16	2.15	2.53	0
▨ 1200-<5000	56	47.37	26.88	24.05	10.47
■ 400-<1200	32	44.21	58.06	56.96	59.3
▨ <400	4	5.26	12.9	16.46	30.23

Distance

Figure 5.3   Variation in lead concentration levels within each group

For the last distance category (>16 feet), 70% of the yard averages in that distance group exceeded 400 ppm – 59% ranged between 400 and 1200 ppm, 11% ranged between 1200 and 5000 ppm, and none exceeded 5000 ppm.

Urban Baseline

To capture the impact of lead in yards from all historic and present sources, we evaluated arithmetic and geometric mean concentrations of lead by distance from building structure (n=102 yards). Figure 5.4 shows the arithmetic and geometric mean values for lead concentration averages in residential yards by five distance categories. The arithmetic mean values are shown to illustrate important excursions in lead levels that may exist in residential areas. For example, within the drip line of the house (0–3 feet), the arithmetic mean was 2247 ppm. The minimum value was 173 ppm and the maximum value was 7495 ppm. The geometric mean value within the drip line was 1668 ppm. In contrast to the drip line of the house, at distances greater than 16 feet from the building structure, the arithmetic mean was 712 ppm. The minimum value was 65 ppm and the maximum value was 3238 ppm. The geometric mean value at distances greater than 16 feet was 580 ppm.

Discussion

The EMPACT pilot study set out to design affordable interim controls for soil lead can be implemented in a timely and cost-efficient manner. The FPXRF in-situ

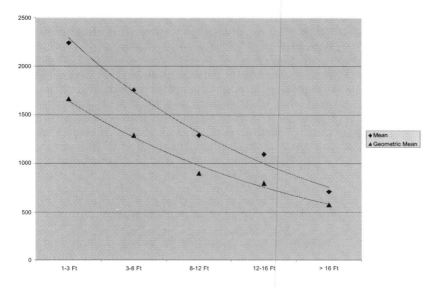

Figure 5.4   Statistical averages for lead concentrations in residential yards, by distance categories

analysis was an effective tool for the measurement of lead in urban soils. The technology allowed field staff to measure up to 30 samples per property in a relatively short period of time. It also aided on-site decision-making regarding sampling location, remedy selections, facilitated feedback to program participants, and guided long-term yard management strategies. Moreover, field personnel were able to respond to extreme lead concentration readings by re-sampling that same day to determine whether the values were real or spurious (U.S. Environmental Protection Agency, 1998).

This project also shed light on lead in soil as an urban hazard. The yard results support the widely held assumption that the highest concentrations of soil-lead concentrate in areas closest to the foundation of the house, referred to as the "drip line" of the housing structure. On average, geometric mean lead levels ranged from 1668 ppm within three feet from building structure to 899 ppm at 8–12 feet from building structure to 580 ppm at 16 feet away from the building structure. Overall, the data support the notion that soil lead concentrations decline over increasing distances from the building foundation.

Notwithstanding this decline, soil lead levels across all distances from building structures exceeded on average the EPA action level of 400 ppm, for both the log-transformed and unadjusted data. Approximately 87% of yards in the pilot neighborhoods have soil lead levels above 400 ppm and approximately 37% of these residential yards have soil lead levels above 1200 ppm, suggesting that, in an urban setting like Boston, 1) residential soil is an important pathway for adverse exposures to lead; and 2) all areas of the yard can pose risks to affected families given the blend of historic point sources (e.g., household exterior paint) and area sources (e.g., ambient deposition of lead from automobiles, local auto body shops and smelting operations). The National Survey of Lead and Allergens in Housing found that an estimated 21% of homes have soil lead levels above 400 ppm and 12% have soil lead levels above 1200 ppm. These data, which reflect the maximum soil values for each housing unit (Clickner et al., 2001), convey the disproportionate burden of lead-contaminated soil in older, low-income residential neighborhoods.

The geometric mean soil lead concentrations for the 102 yards studied in the EMPACT pilot project was 1064 ppm, which is consistent with other studies in the Boston area and beyond (Weitzman et al., 1993). Lanphear and others found that the geometric mean lead concentration for foundation soil was 1000 ppm in Rochester, NY (Lamphear et al., 1998). Rabinowitz and others (*34*) reported a mean surface soil lead concentration for Boston of 600 ppm and "emergency lead poisoning area" average lead concentration of 2000 ppm.[5] Shinn and others reported a median soil lead level of 1773 ppm in a Chicago residential study area (Shinn et al., 2000). While these data suggest the range of lead concentration in urban soils is high enough to warrant concern about its bioavailability as an urban health hazard, caution must be exercised when comparing these values for the purposes of generalizing about ambient lead levels in residential areas given the different metrics used for representing lead concentrations (e.g., arithmetic means, medians, geometric means).

National studies of element concentrations in soils of the conterminous United States have shown that lead levels in virgin soil are estimated to range from 10 to 80 ppm but are subject to variation, from <10 to 700 ppm, when factoring in soil type and geographic location (Shacklette and Boerngen, 1984). In Boston, our study results suggest that estimates of an urban baseline, which reflects multiple sources of lead contamination, range from 580 to 712 ppm at distances greater than 16 feet from building structures. These values fall into the high end of the soil background ranges measured by Shacklette and others (Shacklette and Boerngen, 1984). Also noteworthy is that our urban baseline estimates are above the EPA "safe" level of 400 ppm for children's play areas. These data underscore the importance of lead in soil as a potential source of lead exposure and the need to integrate such information into local public health strategies to reduce population exposures to lead.

Other Project Benefits

The Lead-Safe Yard Project, as a community-based environmental health intervention that results in informed residents and treated properties, has the potential for multiplier effects. In order to document additional and on-going benefits that have accrued to the communities and community partners involved in the Lead-Safe Yard Project, we interviewed three members of the team who were involved in different project aspects. Nicole Flynt, a staff person at DSNI and the outreach and education coordinator for Phase III of the project, pointed to four on-going community benefits from the Lead-Safe Yard Project: 1) residents' sharing knowledge about lead poisoning with their relatives and friends, 2) the expansion of lead soil testing, 3) the network of resources that she can access, and 4) the contagiousness of the project among neighbors. Ms Flynt, who is also responsible for the development and maintenance of open space within the DSNI area, now ensures that lead-soil testing is done in parks and community gardens. In organizing neighborhood clean-ups and planning the creation of a memorial community garden for a resident who was recently killed, she tapped her partners in the Lead-Safe Yard Project for soil testing, donation of materials (including plants, bulbs, mulch, and filter fabric) and funding. Speaking of the project's contagious appeal to residents, she told of one lead-safe yard homeowner who initiated a friendly competition with her neighbors, motivating them to create their own lead-safe yards using methods and design ideas learned from her yard.

Tom Plant, director of the Boston Childhood Lead Poisoning Prevention Program was project manager for combined home de-leading and lead-safe yards in a neighborhood plagued by lead poisoning. He observed that the combined program had numerous impacts beyond the interventions. Homeowners took their own initiatives based on what they learned about lead soil hazards. For example, one homeowner installed an asphalt sidewalk in a heavily used yard area and another built a fence to prevent the runoff of soil from his yard toward a neighbor's yard. He also noted that residents who participated in the project made inquiries about low-interest loans offered by the city for other home improvements, indicating that the combined lead-safe program was a catalyst for neighborhood betterment.

Sandra Duran, a construction manager for Lead-Safe Boston, attracted five community and city-wide landscape companies to Phase III of the Lead-Safe Yard Project. All were trained in occupational health and safety on the job by the team industrial hygienist. According to Ms Duran, the project helped one new community contractor launch and structure his business, and all the companies learned valuable health and safety information which they are passing on to their present clients. "They learned that virtually every property in the city of Boston has contaminated soil and the hazards extend not only to their workforce but also to their client base."

Part IV: Concluding Issues

The Evaluation Process

The National Center for Healthy Housing evaluated the project in 2001 and 2002, looking at the original 39 EMPACT pilot properties and 47 other properties enrolled in 2000. The U.S. Housing and Urban Development Agency (HUD) and USEPA Region 1 provided funding for this evaluation. Key evaluation issues included:

1   Were treatments durable two to twelve months after construction?
2   Did residents' exposure to lead dust decline after treatment?
3   Were participants satisfied with the program?
4   What did participants know about how to reduce soil lead exposure, and did they continue to maintain the treatments after construction?

Evaluation data for all properties included face-to-face interviews with participants, pre-intervention FPXRF measurements, and field observations of the treatments one year after construction. For properties enrolled in 2000, the evaluation also collected floor dust wipe and floor mat dust lead samples before and after treatment. A limited number of properties enrolled in 2000 also had FPXRF measurements taken one year later.

Durability

The vast majority of treatments in all the properties continued to prevent exposure to leaded soil at one year. Some types of treatment, notably grass treatments and areas where wood chips or mulch were not confined to a box, were more likely to have bare soil one year later, but the square footage of exposed soil remained small relative to the total size of the yards. The activity of pets or other animals may help explain why some areas had bare soil. Interview data at the one-year visit suggested that 46% of the properties had pets in the home and that, in the majority of these cases, animals had access to areas in the yard that were treated. In fifty percent of the EMPACT pilot properties with pets and 31% of the properties enrolled in 2000 with pets, soil in the areas to which pets had access was more than half bare.

Effectiveness of Soil Treatments

All three measures of treatment effectiveness (in situ FPXRF soil surface measurements, dust lead loadings on exterior floor mats, and floor dust lead loadings) showed statistically significant reductions in lead levels at one year for the properties enrolled in 2000.

At one year, for a sub-sample of 26 properties, the per property geometric mean for in situ surface readings had dropped from 1714 to 321 ppm, below the 400 ppm EPA lead hazard standard for bare soil in children's play areas. Over 90% of the samples fell below the new 1200 ppm standard for bare soil in areas other than children's play areas.

Treatments were associated with a statistically significant reduction in the amount of lead soil tracked into the home as measured in the amount of lead/square foot (loading) on floor mats. At one year, the mat loading rate, or the amount of lead dust expected to accumulate on a mat per day, was 30% lower than at pre-intervention.

Treatments were also associated with a statistically significant reduction of floor dust lead loadings in the front of the property, but the magnitude of reduction was not as great as seen with mat loadings or *in situ* soil surface readings. In general, rear floor dust lead loadings were roughly twice as high as those on front floors both before intervention and one year after. Statistically significant reductions in the geometric mean dust lead loadings were found at the front exterior and front main entry.

Homeowners' Maintenance, Satisfaction, with Treatments and Knowledge

Low-income property owners are often stereotyped as lacking the skills or desire to undertake regular yard maintenance. The interview data collected do not support this view. Respondents from both groups of properties reported considerable yard maintenance and exterior construction activities. The most frequently reported yard maintenance activities closely corresponded to the recommendations in the project maintenance plans.

The vast majority of participants expressed satisfaction with the landscaping treatments. Those in the later phase reported increased use of their yards for children's play activities and socializing after the landscaping work was complete.

Recall of specific educational messages, as well as beliefs about whether they pertain to the household's situation, may affect homeowner maintenance practices. The majority of households could recall a variety of educational messages related to lead at one year. However, nearly one third of the later phase respondents reported that they did not need to take continuing action to protect children from lead exposure because their houses and yards had been made "safe". (Respondents in the earlier phase were not asked a comparable question.) Since the majority of respondents from both projects also reported performing exterior maintenance activities that could generate large amounts of lead dust, this comment raises concern that participants could inadvertently generate lead hazards in the future.

Lessons Learned

The evaluation identified several key "take home messages" for primary prevention efforts tailored to lead in soil:

1   Low cost soil treatments can significantly reduce the track-in of lead dust from the yard.
2   Continuing maintenance of soil treatments is as important to the success of this intervention as the initial treatments. On-going efforts should be made to reduce or eliminate bare soil in the yard. Essential yard maintenance includes gutter and downspout repair to prevent treatment washout, renewing mulch, watering and reseeding grass, and preventing animals from digging in the yard.
3   Floor mats can play an important role in reducing soil track-in. For maximum effect, mats should be placed outside and inside the front and rear entrances to the structure.
4   Prevention programs must reinforce the message that successfully managing lead dust and lead soil hazards in older homes requires on-going maintenance and vigilance on the part of owners and tenants. Lead Safe Work Practice training for owners and renters who engage in home maintenance is an important component of the prevention message.

Future Directions

A promising plant-based remedial solution for lead in residential soil is a process called phytoextraction or phytoremediation, the uptake of metal contaminants from soil by plants. Recent research has shown that, with the addition of synthetic chelates such as EDTA, lead in soil can be solubilized and transported from the roots to the shoots of specific plants, such as sunflowers and Indian mustard. At elevated levels, lead in the plant tissue corresponds to the concentration of soil lead and the amounts of EDTA soil additive (Blaylock et al., 1997).

With additional feasibility studies, it may be possible to develop a combination of approaches to using phytoextraction, including turf grass and other selective plants in open sunny land areas; portable growing bins in more shaded areas; and a central, municipally managed bio-treatment site with greenhouses where contaminated residential soil could be deposited for phytoremediation and returned to yards when clean. This innovative, yet appropriate-in-scale biology-based technology would enable urban communities to advance beyond interim controls for lead-safe yards, gardens, and play spaces to permanent solutions.

Notes

1   Community capacity is the "interaction of human capital, organizational resources, and social capital existing within a given community that can be leveraged to solve collective problems and improve or maintain the well-being of a given community. It may operate through the informal social processes and/or organized effort" (Chaskin, 2001).
2   Current action levels for lead poisoning, as set by the Centers for Disease Control and Prevention, is 10 mg/dl of blood. Recent studies by Lanphear and others have shown that lead causes cognitive deficits in children at levels as low as 5 mg/dl of blood (Lanphear et al., 2000).
3   QA/QC results from Phase I, II, and III of this project can be obtained from Mr. Paul Carroll of the US Environmental Protection Agency New England Regional Laboratory. Mr. Carroll can be reached by email at Carroll.Paulr@epamail.epa.gov.
4   In total, 103 residential yards were sampled, and results from 102 yards are included in the data analysis. Data for one house were not available for analysis at the time of publication.
5   Emergency Lead Poisoning Areas (ELPAs) were designated by the city of Boston during the late 1980s. They were neighborhoods with the highest prevalence of lead poisoning among young children.

References

Ambler, J. (2001), "Attacking Poverty While Improving the Environment: Towards Win-Win Policy Options", New York: Poverty and Environment Initiative, United Nations Development Programme and the European Commission.
Anonymous (1997), "Update: Blood Lead Levels – United States, 1991–1994," *Morbidity and Mortality Weekly Report*, **46**, 141–6.
Asante-Duah, D.K. (1996), "Investigating Potentially Contaminated Sites", *in Managing Contaminated Sites*, Chichester: John Wiley & Sons, 13–35.
Aschengrau, A., Beiser, A., Bellinger, D., Copenhafer, D. and Weitzman, M. (1994), "The Impact of Soil Lead Abatement on Urban Children's Blood Lead Levels: Phase II Results from the Boston Lead-In-Soil Demonstration Project," *Environmental Research*, **67**, 125–48.
Bellinger, D. and Needleman, H. (2003), "Intellectual Impairment and Blood Lead Levels," *The New England Journal of Medicine*, **349**, 500–502.
Blaylock, M., Salt, D., Dushenkov, S., Zakharova, O., Gussman, C., Kapulnik, Y., Ensley, B. and Raskin, I. (1997), "Accumulation of lead in Indian mustard by soil-applied chelating agents," *Environmental Science and Technology*, **31**, 860–65.
Boyce, J.K. and Pastor, M. (2001), "Building Natural Assets: New Strategies for Poverty Reduction and Environmental Protection", Amherst, MA: Political Economy Research Institute, University of Massachusetts.
Calabrese, E. and Stanek, E.J. (1992), "What Proportion of Household Dust is Derived from Outdoor Soil?" *Journal of Soil Contamination*, **1**, 253–63.
Canfield, R.L., Henderson, C.R., Cory-Slechta, D., Cox, C., Jusko, T.A. and Lanphear, B.P. (2003), "Intellectual Impairment in Children with Blood Lead Concentrations below 10 ug per Deciliter," *New England Journal of Medicine*, **348**, 1517–26.

Centers for Disease Control and Prevention (1997), "Screening Young Children for Lead Poisoning:Guidance for State and Local Public Health Officials," Atlanta, GA: CDC.

Chaskin, R.J. (2001), "Building Community Capacity: A Definitional Framework and Case Studies from a Comprehensive Community Initiative," *Urban Affairs Review*, **36**, 291–333.

Clark, S., Menrath, W., Chen, M., Roda, S. and Succop, P. (1999), "Use of a Field Portable X-Ray Fluorescence Analyzer to Determine the Concentration of Lead and Other Metals in Soil Samples," *Ann Agric Environ Med*, **6**, 27–32.

Clickner, R.P., Marker, D., Viet, S.M., Rogers, J. and Broene, P. (2001), "National Survey of Lead and Allergens in Housing: Final Report – Volume 1: Analysis of Lead Hazards. C-OPC-21356", Rockville, MD: WESTAT, Inc.

Federal Register (1-5-2001), "Identification of Dangerous Levels of Lead: Final Rule", **60**, 4.

Fergusson, J.E., Forbes, E.A., Schroeder, R.J. and Ryan, D.E. (1986), "Lead: Petrol Lead in the Environment and its Contribution to Human Blood Lead Levels." *Science in the Total Environment*, **50**, 1–54.

Fullilove, M.T. and Fullilove III, R.M. (2000), "Place Matters", in *Reclaiming the Environmental Debate: The Politics of Health in a Toxic Culture* (Hofrichter R, ed.), Cambridge, MA: Massachusetts Institute of Technology, 77–91.

Goldman, L., Apelberg, B., Koduru, S., Ward, C. and Sorian, R. (1999), "Healthy from the Start: Why America Needs a Better System to Track and Understand Birth Defects and the Environment". Baltimore, MD: The Pew Environmental Health Commission.

Hynes, H.P., Maxfield, R., Carroll, P. and Hillger, R. (2001), "Dorchester Lead-Safe Yard Project: a Pilot Program to Demonstrate Low-Cost, On-Site Techniques to Reduce Exposure to Lead Contaminated Soil", *Journal of Urban Health*, **78**,198–210.

Institute of Medicine (1988), "The Future of Public Health", Washington D.C.: National Academy Press.

Institute of Medicine (1999), "Toward Environmental Justice: Research, Education, and Health Policy Needs". Washington, D.C.: National Academy Press.

Institute of Medicine (2001), "Rebuilding the Unity of Health and the Environment: A New Vision of Environmental Health for the 21st Century", Washington, D.C.: National Academy of Sciences.

International Healthy Cities Foundation (7-16-2001), "Overview and History of Healthy Cities".

Israel, B., Schulz, A.J., Parker, E.A. and Becker, A.B. (1998) "Review of Community-Based Research: Assessing Partnership Approaches to Improve Public Health," *Annual Review of Public Health*, **19**, 173–202.

Kretzmann, J.P. and McKnight, J.L. (1993), *Building Communities from the Inside Out: A Path Toward Finding and Mobilizing a Community's Assets*, Evanston, IL: ACTA Publications.

Lanphear, B.P., Burgoon, D.A., Rust, S.W., Eberly, S. and Galke, W, (1998), "Environmental Exposures to Lead and Urban Children's Blood Lead Levels", *Environmental Research*, **76**, 120–30.

Lanphear, B.P., Dietrich, K., Auinger, P. and Cox, C. (2000), "Cognitive Deficits Associated with Blood Lead Concentrations <10 ug/dL in US Children and Adolescents", *Public Health Reports*, **115**, 521–9.

Mahaffey, K., Annest, J.L., Roberts, J. and Murphy, R.S. (1982), "National Estimates of Blood Lead Levels: United States, 1976-1980: Association with Selected Demographic and Socioeconomic Factors", *New England Journal of Medicine*, **307**, 573–9.

Mielke, H.W., Anderson, J.C., Berry, K.J., Mielke, P.W., Chaney, R.L. and Leech, M, (1983), "Lead Concentrations in Inner-City Soils As a Factor in the Child Lead Problem", *American Journal of Public Health*, **73**, 1366–9.

Mielke, H.W. and Reagan, P.L. (1998), "Soil is an Important Pathway of Human Lead Exposure", *Environmental Health Perspectives 106, Supplement*, **1**, 217–29.

National Research Council (1996), "Understanding Risk: Informing Decisions in a Democratic Society".

Pirkle, J.L., Brody, D.J., Gunter, E.W., Kramer, R.A., Paschal, D.C., Flegal, K.M. and Matte, T.D. (1994), "The Decline in Blood Lead Levels in the United States", The National Health and Nutrition Examination Surveys (NHANES), *Journal of the American Medical Association*, **272**, 284–91.

Presidential/Congressional Commission on Risk Assessment and Risk Management (1997), Framework for Environmental Health Risk Assessment (Volume I).

Presidential/Congressional Commission on Risk Assessment and Risk Management (1997), "Risk Assessment and Risk Management in Regulatory Decision-Making (Volume II)".

Rabinowitz, M., Leviton, A., Needleman, H., Bellinger, D. and Waternaux, C. (1985), "Environmental Correlates of Infant Blood Lead Levels in Boston", *Environmental Research*, **38**, 96–107.

Shacklette, H.T. and Boerngen, J.G. (1984), "Element Concentrations in Soils and Other Surficial Materials of the Conterminous United States", *US Geological Survey Professional Paper,* **1270**, 1–63.

Shinn, N.J., Bing-Canar, J., Cailas, M., Peneff, N. and Binns, H.J. (2000), "Spatial Continuity of Soil Lead Levels", *Environmental Research*, **82**, 46–52.

U.S. Department of Health and Human Services (2000), "Healthy People 2010: Understanding and Improving Health", Bethesda: DHHS.

U.S. Environmental Protection Agency (1993), "Integrated Report of the Urban Soil Lead Abatement Demonstration Project", EPA/600/P-93/001a. Washington, D.C.

U.S. Environmental Protection Agency (1997), "Test Methods for Evaluating Solid Waste, Physical/Chemical Methods", EPA Method SW-846.

U.S. Environmental Protection Agency (2001), "Lead-Safe Yards: Developing and Implementing a Monitoring, Assessment, and Outreach Program for Your Community", EPA/625/R-00/012. Washington, D.C.

U.S. Environmental Protection Agency (7-12-2001), "What is EMPACT?"

U.S. Environmental Protection Agency New England Regional Laboratory (1998), "Quality Assurance Project Plan for a Community Based Environmental Lead Assessment and Remediation Program", Lexington, MA.

van Oers, J.A.M. (1993), "A Geographic Information System for Local Public Health Policy", Assen, Netherlands: Van Gorcum.

Weitzman, M., Aschengrau, A., Bellinger, D., Jones, R., Hamlin, J., Beiser, A. (1993), "Lead-Contaminated Soil Abatement and Urban Children's Blood Lead Levels", *The Journal of the American Medical Association*, **269**, 1647–54.

Chapter 6

"We don't only grow vegetables, we grow values": Neighborhood Benefits of Community Gardens in Flint, Michigan

Katherine Alaimo, Thomas M. Reischl, Pete Hutchison
and Ashley E. Atkinson

Me and Mrs. Odom, we sit on our porch in the summertime and let people know we're watching them. They got very conscious of the fact that we were concerned. I had a little problem with the little ones pulling up my flowers, and I told their mother. And now they say to each other, "You can't pull them flowers up, that lady will see you." They think I can see them, but I don't need to see them now.

We've had people come off of other streets and come down our street and say, "Y'all really got it going on – this is beautiful! I wouldn't mind coming over and living on this street. You guys got it going." You know that makes you feel good when you've done something that impresses peoples enough to say, 'Hey, I wouldn't mind living over here."

Lillie Neal, East Eldridge Block Club Community Garden, *From Seeds to Stories: The Community Garden Storytelling Project of Flint*, p. 78.

Introduction

The citizens of Flint, Michigan face a number of economic and social challenges. Once one of the wealthiest cities in the nation, the birthplace of General Motors and the United Auto Workers currently wrestles with the radiating impacts of losing over 60,000 jobs at local General Motors factories since 1970. One impact has been a loss of population from 196,940 in 1960 to 124,943 in 2000 (a 37% decline) (U.S. Census Bureau). The loss of population is related to increases in housing vacancies, decreases in local tax revenues and city services, and increases in crime. Currently, over 12% of the city's property is abandoned or vacant, and in 2000, Flint, was ranked 7th nationally in overall serious crime, and 1st in burglary and assault (Detroit Free Press). The city's budget deficit was the impetus for a successful recall of the city's mayor and of the State of Michigan placing the city into financial receivership in 2002.

Despite these challenges, many Flint citizens express their hopes for a better future by investing their time along with their neighbors to address city and neighborhood concerns. Their efforts are supported and directed by over 100 neighborhood associations, local foundations, and community and faith-based organizations whose focus area is Flint and Genesee County.

One concrete expression of these hopes is an urban gardening and beautification movement that is currently gaining momentum. Community gardens and beautification projects can play a significant role in the restoration and revitalization of distressed communities like Flint by transforming neglected land into attractive parks and gardens. Engaging individuals with community gardens can also contribute to the health and well-being of gardeners through increased physical activity and the consumption of fresh fruits and vegetables (Hynes, In Press; Blair, 1991; Relf, 1996). Community gardens can create positive opportunities for youth activities and learning, foster environmental stewardship, and contribute to neighborhood cohesiveness (Hynes, In Press; Armstrong, 2000; Krasny, 2002). These benefits have been studied; however, the number of studies is small.

This chapter describes the community garden movement in Flint and how community gardens can transform urban spaces and improve the conditions of distressed neighborhoods. We present selected findings and lessons learned from "The Community Garden Storytelling Project of Flint," a community-based participatory research project. The project was guided by a community committee, the Flint Urban Gardening and Land Use Corporation Storytelling Committee, and used a case study approach. In this chapter, the following research question is addressed: What are the neighborhood benefits of community gardens in Flint, MI?

The Setting: Flint, MI

Since the founding of Flint in 1855, the city has been a one industry town. During the 19th century, Flint's economy relied on the harvesting of lumber, and eventually on the manufacturing of carriages. Flint became known as "Vehicle City" and became the largest carriage-making center in the world. In 1908, General Motors Corporation was founded in Flint and the growth of the automotive industry became the predominant economic and social influence of the region. The growth in manufacturing jobs attracted European immigrants and African Americans from southern states to Flint throughout the first half of the 20th century.[1] The aspect of Flint history is rich with important events, such as the Flint Sit-Down Strike of 1936–37, which resulted in the recognition of the newly formed United Auto Workers Union by the General Motors Corporation.

Over the past 30 years, however, because of lost market share and aging production facilities, General Motors Corporation has reduced the number of jobs at Flint production plants. Like many other industrial centers in the Northeastern and Midwestern states, Flint has been forced to manage with this declining economic base and the exodus of citizens seeking jobs elsewhere. The City of Flint, for instance, is coping with large budget deficits and the need to downsize its infrastructure and support services because of rapidly declining local tax receipts.

Flint's dependence on the auto industry also influenced Flint's housing and neighborhood structures. Although leagues of workers came to Flint for jobs in the auto factories, they oftentimes did not come to Flint to live and maintained homes and families in the South and other regions. Many workers believed their move was temporary, creating a transient mindset, even within residents who stayed in the city for over thirty years. In addition, with a few notable exceptions, the interaction and interpersonal relationships traditionally associated with neighborhoods was found instead within the United Auto Workers Union and in the automobile factories where residents worked. The exodus of workers has only exacerbated neighborhood decline and in many ways, the efforts to build Flint neighborhoods are in the formative stages of residents building trust, commitment, and a shared concept of neighborhood.

The mass exodus, the budget deficits, lack of neighborhood cohesion, and declining city infrastructure are evidenced by the fact that today there are over 6,700 abandoned properties in the City of Flint, comprising approximately 12% of the city's total real estate market. This massive number of abandoned and blighted properties gives visitors to Flint the impression that nobody cares about the community, makes it extremely difficult to attract new homeowners and businesses to the city, and invites more serious disorder and crime. In addition, blighted and abandoned properties are a tremendous drain on dwindling city resources and Flint's ability to abate public nuisances, and social ills associated with these properties including, illegal dumping, graffiti, arson, and prostitution. For these reasons, vacant and abandoned property is one of the most pressing obstacles to achieving stability and vitality in many Flint neighborhoods.

The Urban Gardening Movement in Flint

> Vicky Hurley and I and some others all went down to Angelo's one day, and talked, and started this group called Neighbors. And Cindy Cheshier – she's a Master Gardener– came up to me and said there was an article in the Smithsonian about this gentleman in Oregon who is doing raised bed vegetable gardens, and he got his grant from the Mott Foundation. So I went to Pete Hutchison at Violence Prevention here, and he went ballistic! He said, "This is what I want. This is what I want in Flint! You've got the grant if you write it up. You've got it." So we did. And we started twelve raised bed gardens in the old ice rink behind the Williams-Edison School ...
>
> That fall, or maybe it was the next spring, Pete called and wanted to have a meeting, and he said, "There are people from all over the city and they want to have gardens." And then Ashley Atkinson came in and that was the start of the Flint Urban Gardens.
>
> Mary Alyce Stickney, *From Seeds to Stories: The Community Garden Storytelling Project of Flint*, p. 17.

The community and urban gardening movement in Flint grew through multiple influences and a series of events that resulted in a community-wide interest in beautification, gardening and land use issues. In 1996, the Flint Neighborhood Violence Prevention Collaborative (NVPC), a program of the Community Foundation of Greater Flint, began awarding small grants to neighborhood organizations and block clubs to implement community projects in their neighborhoods. Some examples of these projects were crime watch projects, youth enrichment programs (e.g., sports teams or performing arts), and neighborhood events, such as summer picnics. In addition, many neighborhood groups applied to the NVPC to receive funding for neighborhood gardening and beautification activities.

In 1997 Flint's Mayor, Woodrow Stanley, organized a bus trip for community leaders to visit the Farm-A-Lot program in Detroit, a program that encourages neighborhood residents to adopt vacant lots in the city and plant gardens on the land. Inspired by the Detroit experience, the community leaders who visited Detroit continued to meet about creating a similar program in Flint. The next year a request was made from the group to Pete Hutchison, the Director of the NVPC, to invite neighborhood groups interested in beautification to their meetings. NVPC grantees that received funding for beautification projects were invited and two meetings occurred.

During the same time period, Ashley Atkinson, a volunteer interested in gardening and land use issues in Flint was working with Salem Housing Task Force, a Flint non-profit housing organization. Ms. Atkinson was holding meetings at Salem Housing with neighborhood residents, Michigan State University Extension, and other groups about urban gardening and vacant land use issues.

In the fall of 1998, the two groups led by Mr. Hutchison and Ms. Atkinson joined together and formed a committee called "Flint Urban Gardens", which later evolved into the Flint Urban Gardening and Land Use Committee (FUGLUC) in the Fall of 1999, and the non-profit organization, the Flint Urban Gardening and Land Use Corporation in Fall of 2001. In January of 1999, Ms. Atkinson became a paid Americorp volunteer and from 1999 until 2000, served as the Coordinator of FUGLUC.

The support of FUGLUC enabled many block clubs to successfully write NVPC grants and carry to out beautification and gardening projects. Flint's urban gardening movement has grown from three community gardens in 1997 to approximately 20 gardens in 2003. FUGLUC has received over $100,000 in grant assistance, and has a paid full-time Executive Director and three staff members. In addition, the Applewood Initiative for Gardening and Community, funded by the Ruth Mott Foundation of Flint, was initiated in the Fall of 2003 to train technical assistants to work with Flint and Genesee County neighborhood organizations to improve neighborhood environments and establish sustainable community gardens.

It is important to note the distinctions between the Flint community gardens and community gardens in many other cities. In many cities, community gardens are maintained by non-profit gardening organizations that divide up land and allocate it to individuals and families for personal gardening. Often a fee is charged of garden members for garden maintenance, watering, and plowing. In contrast, the Flint community gardens consist of neighbors coming together, taking over one or several abandoned vacant lots, clearing and cleaning the lot of brush and trash, plowing the land, and collectively planting vegetables, fruit and flowers. They may be assisted in these tasks by other organizations, such as FUGLUC, but the primary responsibility for the gardens usually is with the neighborhood residents, neighborhood block club, or neighborhood organization. Distribution of the produce tends to be somewhat unregulated. Although a few neighborhoods attempted assigning rows to individual neighbors or families, most neighborhoods work and share the produce collectively.

Because of the large availability of vacant land, Flint block clubs and residents often adopt more than one parcel for their gardens; some gardens have eventually taken up most of the unused land on their block. Much of the vacant land in Flint is owned by one of three levels of government – the City of Flint, Genesee County, or the State of Michigan. Most Flint community gardeners tend land owned by the state/county/city government or a local institution such as a school or church. Nearly all of the vacant land in the city had a house or other structure on the property at one point in time. As a result, buried debris and soil contamination are always a concern.

Since 2002, FUGLUC has been helping gardeners conduct and pay for soil samples to ensure the site is safe for planting. If borderline levels of toxins, such as lead, are found on the site, FUGLUC assists gardeners in building raised bed gardens.

Benefits of Community Gardens

Throughout the history of the Neighborhood Violence Prevention Collaborative (NVPC), Mr. Hutchison became increasingly interested in community gardening and beautification as a vehicle to enhance neighborhood cohesion, encourage civic engagement, and prevent violence in the community. He witnessed the community gardens become focal points for many of the gardening neighborhoods, and become an opportunity for neighbors to come out of their houses and begin to interact with one another. Because many Flint residents originally came from a Southern farming background, gardening was an activity that many neighborhood residents felt they had some expertise, which created a comfort zone that allowed for social interaction. Being an expert also conferred status to the gardeners (many of whom are senior citizens) and gave them the courage to get involved not just in the gardens, but also in other areas of concern in their neighborhoods. Mr. Hutchison believed that the gardening and beautification projects enabled neighborhood residents to meet each other, work together toward a common goal and, in turn, share the responsibility for monitoring the neighborhood to prevent incidents of dumping, crime, and violence.

There have been few research studies specifically on community gardens, but there is some indication in the literature that community gardens can increase neighborhood social capital and assist with crime prevention. A study of community gardens in Philadelphia found that gardeners were more likely than matched controls to regard their neighbors as friendly and were more likely to participate in food distribution projects, neighborhood clean-ups and neighborhood social events (Blair, 1991). Armstrong found that through providing space for neighborhood interaction, community gardens in low-income areas can be catalysts for neighbors addressing other pressing issues such as crime and property maintenance (Armstrong, 2000).

Further, there is an extensive literature on the beneficial effects of nature and natural settings on human well being (Kaplan, 1989; Ulrich, 1981), and a growing literature on the benefits of green common spaces in urban areas for crime prevention, social cohesion, and civic engagement. For example, studies of public housing residents in Chicago have found that apartment buildings surrounded by trees and greenery are safer than those devoid of green (Kuo, 2001). One reason may be because greener, more natural settings encourage social interaction. The researchers found that residents living closer to greener spaces report more social activities, have more visitors, know more of their neighbors, and have stronger feelings of belonging than residents who live near spaces devoid of greenery (Kweon, 1998).

The Community Garden Storytelling Project of Flint

The Community Garden Storytelling Project of Flint is a community-based public health project that engaged the Flint Urban Gardening and Land Use Corporation

(FUGLUC), members of neighborhood associations, and university-based public health researchers, to research and advocate for the community gardens in Flint. The project was initiated after discussions among the Director of the NVPC (Pete Hutchison), the NVPC evaluation team at the Prevention Research Center of Michigan (Thomas Reischl, Katherine Alaimo), and the Director of FUGLUC (Ashley Atkinson) suggested that a focused qualitative and quantitative evaluation of community gardens would be of great value to the NVPC project and to the greater Flint community. The project was supported by Dr. Alaimo's postdoctoral fellowship funded by the WK Kellogg Community Health Scholarship Program, with funds from the Prevention Research Center of Michigan (PRC),[2] and grants from Flint foundations including the Ruth Mott Foundation.

As a project of the PRC, the participants followed the Community-Based Principles adopted by the PRC Community Board. Community-based participatory research is a collaborative approach to research that:

- equitably involves stakeholders (community members, organizational representatives, etc.) and researchers in multiple aspects of the research process,
- recognizes all partners unique contributions,
- shares responsibility for the project among the partners,
- enhances understanding of a given phenomenon and the social and cultural dynamics of the community,
- uses knowledge gained to take action to improve the health or social well-being of community members (Minkler, 2003; Israel, 1998; Reardon, 1998).

The first meeting of the Community Garden Storytelling Project of Flint, as the project came to be named, was in January of 2001. Initial meetings involved setting policies and procedures, and planning. Brainstorming of "hopes" for the project were written up as a mission statement, research questions and anticipated products. Later meetings involved planning and work distribution for data and story collection procedures, data analyses, book and other product editing and distribution, and presentation creation and practice sessions. The Mission statement included language about sharing stories and knowledge about community gardens for the purposes of gaining resources for FUGLUC, and Flint community gardens, land use and beautification projects; advocating for garden-friendly city policies and supportive community norms and mind frames; and to "help the Greater Flint area be seen in a more positive light." Products hoped-for and actualized throughout the tenure of the project were a story/picture book about the Flint community gardens, a FUGLUC Brochure, an NVPC Evaluation Report on the community gardens, research papers, presentations, and maps of the locations of the community garden and beautification projects in Flint.

Community-Based Research Methods

The Community Garden Storytelling Project of Flint was guided by the Flint Urban Gardening and Land Use Corporation (FUGLUC) Storytelling Committee, composed of a diverse group of community leaders, community gardeners, and neighborhood residents. Forty percent of the Committee was African American, 60% were European American, and ages ranged from 20s to 80s. Eighty-two percent of the Committee were women. The Storytelling Committee met bi-monthly for 2.5 years; the committee decided on research questions, data collection procedures, interview questions, and assisted with data collection and interpretation.

To ascertain benefits of community gardens for Flint neighborhood, a case study approach was employed and focused on four Flint neighborhoods with community gardens. The community gardens in these neighborhoods were either funded by an NVPC small grant, or the neighborhood organization had received an NVPC small grant in the past for a gardening project. Two gardens were initiated during the spring of 2001, while two had been in existence for at least three years. The neighborhood organizations in each neighborhood were given $300 gift certificates to a local hardware store at the end of the 2001 gardening season for their participation in the study.

Data collection integrated both qualitative and quantitative methods including participant observation, personal interviews, photography, a survey of neighborhood residents in three of the four case study neighborhoods, and storytelling. Steckler argues that the integration of both qualitative and quantitative methods can enhance understanding of the phenomenon studied, and complement the weaknesses of each approach (Steckler, 1992). While quantitative methods produce reliable information often generalizable to a broad population, qualitative methods, and storytelling in particular, offer rich, detailed, individualized narratives that can inform interpretation of the quantitative results, and "usually leaves the study participants' perspectives in tact" (Steckler, 1992). For this chapter, we have chosen to illustrate the results of the quantitative survey with illustrative stories.

Three of the four neighborhoods were surveyed with a standard survey instrument. The Eastside neighborhood was not selected for quantitative study because of its large geographic area. Phone numbers and addresses for every listed resident in Carriage Town Historic District, East Bishop/East Flint Park neighborhood, and Lakewood Village were obtained from a year 2000 reverse-listing phonebook and from lists kept by block clubs and neighborhood associations operating in the neighborhoods. Each valid phone number was called multiple times until the respondent answered the survey, refused, or the study time period ended. In addition, paper or telephone versions of the survey were given to known community gardeners in each of the three neighborhoods.

Completion rates for the survey – completed surveys divided by operating residential phone numbers obtained, and response rates – completed surveys divided by number of answered phone calls – are shown in Table 6.1.

During the survey interview, respondents indicated whether or not they had engaged in ten different civic activities to improve their neighborhoods including:

1 Attended meetings held by the police precinct.
2 Participated in a neighborhood clean up or beautification project.
3 Participated in a community or neighborhood garden.
4 Participated in a crime watch.
5 Spoke to local politicians.
6 Talked to a person causing a problem in the neighborhood.

Table 6.1   Neighborhood survey completion and response rates

Neighborhood	Completed Surveys	Operating Phone Numbers	Answered Phone Numbers	Completion Rate	Response Rate
Carriage Town Historic District	35	100	48	35%	73%
East Bishop/ East Flint Park	27	66	33	42%	82%
Lakewood Village	15	36	22	47%	68%
Total	**77**	**202**	**103**	**38%**	**75%**

7   Attended a block club or neighborhood meeting.
8   Spoke with a religious leader.
9   Got together with neighbors to do something about a neighborhood problem.
10   Served as a neighborhood leader.

Respondents were also asked: if they feel responsible for making sure that other properties in their neighborhood (such as a park, vacant lot or other people's homes) look good, whether they had made an effort to get to know the police in their area, and a series of questions that were combined into scaled items, including:

- *Satisfaction with Neighborhood.* This five-item scale assessed the respondents' beliefs about the general quality of their neighborhood.
- *Trust and Cooperation.* This two-item scale assessed the respondents' beliefs about their neighbors' willingness to trust and help other people in the neighborhood.
- *Social Support.* This five-item scale assessed the respondents' beliefs about how often neighbors provide assistance to each other and how often neighbors gather for social events.
- *Informal Social Control.* This four-item scale assessed the respondents' beliefs about the likelihood that one of the neighbors would take action to stop a burglary, a drug sale to children, an assault, or children getting into trouble.
- *Neighborhood Influence.* This three-item scale assessed what influence the respondents felt they had in their neighborhood and the efficacy of the neighborhood to solve problems.
- *Know Your Neighbors.* This two-item scale assessed how well the respondents recognized their neighbors and how well the neighbors know the respondent.
- *Intergenerational Relationships.* This two-item scale assessed the respondents' interactions with teenagers and with younger children in their neighborhood.
- *Poor Physical Environment.* This six-item scale assessed the respondents' beliefs about poor environmental conditions in their neighborhood including abandoned cars or buildings, rundown buildings, poor lighting, overgrown shrubs or trees, unattended trash, and empty lots.

- *Neighborhood Crime.* This four-item scale assessed the respondents' beliefs about the occurrence of crime in their neighborhood including illegal drug use, drug sales, vandalism, and prostitution.
- *Neighborhood Loitering.* This four-item scale assessed the respondents' beliefs about the occurrence of panhandling, truancy, loitering, and transients sleeping in their neighborhood.

The analyses for this chapter used the survey data to discern differences in various outcomes described above, such as social support, between neighborhood residents who participated in the community garden and those who did not participate in the community garden. Initial analyses employed SAS PROC MIXED (Littel, 1996) to test for neighborhood level effects (variation in outcomes between neighborhoods, and variation among residents within neighborhoods). Neighborhood level effects were not detected and data from all three neighborhoods were pooled together for the final analyses. Using Stata, linear regression, for continuous variables (scale scores), and logistic regression for binary variables (getting to know police, and feeling responsible for neighborhood upkeep) were employed to assess differences between garden participants and non-participants after controlling for age, gender, education, home ownership, presence of child/children in the home, and length of residence in the neighborhood (StataCorp, 2003).

Results from the survey are illustrated with selected stories. Data analyses were conducted by Dr. Alaimo. Stories were crafted by members of the storytelling committee, Dr. Alaimo and David Hassler, editor of *From Seeds to Stories: The Community Garden Storytelling Project of Flint.* Interviews for the stories presented here were conducted by members of the storytelling committee and were taped, transcribed and published with consent from the storyteller. All research protocols were approved by the University of Michigan Institutional Research Board.

Limitations

There are some limitations with the methodological approach taken for this study. First, it is possible that the community gardens chosen for study are not representative of the experiences of all community gardens in the city. Also, choices of gardeners, neighbors and children for personal interviews and storytelling was based on their "importance" to the garden and also on how convenient they were to reach. The vast majority of the adult interviews were conducted with homeowners in each neighborhood, not renters. In addition, we were only able to survey residents with listed phone numbers.

Importantly, the results that we present in this chapter are the results of a cross-sectional survey and therefore, we cannot make any conclusions about the causal nature of the associations we find. It is possible that participation in the community garden resulted in an increase in certain outcomes; but the reverse is also possible. For example, an increased satisfaction with the neighborhood may have led to an increase in participation in the community garden, and not vice versa.

Neighborhood and Community Garden Descriptions

In each of the three neighborhoods selected for this study, a neighborhood organization, neighborhood association, or a block club was working to improve the neighborhood: Carriage Town Historic Neighborhood Association, East Bishop/East Flint Park Block Club, and Lakewood Village Block Club.

Carriage Town Historic Neighborhood Association

Begun in 1982, The Carriage Town Historic Neighborhood Association (CTHNA) is an incorporated non-profit organization whose members work to improve the historic Carriage Town district by supporting housing renovation, property upkeep, neighborhood clean-ups, crime watches, and holding social activities. Most members are homeowners in the neighborhood. CTHNA's 1998 NVPC grant application stated that because of the neighborhood association:

> In ten years, [the] crime rate has dropped from [the] highest in [the] City to [the] lowest, prostitution and drug trafficking decreased significantly, housing rehab and home-owner occupancy increased from practically zero to over 50, with 70 houses rehabbed or in [the] process of rehab.

CTHNA received three grants from the NVPC. In 1998 and 2000, they received funding to strengthen their crime watch. In 2001, they were funded to clear neighborhood vacant lots, landscape and plant a community Victorian garden, and plant trees and flowers on neighborhood streets. They also received funding for these projects from the Rotary Club of Flint and Global Re-Leaf of Michigan.

CTHNA chose the site for their community Victorian garden because of the high amount of loitering and illegal activity that occurred on the lot. The lot was used as a shortcut between the Carriage Town Mission, a homeless shelter, and the Barrage Hotel, and the supermarket/liquor store approximately three blocks away. A worn path cut right through the lot, which was also full of trees, brush, overgrown grass and garbage. One resident said that about 100 people pass through on any one day. He said, "They're over there drinkin', sellin', ... and they're using the bathroom back there too."

Because the lot was deep and had overgrown trees, it was easy for people to hide and not be seen in the dark. One neighborhood resident said he called the police about that particular lot a couple times per month, but that the police only responded to the complaints about 10% of the time. Prior to 2001, CTHNA had cleared the lot of the trees with a chainsaw for several years in order to make the lot more visible and to prevent illegal activity on the lot. Each year, the invasive Tree of Heaven grew back and needed to be cut again.

In 2001, the CTHNA succeeded in clearing the lots, but did not landscape the site or do any planting. After further fundraising and volunteer labor, the Victorian garden was landscaped and planted in 2003.

East Bishop/East Flint Park Block Club

The East Bishop/East Flint Park Block Club is an association of residents on parallel streets. Approximately 20 families of approximately 100 households in the neighborhood participate in the block club. The organization began in 1996 and they received two grants from the NVPC. In 1997, they received funding for a community garden, stipends for youth to do yard care, a crime watch, and a youth mentoring program that included etiquette classes and a drill team. In 1999, they received another grant for the garden and youth program.

The Block Club holds meetings at a local police mini-station, has a picnic every August, sponsors youth activities, marches in parades, holds clean-ups and beautification contests, and has community gardens on two lots in the neighborhood. Food from the gardens is available to all neighborhood residents, although some rows are designated for the "Plant a Row for the Hungry" program and food is donated to a Flint soup kitchen.

The vacant lots that became the two East Bishop/East Flint Park Block Club community garden sites were unsightly. Trash, broken glass, toilets and other garbage were found on one of the lots and the other was a mess of trash, weeds, and overgrown grass, trees and bushes. The residents believe the dumping is done by people who don't live in the neighborhood, who come in at night to dump their garbage. Unlike the Carriage Town lot, people did not "hang out" on the lots prior to the cleaning. As one resident said, this was because "there was too much garbage".

The Block Club also maintains Simmons Park, an island park on Martin Luther King Avenue. Members plant flowers, mow the grass, and in 2001, hung a new American flag on the flagpole.

Lakewood Village Block Club

Begun in 1995, Lakewood Village Block Club is an association of residents of three streets situated next to Flint Park Lake, or what used to be referred to as "Devil's Lake". There are approximately 50 families in the neighborhood and most participate in the block club in one way or another. They have received three grants from NVPC, in 1997, 1998, and 2000. The grants were for beautification and a community garden, intergenerational bowling and softball teams, a youth program to pay kids for yard maintenance, neighborhood trips to a Detroit Tigers baseball game and the zoo, and a crime watch. The block club has monthly meetings at a neighborhood elementary school in cold weather and on a neighborhood vacant lot during the summer, sponsors bowling nights for kids and adults, has a beautification contest and clean-ups, and has a community garden on a dead-end lot next to the lake.

Prior to the initiation of the block club, neighborhood residents were afraid of crime and violence in the neighborhood. According to one resident,

> ... we had teenagers that were taking over and there were gangs... They had the young children fighting all the time ...

Residents didn't know or trust one another:

> ... because a lot of time we figured that [if we got] to know the neighbors, or their kids, that they would be the [ones to] rip us off... Practically everyone had bars and burglar alarms... We were isolated with fear, and [were afraid] to even associate with each other.

The lot chosen by the block club for the community garden was next to the lake that was known as a disposal place for dead bodies. The lot also was used for dumping, and there were garbage, refrigerators, and other junk on the lot before they cleaned it up.

Results

For this chapter, we were interested in discerning differences in various outcomes between garden participants and non-participants, after adjusting for age, gender, length of residence in the neighborhood, presence of a child/children in the home, home ownership, and education. This section discusses the results from the linear and logistic regression analyses (see Table 6.2) by categories: social capital, intergenerational relationships, crime and disorder prevention, and perceptions of neighborhood environments. Results from each section are illustrated with portions of stories from *From Seeds to Stories: The Community Garden Storytelling Project of Flint* (Alaimo, 2003).

Table 6.2   Results from the linear and logistic regression analyses by categories

	Participate in Community Garden	
	Coeff[a]	p-value
Satisfaction with Neighborhood	0.31	0.01
Trust and Cooperation	0.12	0.45
Neighbors Social Support	0.44	0.01
Informal Social Control	0.38	0.01
Neighborhood Influence	0.14	0.24
Know Your Neighbors	0.27	0.09
Intergenerational Relationships	0.73	0.01
Poor Physical Environment	0.02	0.80
Neighborhood Crime	0.18	0.11
Neighborhood Loitering	0.02	0.78
	OR[a]	p-value
Get to Know Neighborhood Police	8.12	0.05
Feel Responsible for Neighborhood Upkeep	5.36	0.00

Coeff=Coefficient for linear regression analyses
OR=Odds Ratios for logistic regression analyses
[a] Coefficient and odds ratios are adjusted for: age, gender, education, home ownership, presence of child in home, and length of residence in neighborhood.

Social Capital

Neighborhood residents who participated in the community gardens reported more social support and satisfaction with their neighborhoods:

> There used to be different things going on in the neighborhood. Like little parties and parades, games you can play, group meetings. It didn't change nothing. But when the garden started, you know, that's when it really changed. People started to help more and get along. That's when people started focusin'.
>
> Shawn Williams, East Bishop/East Flint Park Block Club Community Garden, *From Seeds to Stories: The Community Garden Storytelling Project of Flint*, p. 40.

> One … day I was down here at the Dort and Durant statues, working on the perennial flower bed. It was a really hot day, and I was all by myself. I was doing the "martyr thing," thinking like, I know everybody sees me and no one's helping me. And I thought, why even bother? I'm just gonna do this and more weeds are gonna grow in it. I had almost had it, when a lady comes down the street from these apartments. She's quadriplegic, and she came in her wheelchair. She had this little thermos of water. And she came up and said, "Well, it's a really hot day isn't it? You look like you're really kinda overheated." I said, "Yeah." "Well I brought you some water," she said. I started drinking the water, and she looked at me and said, "You know, I want to thank you. I don't get out much. But when I come down and look at these beautiful flowers, it's entertainment for me. And I want to thank you." I literally got choked up. I couldn't believe it.
>
> Michael Freeman, Carriage Town Historic Neighborhood Association Community Garden, *From Seeds to Stories: The Community Garden Storytelling Project of Flint*, p. 70.

After adjusting for respondent age, gender, educational attainment, home ownership, length of residence in the neighborhood, and the presence of children in the home, participating in the community garden was associated with increased satisfaction with the neighborhood and social support (see Table 6.2). Scale scores for these items were significantly higher for garden participants. There were no significant differences by garden participation in perceptions of trust and cooperation, knowing your neighbors, nor neighborhood influence.

Intergenerational Relationships

The community gardeners were more likely to report important intergenerational relationships in their neighborhoods:

> A lot of people say, "Don't those kids drive you crazy?" I say, "Yes, sometimes they do. Sometimes they drive me up a wall and around the corner." But I still enjoy working with 'em. I like to see their enthusiasm.
>
> There's a lot of kids around here, and I can't turn any of 'em away. I'm like the Pied Piper, when I say, "Okay, we're going down to look at the garden to work." I've got four kids sitting out there, and we go down and I look up and then I see kids comin' from everywhere. The last evening I went down there, I had about thirteen kids with me in the garden."
>
> Elizabeth Perry, East Bishop/East Flint Park Block Club Community Garden, *From Seeds to Stories: The Community Garden Storytelling Project of Flint*, p. 44.

I'm a kid person. I love working with kids. I got more kids than anybody in the world. I can be out somewhere and someone will call, "Hi Mom!" and they got to come over and hug me. "That's yours?" someone might ask. "No, that's one of my adopted sons," I say. All the kids that work in the garden, from the little ones on up, I tell them that's my adopted family. I just love kids around me.

> Fannie Odom, East Eldridge Block Club Community Garden, *From Seeds to Stories:*
> *The Community Garden Storytelling Project of Flint*, p. 77.

As shown in Table 6.2, participating in the community garden was significantly associated with increased intergenerational relationships. After adjusting for respondent age, gender, educational attainment, home ownership, length of residence in the neighborhood, and the presence of children in the home, scale scores for intergenerational relationships were higher for garden participants versus garden non-participants.

Crime and Disorder Prevention

The participants in the community gardens reported higher levels of responsibility for neighborhood upkeep, informal social control in the neighborhood, and making an effort to know the police who patrol their neighborhood:

> We can joke and laugh when we work in the garden and get done a lot faster. A lot of people in the neighborhood been tryin' to take care of their yard this year. I seen a lot more than last year and the year before that. 'Cause now, I see a lot of people willing to plant flowers and they just want their yard to look nice. And they act different, because usually they just be outside arguin'. I think the garden had a lot to do with it – that and other changes goin' on in the neighborhood. To me, it's a symbol of our neighborhood, that our neighborhood somethin', and it just separates us from other neighborhood.
>
> James Brennan, Lakewood Village Block Club, *From Seeds to Stories:*
> *The Community Garden Storytelling Project of Flint*, p. 8.

> This has been a thoroughfare for a lot of transients, but that afternoon people were apologizing for trespassing. I mean, it was almost that quick. [The Victorian garden] and painting the Jackson Hardy House down the street have just changed the transient population. One gentleman was so sweet, he came through the brush and he saw us working [in the garden], and he was like, "I'm so sorry, I'm just gonna trespass this once, just for a minute, just let me get through here." And we were like, "Oh, it's okay." You know, when you live in the neighborhood, you get to know the transients, and even though there's a cycle of them, you know the faces. And brand new faces want to know when the next time we're gonna work out here. You know, "Is there anything we can do?" It's so exciting that we're not the only ones appreciating our hard work. People are giving us the thumbs up. They're thanking us. Thanking us for giving them something beautiful to look at, giving them something positive that's going on.
>
> Leanne Barkus, Carriage Town Historic Neighborhood Association Victorian Garden,
> *From Seeds to Stories: The Community Garden Storytelling Project of Flint*, p. 68.

> The first thing we did was put flowers on the corners. Every cross street between Saginaw and Martin Luther, we put flowers on the corners. It really made a big difference in the community. And then we cleaned up around vacant houses and we put raised beds out. With our grant we built raised beds and gave everybody mums and tulips to put in there.

Then after that, 'cause everybody didn't like mums and tulips, they put in flowers of their choice. It really made a difference in the boom boxes. It made a difference in the profanity that the young peoples was using all the time going up and down the street. You know once you get the young peoples involved in something, and they spend time cleaning it up, they're not going to see anybody just come in and dump and mess things up.

Lillie Neal, East Eldridge Block Club Community Garden, *From Seeds to Stories: The Community Garden Storytelling Project of Flint*, p. 78.

According to the results shown in Table 6.2, participating in the community garden was significantly associated with increased levels of informal social control. In addition, neighbors who participated in the garden were more likely to make an effort to get to know the police who work with their neighborhood, and to feel responsible for neighborhood upkeep. After adjusting for confounding variables, garden participants were eight times more likely to make an effort to get to know the police who work in their neighborhood, and were five times more likely to feel responsible for the upkeep of neighborhood properties.

Perceptions of Neighborhood Environments

The last group of outcomes studied was perceptions of neighborhood environments. We were interested in finding out if garden participants perceived the neighborhood differently than non-participants in terms of neighborhood crime, loitering, and upkeep. As shown in Table 6.2, there were no significant differences in perceptions of the neighborhood environment by participation status.

Gardeners may not perceive their neighborhood differently than those who did not participate in the "gardens", but some reported how participation in neighborhood associations may have changed the way neighbors thought about the benefits of their collective action:

The dead end [where the community garden is now] was known for abandoned and stolen cars. And it was known for dead bodies. In fact, my grandson was staying with me one weekend and I said, "Oh, that car's still out there. We got to call the police. Maybe a dead body is in there." I just said it, but I didn't have no idea it was true. And it turns out there was a girl's body in the trunk of the car. But after we got the block club, we was more alert and more aware of what was going on. We could call the police, and we had a patrol officer walking around here. And that was a great help, because know we had the law to turn to. We wasn't doing this alone. And it relieved a lot of fear.

Ella Aubrey, Lakewood Village Block Club, *From Seeds to Stories: The Community Garden Storytelling Project of Flint*, p. 3.

Participation in Other Neighborhood Activities

The benefits of participating in community gardens noted above are not exclusive for gardeners. Similar patterns of beneficial results were found for activities such as attending a neighborhood or block club meeting, participating in beautification activities, participating in a crime watch, and serving as a leader in a neighborhood-based organization (data not shown).

Reflections/Conclusions

> Whenever I'm in the garden and something needs picking, I'll pick it. And if I don't want to be bothered with it, I take it up the street or down on the corner. I'll pick it and take it to some of the elderly in the neighborhood. I'll come wagging up the street with a bag of stuff. We have a guy who lives on Flint Park, and he belongs to the block club. He likes string beans. So every time the white potatoes need digging or string beans need picking, I'll dig them up, or pick them, and take them to him. And we planted a whole garden for the soup kitchens. They really appreciate it. I even got letters from them. My brother used to tell me, "You'll never have nothing as long as you're here. You give everything away." Yes I do. I really do. But I get a lot out of givin'. Everybody from Saginaw Street to Martin King, if they don't know my name, they say, "That's the lady that work in the garden."
>   Catherine Catchings, *From Seeds to Stories: The Community Garden Storytelling*
>   *Project of Flint*, p. 41.

The results of our study suggest that neighborhood community gardens provide unique opportunities for neighborhood interventions. Participating in community gardens is associated with increased social capital measures such as satisfaction with the neighborhood and social support. Community gardens provide multiple opportunities for neighbor interaction and social contact through working in the garden, through neighborhood festivities that often occur at the garden sites, and by drawing neighbors to the site for harvesting. One of the strengths of a community garden as a neighborhood intervention is that it is not a one-time event (such as a neighborhood clean-up or a neighborhood party) but a continuous activity. Gardening and harvesting occurs over a series of months and there is continuous potential for neighbors to get to know one another.

Gardens can also be places for neighborhood adults and children to interact in positive and meaningful ways, and the relationships that form can be mentoring relationships. We found that neighbors who participate in the community garden were more likely to spend time with neighborhood children and teenagers. Several of the narratives we heard from both adult and children gardeners demonstrated the importance of these new relationships to the new sense of community that could be found in several of the neighborhoods after the garden was formed.

Further, garden sites can become community-owned and used spaces, as contrasted with abandoned and un-used places that attract dumping or illegal activity. Along with increased familiarity with their neighbors, having these used and owned spaces encouraged and enabled many gardeners to monitor neighborhood behaviors and dumping, and make an effort to get to know the police who work in the neighborhood.

Interestingly, garden participants and non-participants shared a common sense of their neighborhood conditions. While it was not possible for us to measure perceptions of neighborhood conditions prior to the initiation of the community gardens, this result can be interpreted to mean that after the initiation of the garden, neighborhood residents perceived their environment in a similar manner, regardless of their participation in the garden. This makes sense, as all neighbors, regardless of their garden participation, are assessing the physical conditions of the same neighborhood places.

An important limitation of this study is that the quantitative results presented here are the results of a cross-sectional survey and do not give indications as to the causal direction of the associations found. It is possible that participation in the community garden resulted in an increase in neighborhood social capital, intergenerational relationships, and prevention of disorder and crime, but the reverse is also possible. For example, an increased satisfaction with the neighborhood may have led to an increase in participation in the community garden, and not vice versa. However, indication that participation in the community garden preceded improved neighborhood outcomes can be found through the narratives (Alaimo, 2003) and the qualitative analyses of the neighborhood case studies (Alaimo, 2002; Alaimo, 2003; Alaimo, Reischl, in Preparation). Qualitative analyses of the case study texts (data not shown) suggest that participation in the community garden preceded many neighbors' feelings of satisfaction with and pride in their neighborhood, knowing more of their neighbors, feelings of social support, and relationships with the neighborhood youth in at least some of the community gardens. Further, in some cases, through their participation in the community garden and beautification activities, some neighbors were encouraged to monitor the neighborhood for crime and disorder.

In addition, the results of this study corroborate other studies that have found that green common spaces created by community gardens can function as sites for neighbor and intergenerational interaction, can foster neighbor social support and informal social control, and can encourage prevention of neighborhood disorder and crime (Hynes, in Press; Blair, 1991; Armstrong, 2000).

Community-Based Approach to Research

The W.K. Kellogg Community Health Scholars Program defines community-based participatory research as "a collaborative approach to research that equitably involves all partners in the research process and recognizes the unique strengths that each brings. Community-based participatory research (CBPR) begins with a research topic of importance to the community with the aim of combining knowledge and action for social change to improve community health and eliminate disparities" (Minkler, 2003). While not a research methodology in the traditional sense, CBPR necessitates bringing the ideals and principles of social justice, equality, respect for individuals and community, and collaborative partnerships to the research process (see for example, Minkler and Wallerstein, 2003; Israel et al., 1998; Reardon, 1998). Research that takes a CBPR approach can simultaneously build our knowledge base about a certain topic, such as community gardens, and engage citizens to be involved in promoting healthy communities.

In many ways, the research results, stories, and advocacy that resulted from the Community Garden Storytelling Project of Flint were shaped and determined by the community-based participatory approach and partnerships. In essence, the participants' relationships, respect, trust, and shared commitment to building a better Flint were the foundations through which all research results, products, and advocacy emerged. The relationships and trust facilitated the storytelling committee members' participation in aspects of the research process about which they were previously unfamiliar, and facilitated the learning process for the researcher. In addition, it enabled all participants to recognize the relevance of the research and stories to neighborhood development work.

Strong relationships also strengthened the possibilities for the use of the research results to be translated into the work of the organization and the advocacy of the organization's purpose to other members of the community. Within the time frame of the Storytelling Project, FUGLUC grew from a grassroots committee to a fully funded non-profit organization. While not the only reason for this transformation, the organization's participation in the research and storytelling project, its collaboration with the University of Michigan School of Public Health and the Prevention Research Center of Michigan, and its association with high quality products, such as *From Seeds to Stories*, led to a belief by funding agencies, City of Flint departments, neighborhood organizations, political leaders that FUGLUC was worth supporting and sustaining for the future.

This development of the Flint community gardening movement and FUGLUC were further enhanced by the use of mixed methods; both the quantitative research results and the illustrative stories served different purposes, but both were beneficial. The quantitative results served the needs and assurances of specific funding agencies, while the qualitative work enabled individual gardeners to own the research findings in a personal way and provided a rich personal and cultural context within which researchers could understand and interpret the quantitative findings.

From Seeds to Stories: The Community Garden Storytelling Project of Flint was published in May 2003. The book is a collection of narratives and photos from 14 community and school gardens throughout the city. Over 1400 copies of the book have been distributed free-of-charge to Flint community-based organizations, city and county officials and politicians, block clubs and neighborhood organizations, business leaders, and schools. Numerous presentations of the book have taken place throughout the city including a book reading/reception that was held at the Flint Public Library. While the specific impact of the book on the community gardening movement is yet to be determined, the anecdotal positive feedback and enthusiasm has been encouraging.

In his work with narratives, Rappaport discusses how individual narratives can empower communities by becoming collective community narratives that define how citizens see themselves, their community, and how they can or cannot influence their community (Rappaport; 1995). Individual voices within stories have the potential to become narratives for the future transformation of the city. In the words of one storytelling committee member, it is "the people in this city that help keep its image strong and vital". Beyond the community gardening movement, the book enabled other community organizations and foundations to witness the importance of storytelling for sustaining organizations.

According to the American Community Gardening Association, approximately 250 U.S. cities and towns have community gardens and the 1996 survey of 38 cities estimated the existence of over 6,000 community gardens (American Community Gardening Association). Community gardening has been gaining in popularity in recent years and can fulfill cities residents' desires for fresh produce, exercise, social interactions, youth development, educational opportunities, environmental activism, recreation, and green space (Hynes, in Press). The numerous positive aspects of community gardens, including those demonstrated here along with youth development, neighborhood stability, and fruit and vegetable consumption (Krasny, 2002; Blair, 1991; Hynes, in Press) establish that community gardens provide unique opportunities for neighborhood development and restoration.

Through research, storytelling and advocacy, community-based participatory research projects such as the Community Garden Storytelling Project of Flint can participate in the development of distressed communities. The Flint community garden movement, and the Storytelling Project, represent and reflect both the current struggle and the beauty that can be the future of Flint. In the words of the Storytelling Committee: "If you want to get a know a city – its people and soul – get to know its gardeners and listen to their stories. It is the gardeners who understand how faith can grow, and who nurture and cherish the land that sustains us and connects our lives" (Alaimo, 2003).

Notes

1 The US Census population counts in Flint grew from 13,103 in 1900 to 156,492 in 1930 and peaked at 196,940 in 1960 (U.S. Census Bureau).
2 The PRC of Michigan is located at the University of Michigan School of Public Health and is supported by the Centers for Disease Control and Prevention.

Acknowledgments

The Community Garden Storytelling Project of Flint was generously funded by the Ruth Mott Foundation, the Neighborhood Violence Prevention Collaborative/ Community Foundation of Greater Flint, the W.K. Kellogg Foundation's Community Health Scholars Program, the University of Michigan Institute for Research on Women and Gender, the Greater Flint Arts Council, and the Prevention Research Center of Michigan. Members of the Flint Urban Gardening and Land Use Corporation Storytelling Committee included: Katherine Alaimo (Co-chair), Mary Alyce Stickney (Co-chair), Ella Aubrey, Ashley Atkinson, Lee Bell, Edna Chaney, Constance Cobley, Dorris Elam, Craig Farrington, Jennifer Farrington, Pete Hutchison, Pat Legg, Lillie Neal, Fanny Odom, Julie Parsons, Elizabeth Perry, Janelle Powell, Erma Pugh, Stephanie Shumsky, and Andrew Younger.

References

Alaimo, K. and Hassler, D. (eds) (2003), *From Seeds to Stories: The Community Garden Storytelling Project of Flint.* Flint Urban Gardening and Land Use Corporation and the Prevention Research Center of Michigan.

Alaimo, K. and Stickney, M.A. (March 2002), *Neighborhood Violence Prevention Collaborative Evaluation Report: Community Gardens,* submitted to the Community Foundation of Greater Flint.

Alaimo, K. and Reischl, T. et al. (in preparation), *Neighborhood Community Gardens, Defensible Space, and Fear of Crime: Results from the Community Garden Storytelling Project of Flint.*

Alaimo, K. and Reischl, T. et al. (in preparation), *Neighborhood Beautification, Community Gardens and Social Capital.*

American Community Gardening Association (1998), *National Gardening Association Survey: 1996*, Philadelphia, PA: American Community Gardening Association.

Armstrong, D. (2000), "A survey of community gardens in upstate New York: Implications for health promotion and community development", *Health and Place*, **6** (319–27).

Blair, D., Giesecke, C.C. and Sherman, S. (1991), "A dietary, social and economic evaluation of the Philadelphia urban gardening project", *Journal of Nutrition Education*, **23** (161–7).

Detroit Free Press (May 8, 2000), *Crime rate rankings in Detroit, Flint, and across the U.S*, Detroit Free Press.

Hynes, H.P. (2002), *Urban Gardens and Farms: Community Benefits and Environmental Risks*. Urban Agriculture online: httl://www.urbanag.info

Hynes, H.P. and Howe, G. (in press), "Urban Horticulture in the contemporary United States: Personal and community benefits", *Acta Horticulture*.

Israel, B.A., Schulz, A.J., Parker, E.A. and Becker, A.B. (1998), "Review of community-based research: Assessing partnership approaches to improve public health", *Annual Review of Public Health*, **19** (173–202).

Kaplan, S. (April 19–21, 1990), "The restorative environment: nature and human experience", *Proceedings of the Role of Horticulture in Human Well-being and Social Development: A National Symposium*, Arlington, VA: 134–42.

Kaplan, R. and Kaplan, S. (1989), *The experience of nature: A psychological perspective*, New York: Cambridge University Press.

Krasny, M. and Doyle, R. (2002), "Participatory approaches to program development and engaging youth in research: The case of an inter-generational urban community gardening program", *Journal of Extension*, **40** (5).

Kweon, B.S., Sullivan, W.C. and Wiley, A. (1998), "Green common spaces and the social integration of inner-city older adults", *Environment and Behavior,* **30** (6):832–58.

Kuo, F. and Sullivan, W. (2001), "Environment and crime in the inner city: Does vegetation reduce crime?" *Environment and Behavior*, **33** (3):343–67.

Littell, R.C., Milliken, G.A. and Stroup, W.W. et al. (1996), *SAS, System for Mixed Models*, Cary, NC: SAS Institute Inc.

Minkler, M. and Wallerstein, N. (eds) (2003), *Community-based participatory research for health*, San Francisco, CA: John Wiley and Sons.

Rappaport, J. (1995), "Empowerment meets narrative: Listening to stories and creating settings", *Am J Community Psychology*, **23** (5):795–807.

Rappaport, J. (1998), "The Art of Social Change: Community narratives as resources for individual and collective identity", in Arriage, X.B. and Oskamp, S. (eds), *Addressing Community Problems: Psychological research and interventions*, Thousand Oaks, CA: Sage Publications.

Reardon, K.M. (1998), "Enhancing the capacity of community-based organizations in East St. Louis", *Journal of Planning Education and Research*, **17**: 323–33.

Relf, D. (1996), "Gardening really is good exercise", Virginia Polytechnical Institute. www.ext.vt.edu/departments/envirohort/articles/misc/exercise.html.

StataCorp. Stata Statistical Software: Release 8.0. (2003), College Station, TX: Stata Corporation.

Steckler, A., McLeroy, K.R. et al. (1992), "Toward integrating qualitative and quantitative methods: An introduction", *Health Education Quarterly*, **19** (1): 1–8.

Ulrich, R.S. (1981), "Natural versus urban scenes: Some psychophysiological effects", *Environment and Behavior*, **13** (5): 523–56.

U.S. Census Bureau. http://www.census.gov

SECTION C:
URBAN DEVELOPMENT AND TRANSPORTATION

Chapter 7

An Environmental Health Survey of Residents of Boston Chinatown

Doug Brugge, Andrew Leong, Abigail Averbach and Fu Mei Cheung

Introduction

The Asian Pacific Islander (API) population represents a relatively small segment of the US population (3.8% as of 1998 Current Population Survey, US Census). It is a community that is comprised of many different groups, with some having a history of more than 150 years in the US while others are recent immigrants. Considering a 1996 US Census Bureau estimate that 94.2% of the APIs reside within metropolitan areas, too little is known about the impact of urban living and environmental factors on the health status of this population. A cursory examination of health-related articles in various newspapers and scholarly journals indicate that APIs are rarely mentioned. A recent search by the authors in both Medline® and Lexis/Nexis® revealed even less information within the specific area of environmental health. There is virtually nothing written about the environmental health of highly urbanized API immigrant communities, such as Boston Chinatown, the subject of this study.

Indeed, in the course of our investigation, we collected the available data from the City of Boston for Chinatown. Health data, primarily hospital discharge data and mortality data, did not shed much light on the issues that we sought to investigate. Environmental data mostly consist of modeling exercises for environmental impact statements. Neither ruled out the potential for environmental health problems, nor did these data provide strong indications of a problem. Because the population in Chinatown is small, the rates of diseases and deaths in most age groups were also small, bringing into question the statistical stability of such estimates and the validity of making comparisons with other populations. Standard disease and vital statistics registries are inadequate for describing the potential health impact of environmental exposures. Furthermore, many of them are not geo-coded to allow for analysis at the neighborhood level. Ultimately, we hoped that collecting survey data would provide data about environmental conditions and more depth of information about health status.

One reason for the absence of APIs in health research is the general perception of the US population as a black/white paradigm. With the increasing Latino population, more studies are including Latinos. However, despite APIs being the fastest growing minority group in the US (Ong and Hee, 1993) they largely remain outside of the scientific research arena. For present and future health studies not to acknowledge this group's existence would be not only a public policy failure but also an acceptance of the "model minority" myth associated with this group. According to this myth, APIs "are a racial minority that has succeeded through education and hard work, and whose income and wealth match or exceed that of White Americans" (Chin, Cho, Kang, and Wu, 1996). This begins a vicious cycle where APIs are seen as not having any problems and therefore are excluded from health studies. Consequently, there are no data to demonstrate the presence of risk factors in these communities and, thus, no incentive to study the population.

While APIs, in general, are absent from the literature, communities such as Boston Chinatown tend to be overlooked even more so because they are poor. Urban, low socio-economic status communities, which also tend to be largely minority, face disproportionately higher burdens of environmental pollution and consequent health risks (Institute of Medicine, 1999). The "environmental justice" movement has developed with the specific goal of focusing attention on these communities. Among other things, the movement aims to change the national research agenda by advocating for new approaches to evaluate environmental risk to minority and poor populations (Institute of Medicine, 1999). Such research may require adaptation of existing methods as was recently noted by the Institute of Medicine, "[c]onventional epidemiology will encounter difficulties ... [in studying these populations] ... because of shortcomings in existing databases, the small populations typically involved, and the cultural differences of researchers with residents of the communities of concern" (Institute of Medicine, 1999). The realization of environmental justice will require creative means to overcome these barriers. The study described below is a first stage attempt to answer environmental health questions in the face of these challenges.

Boston Chinatown

Chinatown is distinct from neighboring communities in the downtown Boston area (and, indeed, in many ways from all other communities in Massachusetts) through the combined effect of the physical nature of the area and the population that lives there. Chinatown is the only neighborhood at the juncture of the two major highways transecting Boston, highways that combined account for a quarter of a million vehicle trips daily. In addition, traffic clogs Chinatown streets seven days a week and virtually 24 hours a day due to the work day commuters, evening theater goers, non-working hour shoppers and restaurant goers and late night drug dealing and prostitution (Brugge, Leong, and Lai, 1999 also, see Chapter 8). These features may spill over, but do not concentrate in neighboring communities. Further, Chinatown has primarily high-rise low-income housing developments compared to the middle class brownstones that compose adjoining neighborhoods. A visual survey of other Boston downtown neighborhoods (Bay Village, Beacon Hill, North End) reveals that, in general, they have less traffic, fewer businesses and/or more of a residential character. Since both housing conditions and the environmental effects of traffic can be expected to exert influence on environmental health, it seemed important to the authors that they investigate environmental health in this community.

Besides the physical environmental features particular to Chinatown there are factors related to the population that were expected to influence our findings. The Chinatown population tends to be first generation immigrant – as such, their language and culture was expected to influence their reaction to and concern or lack of concern about environmental factors. In particular, their level of education and degree of acculturation might affect their perception of the connection between the environment and their health. Furthermore, the use of home, herbal, or non-western medicine may enter into play regarding their perception of whether they are ill. In turn, the various medical statistics that are gathered on a citywide basis would be reduced if, for instance, the resident chose to treat their condition in a non-western way.

Language and culture also limit mobility outside of Chinatown and access to political power within the city. Since most of the residents in Chinatown are first generation immigrants many are ineligible to vote since they have not yet naturalized. People from other Downtown Boston communities have greater opportunities to move into a suburb or to preserve residential aspects of their neighborhood through political action. This is in part because the population in Chinatown is predominately working class and within or near the poverty threshold whereas most of Central Boston is of considerably higher income. Furthermore, race might also enter into play as a factor since the rest of Central Boston is predominately white.

The historical experience of Chinatown was also expected to be a contributing factor to the uniqueness of responses that we elicited with our survey. There are a significant number of life long residents residing in Chinatown who have seen the long and dramatic changes that their community has experienced from urban renewal to the present. Their historical experience probably affects their current level of dissatisfaction. In addition, the community has developed into a cultural center for Asians in the Greater Boston area. The survey asks opinions as well as questions about concrete conditions, opinion questions could be influenced by respondent's sense of how Chinatown reflects on the condition of Asians more broadly.

The co-authors initiated this and other studies (Brugge, Leong, and Lai, 1999) out of necessity in the struggle for community survival. Boston Chinatown (which is roughly 10 by 9 city blocks in its longest dimensions) has been ravaged for decades by urban renewal policies and by institutional expansion (Leong, 1995/1996). Over the course of the last several decades Chinatown has lost over 1200 units of housing and had 1/3 of its land taken over by neighboring institutions. It has also suffered the legacies of poor public land use and transportation policies – living next to the intersection of two major interstate highways built during the 1950s and 1960s, as well as the City's only red light district (having been rezoned specifically next to Chinatown in 1973).

In an attempt to counteract further commercial and government developments in and adjacent to Chinatown, community groups have been waging a long war to preserve and improve the community's residential aspects. These groups often face responding to the reams of documents that development proponents have generated to fulfill environmental review procedures. These documents invariably conclude that the proposed development would have little or no deleterious effects on residents. Having reacted long enough to the "facts and figures" from the proponents, the community has recently undertaken the task of conducting field studies to generate data of its own.

Chinatown residents currently endure the effects of the largest construction project in the US (the depression of the Central Artery, the North-South highway through

Boston). They tolerate daily commuter traffic jams from neighboring institutions, and experience the nightly noise and congestion of both the adult entertainment district and the theater district. Based on this, we wanted to examine the residents' health status from the environmental perspective. The goal was to begin an exploration into the connections between the environment and health in Chinatown, with a particular focus on developing research methods that work in this particular community, but that might also shed light on research in similar communities elsewhere. Furthermore, we believed that findings from the study would be helpful with respect to assessing the need for and content of further studies.

Methods

Community Collaboration

The research team was formed as a collaboration between the Campaign to Protect Chinatown (CPC), the South Cove Community Health Center (SCCHC) and Tufts University School of Medicine (TUSM). CPC is a grassroots coalition that has led several struggles to oppose or alter development plans in Chinatown. SCCHC is the health care provider for the majority of community residents. It offers staff proficient in Chinese (and other Asian languages) and is located in the heart of Chinatown. TUSM is located in Chinatown and is one source of institutional expansion in the community. Each partner brought unique skills and abilities to the project. CPC contributed bilingual and cultural knowledge and a concern about environmental conditions. SCCHC did likewise, but also brought the respectability of a broadly known and trusted institution. TUSM brought research skills. CPC was the lead party, essentially commissioning the study for the purpose of evaluating issues of concern to its constituency.

Sampling Plan

A sampling protocol was developed based on the work of Loo (Loo, 1991). Names and addresses for residents who were age 18 or older were obtained from the Boston City Hall 1997 Census Report for Chinatown. The study boundary was defined by a range of address numbers along each street within the community. This corresponds to Chinatown boundaries as previously defined by the authors (Brugge, Leong, and Lai, 1999), see Figure 8.3, pp. 177–178. There were a total of 2606 addresses and corresponding names that met our study area definition. The addresses were entered into Paradox, a computer database program. Since the Census Report did not include the residents' telephone numbers, a Boston Telephone Directory was consulted in an attempt add the telephone numbers. We were able to identify only a small percentage (about 20%) of the telephone numbers. The names in the database were put in random order.

Instrument Development

The project team, with members from Tufts University (DB), South Cove Community Health Center (FMC) and the Campaign to Protect Chinatown (AL), developed a first draft of survey questions in English. Questions were worded in simple terms for ease of understanding. We did not aim for a specific grade level since we anticipated reading and explaining the survey questions to interviewees as needed. For example, a complicated medical terminology (arteriosclerosis) might have been more accurate, however the use of the term would not be useful where residents could not understand the term in lieu of a more generic word or phrase (heart disease). These were reviewed, discussed and modified and then translated into Chinese by a bilingual project team member (FMC). Accuracy of translation was confirmed by review by a second bilingual member of the project team (AL). We did not use traditional back translation, choosing instead a more iterative process that we felt would be more likely to encourage discussion about the best translation. Where possible, a verbatim translation was done. It should be noted here that although there are many different dialects of spoken Chinese (e.g. Mandarin, Cantonese, Toisanese, Haka, etc.) they all use a common written form. A consent form was developed by the same procedure. Upon completion, both the Chinese and the English versions of the consent form were approved by the Committee on Clinical Investigations at the Beth Israel Deaconess Medical Center, which is affiliated with SCCHC.

Field Testing

A sample of 15 randomly selected addresses was used to field test recruitment of subjects and the use of the survey and consent forms. An introductory letter in Chinese and English, signed by the director of SCCHC and on the SCCHC letterhead, was sent as the initial contact. Despite having SCCHC's support, the initial response was weak. Three letters returned due to unknown addressee, one resident called the office and responded that they were unable to participate in the survey, three subjects with telephone numbers agreed to participate, and there was no response to the remaining letters. After a two-week wait none of the persons who had indicated that they would complete the survey had sent it back. Our experience led us to conclude that the method in soliciting subjects must change from the original telephone/mail contact approach to a door-to-door solicitation in order to increase our response rate.

Based on the difficulties encountered in recruiting residents, we designed a second method for field-testing the survey and consent forms. Flyers both in Chinese and English were posted in the Chinatown area to solicit participants. Following this, a dozen residents were scheduled for appointments at the health center. As a result of these practice interviews, one of the questions in the survey was changed for clarity.

Letters of Inquiry and Calls

The survey pool of 100 randomly selected addresses had introductory letters sent to them. The letter explained the study and that an honorarium of $10 would be provided for participation. The contact person for the project was listed (FMC) and the letter informed prospective subjects that project teams would visit their home in the near future. We waited two weeks after mailing the letters to begin going door-to-door. Within this period, a total of 15 letters were returned to the office for unknown addressee. These residents, who had moved or changed address, were deleted from our database and were replaced by additional randomized names.

Door-to-Door Canvassing

Two teams of two bilingual high school students each with fluency in both English and Cantonese were recruited from Chinatown to visit the selected subjects at their homes. The teams were trained to be culturally appropriate by the community-relations staff at SCCHC and instructed by one of us (DB) on how to remain objective while conducting interviews. The students were trained to ask questions in a culturally appropriate manner since perception of inappropriate conduct on their part might have ended the interview with the subject. Examples of what would be "culturally appropriate" include properly addressing one's elders with the appropriate title of respect, or not asking questions relating to one's age right at the onset of the interview but waiting until after the student had established a relationship with the resident. Each team was given 50 addresses. They made three attempts to contact an adult at each address and recorded the response that they received or the reason for failure to make contact. If, after three attempts, the subject was not reached, a package containing the consent form and the survey was mailed to the address. Subjects who had agreed to participate either completed the survey in the presence of the team or filled it out later to be collected by the team. In some cases the team read the questions to the subjects.

Statistical Methods

A data entry program was developed in SPSS and data verification systems were incorporated into the program to minimize key entry errors. The survey data were entered and basic frequency distributions were performed to inspect for illegitimate values. Suspicious values were checked on the original survey forms and subsequently some of the data were edited or re-entered. The distribution of continuous values (age, for example) was examined in order to define meaningful groupings for the creation of categorical variables. The data were converted to a SAS data set where two-way cross tabulations were calculated for all relevant combinations of variables. Pearson Chi Square test of independence was used to test for the overall association between two variables. Fisher's Exact Test was used when expected cell frequencies were less than five. Statistical significance was determined when the p-value was less than 0.05. The calculation of a Rate Difference and 95% Confidence Interval were performed in MS Excel and were used to answer the question of whether the observed percentage difference between two groups might have been due to chance alone, assuming no bias or confounding factors.

Results

Responses to canvassing are given in Table 7.1. Excluding those addresses for which there was a barrier that prohibited contact (i.e. no doorbell), those outside of the study area and those the teams were unable to locate despite repeated attempts, we had a response rate of 49% (42 completed surveys). The interview teams often encountered negative reactions and residents who were skeptical about participating. In one case the survey team abandoned an address due to perceived safety concerns. A small number of the residents were completely unwilling to speak with the students. In some instances, even though residents were home, they did not answer their doorbell.

Table 7.1   Responses to survey teams by residents

Completed Survey	42
Rejected Survey	26
Attempted but failed (No Response)	18
No Doorbell	8
Access Problem; locked gate or fence	1
Unable to locate address	3
Out of studied area	2
Total	100

Demographics, Residential History and Employment Status

Most of the respondents identified their race/ethnicity as Chinese (85.7%). The majority of respondents were immigrants to the U.S. (78.6%) and a majority had lived in Chinatown for over ten years (59.5%). There were slightly more females (54.8%) than males (45.2%) and there was a higher proportion of females in the 25-44 age group (Table 7.2). The largest age group was comprised of respondents age 65 and over (40.5%).

Table 7.2   Age distribution by gender

Age Group	Male #	(%)	Female #	(%)
<25 years	2	(10.5)	3	(13.0)
25-44 years	1	(5.3)	7	(30.4)
45-64 years	8	(42.1)	4	(17.4)
65 and over	8	(42.1)	9	(39.1)
Missing	0	(0.0)	0	(0.0)
Total	19	(100.0)	23	(100.0)

Lifestyle and Health

An overwhelming majority of respondents were non-smokers (88.1%) and, of the four who were smokers, all were male. Half of the respondents reported spending more than 16 hours per day at home indoors. These tended to be older respondents, with 80% of them being 60 years old or more. About a third of the respondents

(35.3%) lived in homes where there was less than one room per person. Three respondents reported being diagnosed with asthma (7.1%), one reported having emphysema (2.4%) and two reported having heart disease (4.8%). The most common symptoms that respondents had experienced during the past 30 days were runny nose (36%), headaches (29%), excessive tiredness (26%) and burning/itching eyes (29%) (Table 7.3).

Table 7.3   Symptoms

SYMPTOMS[1]	Percent
Dizziness	16.7
Headaches	28.6
Nausea	9.5
Coughing	21.4
Excessive tiredness	26.2
Nosebleeds	0.0
Trouble breathing (including shortness of breath)	16.7
Lack of concentration	4.8
Runny nose	35.7
Ear pain or infection	7.1
Irregular heartbeat	4.8
Skin rashes/problems	9.5
Tightness in chest	4.8
Burning/itching eyes	28.6
Shakiness/tremors	0.0
Sore or dry throat	16.7
Other	4.8

[1] These percentages may total more than 100% because respondents were asked to check all that apply.

Noise and Air Pollution

Table 7.4 contains information on the experiences and attitudes of Chinatown residents with regard to noise and air pollution. Almost three-quarters of respondents (71.5%) reported that noise from traffic was a bother to them either "often" or "sometimes" while they were inside their homes. Noise was less of an issue while they were outside doing recreational activities in Chinatown, though it still affected the majority of respondents (with 52.4% saying traffic noise bothered them either "often" or "sometimes" while they were outdoors). Furthermore, 57.1% reported hearing the helicopters landing at New England Medical Center while inside their homes. Noise from construction was a problem "often" or "sometimes" inside homes for less than half the respondents (45.3%) and 31.0% said it was "never" a problem.

Table 7.4   Experiences with noise and air pollution (last 6 months)

QUESTION	Percent (n)
How often has noise from traffic bothered you … … while you were inside your apartment? Often or sometimes Rarely or never Missing	 71.5 (30) 23.8 (10) 4.8 (2)
… while you were involved in activities outdoors in Chinatown? Often or sometimes Rarely or never Missing	 52.4 (22) 42.9 (18) 4.8 (2)
While inside your apartment, have you heard the helicopter landing? Yes Missing	 57.1 (24) 2.4 (1)
Has noise from construction bothered you inside your apartment? Often or sometimes Rarely or never Missing	 45.3 (19) 0.0 (0)
While you were inside your apartment, how often has exhaust from vehicles bothered you? Often or sometimes Rarely or never Missing	 35.7 (15) 61.9 (26) 2.4 (1)
While you were outdoors in Boston Chinatown, how often has exhaust from vehicles bothered you? Often or sometimes Rarely or never Missing	 61.9 (26) 38.1 (16) 0.0 (0)
Has dust from construction bothered you inside your apartment? Often or sometimes Rarely or never Missing	 35.7 (15) 61.9 (26) 2.4 (1)
Has dust from construction bothered you when you are outside in Boston Chinatown? Often or sometimes Rarely or never Missing	 28.6 (12) 69.1 (29) 2.4 (1)
Has construction activity interfered with your plans to spend time outdoors in Boston Chinatown? Yes Missing	 11.9 (5) 7.1 (3)

During the six months prior to the survey, air pollution emanating from vehicle exhaust was "often" or "sometimes" a problem for a little over a third of the respondents (35.7%) while they were inside their homes (Table 7.4). A much greater proportion of the residents, 61.9%, said it was a problem while they were outdoors in Boston Chinatown. Dust from construction was also a problem either "often" or "sometimes" for 35.7% of the residents while in their homes. Less than a third of the respondents (28.6%) said that construction dust bothered them "often" or "sometimes" when they were outdoors in Boston Chinatown. About twelve percent (11.9%) of the respondents said that construction activity interfered with their plans to spend time outdoors in Boston Chinatown during the six months prior to the survey.

Respondents under age 60 (who tend to spend more time outside of the home) were more likely to report being bothered by traffic noise while inside their apartment than were respondents age 60 and over (p=0.0003). Age was not related to being bothered by either construction dust or vehicle exhaust. People who reported being bothered at home by construction dust were also more likely to report being bothered by both vehicle exhaust (p=0.043) and traffic noise (p=0.007), although vehicle exhaust and traffic noise were found to be independent of each other (p=0.279). The limited sample size may restrict our ability to adequately address confounding between these reported exposure parameters.

The rate of symptoms by exposure status was evaluated in order to determine whether people who experienced health symptoms in the past 30 days were more or less likely to report being bothered by air and noise pollution in their homes (Table 7.5). Among respondents who reported having experienced burning/itching eyes, 53.9% said they "often" or "sometimes" are bothered by construction dust at home as compared to only 20.0% who "rarely" or "never" are bothered by construction dust at home (RD = 33.9%; CI = 2.5% - 65.2%). Similarly, respondents who reported having headaches were more likely to be bothered by vehicle exhaust (RD = 33.85%; CI = 2.54–65.16%) and respondents who reported having a runny nose were more likely to be bothered by traffic noise (RD = 41.85%; CI = 15.38 - 68.33%).

It was of interest to determine if any of the symptoms were related to age. Respondents who were over 60 years old were somewhat less likely than younger respondents to report headaches (p=0.163) and runny nose (p=0.107).

Motor Vehicle Accidents, Traffic and Pedestrian Safety

Motor vehicle related accidents are common in Chinatown (Brugge et al., 1999). Survey respondents were asked a series of questions about their experiences with accidents, traffic, and pedestrian safety in Chinatown (Table 7.6). The majority of respondents do not own a car (76.2%). Over half (54.8%) reported having difficulty crossing the street when they had the "right of way". Four respondents (9.5%) said they had been in a motor vehicle accident in Boston Chinatown and three of these were pedestrians. Eleven respondents (26.2%) said they knew at least one Boston Chinatown resident who had been in a motor vehicle accident in Chinatown and of these, eight reported these were pedestrian accidents. Furthermore, almost half (45.2%) of the respondents said they "often" or "sometimes" had felt that they were in danger of being in a motor vehicle accident while walking in Boston Chinatown. In

Table 7.5   Rate differences for respondents who are "Often/Sometimes" bothered by pollutants compared to those who are "Rarely/Never" bothered by pollutants, Chinatown Survey Respondents, 1998

How often pollutants are a bother at home:	Reported Symptom:			
	Burning/Itching Eyes	Headaches	Tiredness	Runny Nose
Construction Dust				
Often/Sometimes	53.9%[1]	36.4%	50.0%	58.3%
Rarely/Never	<u>20.0%</u>[2]	<u>26.9%</u>	<u>20.0%</u>	<u>32.0%</u>
Rate Difference (CI)[3,4]	**33.9% (2.5%, 65.2%)**	**9.4% (-23.7%, 42.6%)**	**30.0% (-2.3%, 62.3%)**	**26.3% (-7.0%, 59.7%)**
Vehicle Exhaust				
Often/Sometimes	46.2%	53.9%	33.3%	53.9%
Rarely/Never	<u>24.0%</u>	<u>20.0%</u>	<u>25.0%</u>	<u>33.3%</u>
Rate Difference (CI)	**22.2% (-9.7%, 54.0%)**	**33.9% (2.5%, 65.2%)**	**8.3% (-23.5%, 40.1%)**	**20.5% (-12.5%, 53.5%)**
Traffic Noise				
Often/Sometimes	35.7%	34.6%	33.3%	51.9%
Rarely/Never	<u>20.0%</u>	<u>10.0%</u>	<u>20.0%</u>	<u>10.0%</u>
Rate Difference (CI)	**15.7% (-14.8%, 46.2%)**	**24.6% (-1.5%, 50.7%)**	**13.3% (-17.2%, 43.8%)**	**41.9% (15.4%, 68.3%)**

[1] This represents the percentage of respondents who reported burning/itching eyes who said that construction dust "often" or "sometimes" bothers them at home.

[2] Likewise, this represents the percentage of respondents who reported burning/itching eyes who said that construction dust "rarely" or "never" bothers them at home. NOTE: For the distribution of respondents who did not experience any symptoms, refer to tables A11-A14 in the Appendix.

[3] The Rate Difference reflects the difference between the percentage of respondents who said that the pollutant was "often" or "sometimes" a bother at home compared to those who said it was "rarely" or "never" a bother at home among all the respondents who reported experiencing the specified symptom.

[4] CI= 95% Confidence Interval.

the bivariate analyses, difficulty crossing the street (p=0.757) and fear being in an accident with a motor vehicle (p=0.867) were not significantly associated with age.

Table 7.6   Motor vehicle accidents, traffic and pedestrian safety

QUESTION	Percent (n)
Do you own a car?	
Yes	23.8 (10)
Missing	0.0 (0)
In the last six months in Boston Chinatown, how often have you experienced difficulty crossing the street, at the intersection, on the green or walk signal?	
Often or sometimes	54.8 (23)
Rarely or never	45.2 (19)
Missing	0.0 (0)
Have you ever been in an accident with a motor vehicle in Boston Chinatown?	
Yes[1]	9.5 (4)
Missing	0.0 (0)
If you were in an accident with a motor vehicle in Boston Chinatown, were you …	
A pedestrian?	7.1 (3)
In a vehicle?	2.4 (1)
Missing	0.0 (0)
Do you know any Boston Chinatown residents who have been in a motor vehicle accident in Boston Chinatown?	
Yes[1]	26.2 (11)
Missing	7.1 (3)
If you know someone who was in an accident(s) with a motor vehicle in Boston Chinatown, were they …	
A pedestrian?	19.0 (8)
In a vehicle?	4.8 (2)
Both?	2.4 (1)
Missing	4.8 (2)
In the last six months, while walking in Boston Chinatown, did you feel that you were in danger of being in an accident with a motor vehicle?	
Often or sometimes	45.2 (19)
Rarely or never	52.4 (22)
Missing	2.4 (1)

[1]One of the survey respondents answered "no" for this question, but also responded to the question that followed. For consistency, the "no" response was recoded to "yes."

Open Space

An overwhelming majority (92.9%) of the respondents felt there were not enough parks in Boston Chinatown and nearly as many (88.1%) felt similarly about the lack of playgrounds (Table 7.7). In fact, 61.9% of the respondents said they go to parks or playgrounds outside of Chinatown when they want to spend time outdoors. Nearly forty percent (38.1%) said there were times during the six months prior to the survey when they wanted to go outside but did not because of a lack of open space.

Table 7.7   Open space and outdoor recreation

QUESTION	Percent (n)
In your opinion, are there enough parks in Boston Chinatown?	
No	92.9 (39)
Missing	0.0 (0)
In your opinion, are there enough playgrounds in Boston Chinatown?	
No	88.1 (37)
Missing	2.4 (1)
During the last 6 months, when you want to spend time outdoors, where do you go?[1]	
Park/Playground In Boston Chinatown	33.3 (14)
Park/Playground Outside Of Boston Chinatown	61.9 (26)
Sidewalk/Street In Boston Chinatown	42.9 (18)
Sidewalk/Street Outside Of Boston Chinatown	23.8 (10)
Restaurant Or Coffee Shop In Boston Chinatown	26.2 (11)
Restaurant Or Coffee Shop Outside Of Boston Chinatown	16.7 (7)
Other	9.5 (4)
During the last 6 months, were there times when you wanted to go outside, but because of a lack of open space in Boston Chinatown, you chose not to?	
No	61.9 (26)
Missing	0.0 (0)

[1] These percentages total more than 100% because respondents were asked to check all that apply.

Environmental Risk Factors and Priority Issues

In terms of what Chinatown residents see as agents that can be harmful to their health, automobile exhaust and tobacco smoke were the most commonly cited, with over 70% of the respondents naming these two factors (Table 7.8). Recognition of

Table 7.8   Knowledge about environmental risk factors and responsibility

QUESTION	Percent (n)
Mark each of the following if you think they can harm your health:[1]	
Automobile Exhaust	73.8 (31)
Tobacco	71.4 (30)
Construction Dust	47.6 (20)
Power Plant Smoke	40.5 (17)
Lead Paint	35.7 (15)
Noise From Traffic	31.0 (13)
Compared to other communities in the Boston area, would you say that Chinatown has	
Less pollution?	4.8 (2)
More pollution?	81.0 (34)
The same?	14.3 (6)
Missing	0.0 (0)
Compared to where you lived before moving to Boston Chinatown, do you think that Boston Chinatown has	
Less pollution?	4.8 (2)
More pollution?	76.2 (32)
The same?	14.3 (6)
Missing	4.8 (2)
Who do you think should be responsible for making sure that Chinatown's environment is safe and healthy for residents?[1]	
The MDEP (Department of Environmental Protection)	57.1 (24)
The Boston City Government	42.9 (18)
The US Environmental Protection Agency	40.5 (17)
Boston Chinatown Residents	35.7 (15)
Developers of Buildings and Roadways in or Near Boston Chinatown	31.0 (13)
Boston Chinatown Agencies	23.8 (10)

[1] These percentages total more than 100% because respondents were asked to check all that apply.

construction dust (47.6%) and power plant smoke (40.5%) as health hazards was lower. Only 35.7% of the study population identified lead paint as a harmful agent. There was no statistical correlation between whether respondents experienced the problem in their homes and whether they believed that vehicle exhaust ($p=0.70$), construction dust ($p=0.51$) or traffic noise ($p=1.0$) could harm ones health.

More than three-quarters of the respondents said that Boston Chinatown was more polluted than other Boston area communities and more polluted than their most recent former residence (Table 7.8). Data was not collected on the rural or urban nature of previous residence, thus it is not possible to compare the responses on that basis. Governmental agencies (Massachusetts Department of Environmental Protection, Boston City Government and US Environmental Protection Agency) were on the top the list of who Chinatown residents hold responsible for protecting the environment, although none was indicated by more than 60% of respondents (Table 7.8).

Table 7.9 presents a list of environmental priorities that were rank ordered based on each respondent's opinion of which issues he or she considered most important. The category of mould, insects and other indoor environmental problems was considered the highest priority issue both in terms of the final score and the number of times it was ranked first (seven times). Other highly ranked concerns included vehicle exhaust, environmental tobacco smoke, overcrowding and pollution from construction. There was little association between whether respondents ranked an issue in the top four and whether that respondent had reported personally experiencing that particular problem. An exception was the case of vehicle noise which was more often ranked among the top four by people who were bothered by vehicle noise at home than people who "rarely" or "never" had that problem at home (p=0.036).

Table 7.9   Environmental priorities

Rank	Environmental Issue	Total Score[1]	Times it Ranked 1st
1	Mould, insects and other indoor environmental problems	179	7
2	Exhaust from cars and trucks	217	4
3	Environmental tobacco smoke	227	2
4	Overcrowding	246	3
5	Pollution from construction	269	1
6	Noise from cars and trucks	273	5
7	Smoke from power plant	274	1
8	Pedestrian accidents	293	2
9	Lack of affordable housing	295	5
10	Lack of open/green space	307	2
11	Noise from construction	317	3
12	Lead paint in housing	317	3
13	Scarcity of community gardens	323	3
14	Development of new downtown buildings	347	2

[1] Respondents were asked to rank each of these items, based on their opinion, with "1" being the most important problem, "2" the next most important and so forth. Therefore, the item with the lowest total score represents the highest priority.

Discussion

Study Limitations

Our data were based on self-reporting, were cross-sectional in nature, our sample size was small and there was a low response rate. This limits the interpretation that can be applied to findings. While self-reported indicators of exposure (Hyland et al., 1997) and disease (Boyko et al., 1997) may be reasonably accurate, surveys of Asian populations have been reported to have greater levels of misclassification of responses (Hyland et al., 1997). One of the main limitations of self-reported data is that it may contain selective reporting and bias due to pre-existing opinions of the respondents. In our study there was also the added concern that language and literacy may have introduced misunderstandings and confusion despite our attempts to limit such problems. Nonetheless, we have no a priori reason to believe that respondents were systematically biased in their responses. Indeed, the general lack of knowledge about the environment displayed by respondents suggests that the study population was not very sophisticated about such issues.

The cross-sectional nature of the study means that the associations that we found between exposure and health parameters must not be considered causal. Further, the small sample size limited the statistical power of the study such that we were able to observe only those associations between exposure and health that were robust. We interpret this to mean that the associations we observed to be statistically significant are likely candidates for future investigation. It should be kept in mind, however, that the limited power of the study also means that there may be other associations that, while real, were missed due to their relatively lower magnitude.

The time of day and day of the week during which surveys were collected could have affected the response rate and/or biased the respondent pool. Surveys were done on weekday afternoons and weekend days. These times include those when restaurant workers are less likely to be at work. Nevertheless, it is possible that those who were at home were more likely to be available because they were ill, retired or unemployed. This could bias our results toward overestimation of symptoms. In addition, because very few smokers responded to our survey, we have chosen not to adjust the data for smoking. Finally, the survey was performed in late spring, which is usually allergy season in New England. Therefore it is possible that some of the reported symptoms of runny nose, headaches, and burning/itching eyes were caused by pollen.

Recommendations from Findings

The data presented here are far from conclusive. They do, however, suggest a need to begin to evaluate the environmental health risks faced by inner-city Asian populations such as the residents in Boston Chinatown. It would be fair to conclude that reports of being bothered by environmental factors associated with traffic, construction, lack of open space and crowding represents a documentation of the experience and perception of Chinatown residents.

Noise and air pollution are known to be associated with health effects. Noise levels below 80 dB, that do not cause hearing loss, have been reported to be associated with increased blood pressure, increased cholesterol levels, and impairment of reading and language skills in children (Fay, 1991). Many components of vehicular exhaust and other ambient pollution are toxic and known to be associated with acute and chronic health outcomes. One study correlated physician home visits and acute symptoms with environmental exposures (Medina et al., 1997). In that study particulate matter, sulfur dioxide and nitrogen dioxide were associated with headaches, while ozone was associated with eye conditions. In addition, the same study found that sulfur dioxide and nitrogen dioxide were associated with asthmatic symptoms. Modeling studies for carbon monoxide in Boston Chinatown have suggested that levels could exceed federal limits at some intersections (Mass DPW, 1990), but the limited monitoring conducted to date has not confirmed this (Paino, 1993; ENSR Consulting and Engineering, 1997).

We should be careful about how we interpret our findings of associations between environmental factors and health symptoms. The associations between construction dust and eye symptoms and between vehicle exhaust and headaches are, on their face, plausible. At least some types of dust can affect the eyes (Thriene et al., 1996; Vona, 1997) and components of exhaust (particulate matter and nitrogen dioxide) are associated with headaches (Medina et al., 1997). Another component of exhaust, carbon monoxide, while associated with headaches, appears to do so only at levels well above those in ambient air pollution (American Thoracic Society, 1996). The third association, runny nose and traffic noise, is not so amenable to explanation. Our small sample size prohibits controlling for multiple exposures, lifestyle, age or gender factors. Indeed, we have noted that there is confounding between reported exposure variables.

Fifty percent of our sample spent more than 16 hours and another 36% spent between nine and 16 hours each day indoors at home. It is possible that our sample overestimates time spent at home because those spending more time at home would be more likely to be available to answer the survey. People who are ill may also spend more time at home. Overall, however, our findings were consistent with the observation that other US populations spend 90% of their time indoors, the majority of that time at home (Ott, 1995). Further, it suggests that the home environment is pivotal. Independent of our survey a public debate has begun in Boston Chinatown about the future and status of Housing and Urban Development housing in the community (O'Malley, 1999). Any follow-up study should take housing factors into consideration in two ways. First environmental pollutants should be measured both inside and outdoors. Second, indoor air pollutants, such as mould from water damage, which were not addressed in our survey, should be investigated. The condition of housing stock, the degree of crowding and the relative priority given to indoor factors by respondents all contribute to the need for follow-up on the indoor environment.

Traffic Safety

While few of the Chinatown residents answering our survey owned a car, almost 10% had been in a motor vehicle accident in Chinatown, most as pedestrians. Although it does not make for easy comparison, annual incidence rates for pediatric pedestrian injuries by motor vehicles that have been reports in the literature in the order of one in 1000 (Rivera et al., 1985, Mueller et al., 1990). In our survey, 26% of respondents acknowledged that they know a Boston Chinatown resident who has been in a motor vehicle accident while in Boston Chinatown. Further, our survey suggests that residents experience difficulty crossing the streets in the community regardless of their age.

A recent study of traffic-related injury reports based on police records and 9-1-1 calls in Boston Chinatown documented that there were 110 injuries reported in one year (Brugge, Leong, and Lai, 1999; also see Chapter 8). A subset of 12 injury reports was examined to determine the residence of the parties involved. It was found that two of five pedestrians were residents of Chinatown, while none of the 19 drivers (seven incidents involved two vehicles) were from Chinatown (Brugge, 1998). Thus the responses to the survey, which indicate frequent pedestrian injuries to Chinatown residents, are consistent with police records. A recent study commissioned by the City of Boston has proposed changes to the streets and intersections in Boston Chinatown that would be aimed at addressing safety and congestion problems.

Open/Green Space

There was an overwhelming consensus that there were not enough parks or playgrounds in Chinatown. This finding is consistent with longstanding complaints by community groups and residents (Chinatown Neighborhood Council, 1990). The long hours spent indoors at home (reported above) may reflect an impact of the lack of acceptable outdoor spaces for recreation in the community. Indeed, Chinatown is the most densely populated community in Boston, with a ratio of 111 residents per acre, compared to its neighbors in the South End, which has a ratio of 26 residents per acre (Chinatown Neighborhood Council, 1990). With only 0.6 acres of open space available in Chinatown per 1000 residents – this amounts to the least open space per resident in the city. By contrast, there is no shortage of parking spaces. Where the City of Boston as a whole has 1.7 parking spaces/acre, the South End, adjacent to Chinatown, has 4.6 parking spaces/acre – Chinatown has 34 parking spaces/acre (The Chinatown Coalition, 1994).

Education Needs

Our survey showed that there were large gaps in the environmental health awareness of respondents. Few thought that construction dust, power plant smoke, lead paint or traffic noise could affect their health. While larger numbers thought that automobile exhaust and tobacco smoke could harm health, the response rate was still less than might be expected. In addition, only slightly more than one-half named the Massachusetts Department of Environmental Protection and less than one-half named the municipal government or the US EPA as being responsible for the environmental health and safety of Chinatown residents.

These responses suggest that there are significant environmental health education needs in the community. For a community that is as urbanized as Boston Chinatown and that faces intense development pressures and high traffic volumes, it is a deficit if large percentages of the residents, as indicated by our survey, are unaware of the associations between environmental pollutants and health. Greater awareness would likely influence their opinions about and interest in the changes that their community is experiencing. For residents to be able to participate minimally in the public processes that normally accompany environmental impact assessments they will need to have a deeper understanding of the issues involved. While further research would be interesting, we feel that the results of our survey are sufficient to suggest initiating action on this point. A community-based environmental education program would be a good first step toward addressing this issue.

Priorities

The process of ranking potential environmental concerns did not produce qualitatively distinguishable priorities since all 14 items were bunched together in their scores and every one of the choices had at least one respondent who ranked that issue number one. Nevertheless, some concerns rose to the top of the list. These were, in order from most often ranked as important to less often, the indoor environment (mould, insects etc.), motor vehicle exhaust, environmental tobacco smoke, overcrowding, pollution from construction, and noise from traffic. Clearly the low level of environmental knowledge of Chinatown residents may affect the choices that they made in the prioritization exercise. Lead paint, for example, was ranked low in priority, but it was also a hazard that few respondents thought could affect health. Thus, it is possible, perhaps even likely, that priorities could change following education about environmental issues.

Methodological Lessons

The collection of health related information about APIs is a relatively new phenomenon. The API population is so small that it has been difficult to conduct general studies including APIs that would yield a representative sample. Since APIs have not been included historically in most health studies, we see recently the formation of national groups such as the Asian and Pacific Islander American Health Forum, as well as the Asian Pacific American Community Health Organization that addresses health related issues specific to this community. Supporting the above points is the announcement in 1998 of a major initiative (Asian American and Pacific Islander Initiative) by the US Department of Health and Human Services. Out of the six components within the initiative, two are targeted towards improving data collection and research (Bau, 1999).

We view our study as consistent with these goals. In particular the work reported here is a first step toward an evaluation of environmental health in Boston Chinatown. As a pilot study it has helped us to develop and test survey methods in the context of this highly urbanized, poor and immigrant community. It would be of interest to conduct a future survey in conjunction with collection of comparable environmental and health status data in order to validate the accuracy of responses. There is also a need to test the survey in a larger sample size and to assess whether it is replicable when interviewees are surveyed repeatedly. Despite the preliminary nature of our study, we think that it is important to report both because there is virtually no literature on the experience of urban Chinese communities with respect to environmental health and because of the needs to develop methods for studying environmental justice issues. Indeed the Institute of Medicine (1999) suggests that, "before embarking on large, costly data collection efforts, it is sometimes possible to gain insight into local health risk by conducting preliminary studies...called *preepidemiology*" (emphasis in original).

Our statistical sample was derived using slight variations on standard survey methods and applied to a community that is not standard. The population in Boston Chinatown is very challenging to contact. Language barriers, the predominance of recent immigrants, cultural factors and poverty likely affected our ability to reach and enroll residents in the study. One sector of the Chinatown population is transient, consisting of working age recent immigrants; while another sector of the community has spent their entire lives there. The transient population arrives in Chinatown as a point of entry to the US and later moves out to other communities as they gain cultural and economic footholds. Some of these "residents" may simply have an address in Chinatown, while spending their non-working hours in dorms associated with suburban restaurants at which they work. Others may share one address among several people. There is a need to deepen our quantitative understanding of the micro-demographics of Chinatown.

The low rate of response to our survey skews our sample from being truly representative. In particular, males ages 25–44 were under sampled by our approach, suggesting that there is a need to over sample for this group. This demographic group works long and unconventional hours (nights, weekends) and may be more likely to be asleep or at work during times that we were conducting our survey. Attempts to reach this population at different times and, possible locations other than the home, are warranted. Focus groups with this population could reveal when and where they may be reached with greater success. On the other hand, older men and women of all ages were well represented, which contrasts with attendance at community meetings at which older women are predominate. Our response rate in Boston Chinatown was higher than that of another study recently conducted in the community, which obtained only 17% responses during random sampling before resorting to a convenience sample (Ren and Chang, 1998).

The under-representation of working age men could bias the study. Men in this age group are likely to have stressful lives due to strenuous jobs and long hours of work as well as having different priorities and needs from the elderly. In particular, men are far more likely than women in this population to be smokers (CDC, 1992, USDHHS, 1998). It is likely that working age men would be aware of at least some information available to the general US population because of their interaction with the wage economy and the chance that they will learn English. Compared to the elderly, they would almost certainly be more mobile, either in making use of public transportation or via company/restaurant vans. They would spend more time out doors and in other communities. The fact that these people get out of Chinatown (e.g. to work in suburban restaurants) could give them a greater basis for comparison and therefore increase their level of dissatisfaction with their current living conditions. Thus their inclusion would possibly shift concern to the outdoor environment and would likely increase measured awareness and understanding of environmental problems.

The study method was successful in several respects. The collaboration between the three organizations effectively brought needed skills together with understanding of and respect within the community. It appears to us that this was necessary in order to conduct a study that was both scientifically valid and well received by residents. The formulation of survey questions drew on knowledge of resident complaints, which meant that we managed to ask questions that in many cases elicited strong responses. In other words, we were asking about things that mattered to respondents. The translation of the survey into Chinese, use of bilingual Chinese interviewers and consideration of culturally viable approaches to interviewees, while not raising response rates as far as we would have wished, likely saved us from a much lower response rate. In addition, unlike most surveys done in Chinatown ours was not a convenience sample. It appears that greater resources and time would be needed to gain a larger sample size. Because of low response rates it is not clear that such a sample, however large, would be representative.

A follow-up to our survey should not simply recruit larger numbers of respondents. Over-sampling of working age men should be included. Future surveys should also focus and sharpen the questions asked. For example, more detail could be asked about health status and symptoms, and about exposure experience. Reformulated questions should seek to reduce the confounding associations that we have noted between exposures (construction dust and vehicle exhaust being the most notable). In addition, direct monitoring of dust and chemical exposures could be conducted. Candidates for monitoring would include components of vehicular exhaust such as carbon monoxide and nitrogen oxide. Levels of particulate matter, which is found in both construction dust and exhaust, could be assessed. It would be of interest to measure noise levels. Any follow up to this study should add an emphasis on exposure inside the home, including parameters such as biological growth and environmental tobacco smoke, which we did not assess. Finally, respondents should be asked about allergies in order to control symptom rates for allergy status.

Conclusion

This survey was a first step toward understanding the environmental health of Boston Chinatown residents. It is difficult to draw conclusions about the magnitude or nature of environmental impacts on health in the community based solely on our data and analysis. It is possible, however, to state that the results reported here are suggestive that air pollution from traffic and construction dust and noise from traffic could be associated with negative health outcomes in this population. We suggest that there is a need for further investigation. We further suggest that insights from the methodological lessons be taken into consideration in future studies.

Acknowledgments

The authors wish to thank Kathy Wong, Henry Chow, Betty Lum, Cindy Lau for conducting the door to door surveys, Esther Ang of South Cove Community Health Center for helping with training and supervising and Christina Hill for assistance with preparing the manuscript. The study was funded by a grant from the Jesse B. Cox Foundation. The Chinese Progressive Association served as our fiscal sponsor.

References

American Thoracic Society (1996), "Health effects of outdoor air pollution: Part 2," *Am J Respir Care Med*; **153**, 477–98.

Bau, I. (1999), "We're not all a picture of health". *Asianweek*, **20**, 18.

Boyko, E.J., Ahroni, J.H., Davignon, D., Stensel, V., Prigeon, R.L. and Smith, D.G. (1997), "Diagnostic utility of the history and physical examination for peripheral vascular disease among patients with diabetes mellitus," *J Clin Epidemiol*, **50**, 659–68.

Brugge, D.M. (1998), "An analysis of the impact of traffic on air pollution and safety in Boston Chinatown", Boston, MA: The Coalition to Protect Chinatown.

Brugge, D.M., Leong, A. and Lai, Z. (1999), "Can a community inject public health values into transportation questions?" *Public Health Reports*, **114**, 40–47.

CDC (1992), "Cigarette smoking among Chinese, Vietnamese, and Hispanics – California, 1989–1991," *MMWR – Morbidity & Mortality Weekly Report*, **41**, 362–7.

Chin, G., Cho, S., Kang, J. and Wu, F. (1996), "Beyond self interest: Asian Pacific Americans towards a community of justice," Los Angeles, CA: LEAP Asian Pacific American Public Policy Institute and the UCLA Asian American Studies Center.

ENSR Consulting and Engineering (1997), "Central Artery (I-93)/Tunnel (I-90) Project: Air quality monitoring data report for CO and PM10 at the intersection of Hudson Street and Harrison Avenue (Chinatown)," Boston, MA: ENSR Consulting and Engineering.

Fay, T.H. (1991), "Noise & Health," New York, NY: New York Academy of Medicine.

Hyland, A., Cummings, K.M., Lynn, W.R., Corle, D. and Giffen, C.A. (1997), "Effect of proxy-reported smoking status on population estimates of smoking prevalence," *Am J Epidemiol*, **145**, 746–51.

Institute of Medicine (1999), "Toward Environmental Justice: Research, Education, and Health Policy   Needs," Washington, DC: National Academy Press.

Leong, A. (1995/1996), "The struggle over Parcel C: How Boston's Chinatown won a victory in the fight against institutional expansion and environmental racism," *Amerasia Journal Winter*, **21**, 99–119.

Loo, C.M. (1991), "Chinatown: Most time, hard time," New York, NY: Praeger.

Massachusetts Department of Public Works (1990), "Central Artery (I-93)/Tunnel (I-90) Project final supplemental environmental impact report, Part 1," Boston: The Department.

Medina, S., Le Tertre, A., Quenel, P., Le Moullec, Y., Lameloise, P., Guzzo, J.C. et al. (1997), "Air pollution and doctor's house calls: Results from the ERPURS system for monitoring the effects of air pollution on public health in Greater Paris, France 1991–1995," *Env. Res.*,**75**, 73–84.

Mueller, B.A., Rivera, F.P., Lii, S-M. and Weiss, N.S. (1990), "Environmental factors and the risk for childhood pedestrian-motor vehicle collision occurrence," *Am J Epidemiol*, **132**, 550–60.

O'Malley, R. (April 2, 1999), "Battling for Subsidized Housing", *Sampan*, **3–4**.

Ong, P. and Hee, S.J. (1993), "The Growth of the Asian Pacific American Population: Twenty Million in 2020," in *The State of Asian Pacific America: Policy Issues to the Year 2020* Los Angeles, CA: LEAP Asian Pacific American Public Policy Institute and UCLA Asian American Studies Center, 11–23.

Ott, W.R. (1995), "Human exposure assessment: The birth of a new science", *J Exp Ana Environ Epideol*, **5**, 449–72.

Paino, J.H. (1993), "Carbon monoxide saturation study in Boston," Lawrence, MA: Massachusetts Department of Environmental Protection.

Rivera, F.P. and Barber, M. (1985), "Demographic analysis of the childhood pedestrian injuries," *Pediatrics*, **76**, 375–81.

Ren, X.S. and Chang, K. (1998), "Evaluating health status of elderly Chinese in Boston," *J Clin Epidemiol*, **51**, 429–35.

South Cove/Chinatown Neighborhood Council (1990), "Chinatown community plan," Boston Redevelopment Authority: City of Boston.

The Chinatown Coalition (July 1994), *Report*, 65.

Thriene, B., Sobottka, A., Willer, H. and Weidhase, J. (1996), "Man-made mineral fiber boards in buildings - health risks caused by quality deficiencies," *Tox Letters*, **88**, 299–303.

USDHHS (1998), "Tobacco use among US racial/ethnic groups – African-Americans, American Indian and Alaska Natives, Asian Americans and Pacific Islanders, and Hispanics: A report of the Surgeon General," Atlanta: US Department of Health and Human Services, Center for Disease Control and Prevention.

Vona, I. (1997), "Immunutherapy for house dust allergy", *Cln Otolaryngol*, **22**, 52–6.

Chapter 8

Traffic Injury Data, Policy and Public Health: Lessons from Boston Chinatown

Doug Brugge, Zenobia Lai, Christina Hill and William Rand

On May 7, 1998 a pedestrian was struck and seriously injured just outside of the boundaries for this study (South Station on Figure 3). A legal settlement for $6 million was reported on August 2, 2000 between the Central Artery Project and the driver of the car.
(Palmer, 2000).

Introduction

Chinatowns are some of the most vibrant ethnic neighborhoods in America's landscape. Home to recent immigrants and old-timers alike, a Chinatown is the heart of many urban Asian American communities. However, Chinatowns are often found in city centers and in crowded and polluted environments (Loo, 1991; Brugge et al., 2000, see also Chapter 7; Brown, 2000). Boston's Chinatown (Chinatown, hereafter) is no exception. While this small but densely populated community is for many purely a commercial district of "exotic" shops, markets, and restaurants, which are toured on weekend excursions, it is also a residential community and home to more than 5,000 people.

The causes of the current day traffic patterns in Chinatown lie in the history of the community's development. In the 1950s and 1960s, Chinatown lost one-half of its land and one-third of it's housing to two new highways: the Central Artery and the Massachusetts Turnpike Extension (Boston Redevelopment Authority, 1979). Built between 1953 and 1959, the Central Artery destroyed over fifty multi-unit housing structures as well as half of the celebrated On Leong Merchant Association building. Built in 1963, the Massachusetts Turnpike extension destroyed sixty more multi-unit housing structures (Chinese Economic Development Council, 1975). As a result, Chinatown lost one-half of its land base and over 1000 units of housing (Sullivan, 1970). Cutting off potential routes of expansion, these highways eliminated much affordable housing, reduced the number of commercial venues, and added to traffic congestion, noise, and pollution (Massachusetts Turnpike Authority, 1993). The Boston Redevelopment Authority has conceded that Chinatown suffers from "chronic traffic congestion [and that] pedestrian safety in the heavily concentrated residential areas has been threatened" (Boston Transportation Department, 1999).

In more recent years, Tufts University School of Medicine and New England Medical Center (NEMC) have expanded in the heart of Chinatown, further squeezing space for housing and business (Leong, 1995/1996). In 1993, NEMC proposed building a 455-car garage next to a community day care facility in Chinatown. The garage would generate over 3000 daily vehicle trips circulating within a block of an elementary school, elderly and family housing and would stand within four feet of a community day care facility (Leong, 1995/1996; Liu, 1999; Lai et al., 2000). The Chinatown community organized to oppose the garage, undertook its first traffic study which challenged developer traffic volumes by counting vehicles at intersections near the proposed garage and urged the state Secretary of Environmental Affairs to review the cumulative impacts of all the developments in a longitudinal and cumulative manner.

Within two years of defeating the medical center garage, the community rallied to oppose a more formidable foe. The State's Highway Department revived a plan to build a permanent exit ramp (Ramp DD) into Chinatown, and the Central Artery/Tunnel project planned to build an additional temporary detour ramp (Albany Street Detour) into Chinatown (Massachusetts Highway Department, 1996). If constructed, either of these would generate 25,000 additional daily vehicle trips into the already overloaded roadways of the community. The Chinatown community launched another traffic and transportation study, and worked with the Boston Transportation Department to eventually come up with alternatives that lead to neither ramp being constructed.

In 1997 a private developer proposed building a hotel-condominium-theater-mall complex – now under construction (Vanasse Hangen Brustlin, Inc, 1997a; Vanasse Hangen Brustlin, Inc, 1997b). The community quickly learned that this was only the first in a wave of up to 30 proposed developments slated for the Chinatown area. It became obvious to community activists that they could no longer address the cumulative impacts of all these developments by relying on volunteer-driven small-scale traffic studies. Representatives from the Chinatown community, using political pressure and the findings of preliminary studies (Brugge et al., 1999), pressured the city to conduct a comprehensive transportation study of Chinatown.

The City of Boston responded by commissioning a consultant to undertake a study in 1998 (Boston Transportation Department, 1999). The study produced an extensive set of recommendations that focused both on interventions such as roadway and sidewalk modifications and enforcement of traffic laws and on more rigorous assessment of the impact of new development. It did the later by summing expected traffic increases from all known future development whereas previously developers had measured their traffic impact against existing conditions and ignored the combined impact of other projects. However, despite the fact that the study incorporated input from community representatives in terms of scope and methodology, it failed to address injuries.

Traffic-Related Injuries

Injuries are, however, one of the most tangible and immediate consequences of traffic. In the 1990s, motor vehicles were the leading cause of death from injury nationally and one of the top four causes of emergency department visits (Fingerhut and Warner, 1997; Grossman, 2000). The literature with respect to traffic-related injuries focuses on children (Grossman, 2000; Durbin, 1999), pedestrians (Galloway and Patel, 1982), and especially pediatric pedestrians (Calhoun et al., 1998; Mueller et al., 1988; Roberts et al., 1995; Rao et al., 1997). Studies of injuries to motor vehicle occupants have tended to place greater emphasis on fatalities, the role of alcohol in causing crashes and safety features in the design of automobiles (Rivera and Grossman, 1997). In contrast we choose to look at all injuries to pedestrians and occupants on low speed streets in an urban setting.

Parts of the literature are, however, relevant, if not entirely comparable to our focus. For pedestrians, factors reported to be associated with injuries include traffic volume, high density of parked vehicles, high speeds of travel, inadequate sidewalks, total number of pedestrians and living in multifamily dwellings (Calhoun et al., 1998; Roberts et al., 1995; Agran et al., 1996; Mueller et al., 1990). Many elderly are unable to cross intersections during the time allotted by signals (Langlois et al., 1997) and injury rates for children increase if they have to cross more streets to walk to school (Macpherson et al., 1998). Geographical mapping of pedestrian injuries suggests more injuries closer to downtown (Allard, 1982) and temporal analysis suggests higher fatalities on the weekends and at night (Galloway and Patel, 1982; Haddon et al., 1961).

Massachusetts and Chinatown

In 1998, Massachusetts was reported to have rates of traffic fatalities (6.6/100,000 population) that were less than half the national average (15.34/100,000) (U.S. Department of Transportation, 1998). However, the state has the highest rate of automobile injury claims (2.29/100 insured cars), which is more than twice the U.S. national average (1.17/100 insured cars) (Insurance Research Council, 2000). The state also has the fourth highest proportion of deaths being pedestrians (U.S. Department of Transportation, 1998).

Previously reported was an analysis of Chinatown traffic injury data for one year, 1996 (Brugge et al., 1999). The relatively small sample size (110 injuries) precluded elucidation of temporal or geographic patterns with adequate statistical clarity. Nevertheless, late night and weekend injuries were apparent. It was also observed that injuries rose and fell with commuter traffic peaks during weekdays. A pilot environmental health survey also asked questions about Chinatown residents' experience with traffic (Brugge et al., 2000; see also Chapter 7). Difficulty crossing intersections on the green or walk signal was reported by 54.8% of respondents and 9.5% reported having been in a motor vehicle accident in Chinatown.

We report here analysis of three years of traffic-related injuries in Chinatown and comment on their relevance to land use and transportation policy and to public health interventions. Our primary goal was to analyze injury and vehicle volume data in an exploratory manner that could prompt changes in policy with respect to traffic-related injuries. Our secondary goal was to contribute to general knowledge about the relationship of traffic to injuries.

Methods

Study Area

The study area was defined as the area south of Boylston/Essex Street and north of East Berkeley Street. On the eastern side, the boundary line runs from Atlantic

Avenue to Kneeland Street to the John Fitzgerald Highway ("Central Artery") and Albany Street. In the west, the division is set along Tremont Street (see Figure 8.3).

Traffic Injury Report Databases

Traffic-related injury report data for the Chinatown area was requested in writing from the Boston Police Department (BPD) Office of Research Analysis. Data were provided for the time period from January 1, 1996 through December 31, 1998 in two databases as described in Table 8.1. One data set consisted of calls for service to 9-1-1 and the other of records on file with BPD. The 9-1-1 data identified motor vehicle accidents involving a pedestrian (MVAPED). The BPD report data included the set of all reports listed as "M/V ACC.INJURIES", or motor vehicle accidents with injuries. Each data set consisted of information on the location of the reported injury (street number or intersection), the time (displayed by the hour and minute, AM or PM), date, and day of the week. The data were also indexed according to police-designated reporting areas, which are several square block areas.

The two data sets were cross-referenced to identify overlapping of service responses and to separate pedestrian from vehicle occupant injuries. Reports deemed to be the same incident in the 9-1-1 and BPD data sets were those that occurred at the same location, on the same date, within 1 hour of each other. In most cases, the reports counted as a single injury were within ten minutes of each other. The overlapping data, those incidents listed in both databases, were defined as confirmed pedestrian injuries. These were combined with the 9-1-1 calls without a BPD report to constitute all pedestrian injuries. The remaining BPD reports were defined to be injuries to motor vehicle occupants (see Table 8.1).

Table 8.1   Data used in the study

	Data	**Coded as**
9-1-1 calls	Pedestrian injuries	Pedestrian injuries
BPD Reports	All traffic injuries	All traffic injuries
Study Data Set	All traffic injuries	Pedestrian and occupant injuries

Traffic Volume Databases

TAMS Consulting of Boston provided the only 24-hour traffic volume data available to us. These data describe 24-hour traffic volume at six locations and intersections during Friday, Saturday, and Sunday June 19, 20 and 21, 1999. They were collected as part of the Chinatown Transportation Study commissioned by the Boston Transportation Department (1999). Traffic volumes were assessed under a subcontract by a commercial firm, Accurate Counts using Jamar Technologies Trax II® automatic tube recorders (ATRs) that use pneumatic tubes to record vehicles passing. The recordings were downloaded to a computer in fifteen-minute intervals using the software Tasplus 4®.

Adequate intersection traffic volume data were not available for the years in which we analyzed injuries so we used data from the closest years for which it was available. Two sources were used to generate estimations of traffic volume at intersections in Chinatown. The preferred source of data was a model reported by the Chinatown Transportation Study, which was based on combined data from several studies by developers that overlapped with the time period for our injury data (Boston Transportation Department, 1999). Although not included in the official report, we were provided by the Boston Transportation Department with a map of intersection vehicle volumes from their supporting materials. Unfortunately, this study did not investigate all of the intersections of interest to us since it concentrated primarily on the northern parts of Chinatown. As a supplement, we used New England Medical Center's 1994 draft impact report on traffic in the southern section of Chinatown (Insurance Research Council, 2000). Both data sets reported vehicle volumes for 7–9 AM and 4–6 PM.

The data used were generated by similar modeling methods that were comparable and should give an accurate relative sense of traffic volume. The data do not reflect day-to-day variation in traffic that limits the quality of information on which the study is based. Nevertheless, the data for Boston Chinatown are better than for most communities because of the large number of development impact studies that are available. For each intersection for which data were available, the number of cars driving into the intersection was totaled. If the intersection was shown on both the Chinatown Transportation Study and the NEMC draft report, we used the values from the Chinatown Transportation Study.

The configuration of roadways at intersections was divided into three categories. The first was defined as "simple" which consisted of intersections in which two one-way streets intersected cleanly. The second was defined as "complex" and included combinations of one-way and two-way streets in non-conflicting configurations and intersections of two-way streets. The third category was defined as "confusing" and consisted of two intersections that had one-way streets that met two-way streets head-on.

Analysis of the Injury Data

The injury data were analyzed for variation based on the time at which injuries occurred in order to determine whether there were any temporal patterns to injury risk. Data were stratified along the variables year, month of the year, day of the week, and hour of the day for the complete data set and for both pedestrian and vehicle occupant injury reports. We choose these time parameters both because the data was coded this way and because they are standard units of time. For grouping of weekend days (Friday, Saturday and Sunday) or commuter hours (AM, noon and PM), we choose days and times that both fit our sense of traffic flow from observation of the community and those that corresponded to those frequently used by developers to analyze traffic impacts.

Most of the injury reports provided a location for injuries designated with either two streets (an intersection) or a single street name and address number (occasionally also an intersection). This allowed straightforward mapping of injuries by location for a large majority of injuries. However, there were twenty-nine reports listed only by street name and reporting area. In the case of these injury reports, a cross-reference with reporting area numbers was necessary in order to provide a reasonable estimation of injury location. In these instances, the incident was mapped to a location on the street listed, within the designated reporting area, at the center point of the street as it passed through the reporting area. This method provided accuracy to within two blocks or less.

In 1987, the Boston Redevelopment Authority (BRA) published two physical area maps that included most street numbers. These were used as a reference when plotting injury data. Tiger line files for Boston were obtained from the U.S. Geological Survey and were used as base maps in the computerized mapping system, Map Info, Professional®. The BPD and 9-1-1 data were layered on top of these maps for geographic analysis.

Statistical Analysis

Patterns of injuries with time and location were examined using Chi-squared goodness of fit analysis while the relation between location and type of injury was analyzed with Chi-squared contingency table analysis. The dependence of traffic volume on site and time was analyzed using Analysis of Variance followed by Newman-Keuls post hoc testing and the relationship between traffic volume and number of injuries was estimated with Spearman rank correlation. All data were entered into MS Excel® and transferred to SPSS® for analysis.

Results

Temporal Analysis

Over the three-year period encompassed by the study there were 92 pedestrian injuries and 236 vehicle occupant injuries reported in the BPD databases. The total number of vehicle occupant injuries was 71 in 1996, 87 in 1997 and 78 in 1998. The total number of pedestrian injuries was 39 in 1996, 26 in 1997, and 27 in 1998.

Injury reports did not differ statistically by day of the week ($p=0.496$; $p=0.163$) or month ($p=0.369$; $p=0.440$) for vehicle occupants or pedestrians respectively. The lowest and highest numbers of injuries did not form a pattern (Figure 8.1). The ratio of pedestrian injuries to occupant injuries also did not differ significantly with day of the week ($p=0.309$) or with month ($p=0.643$). Assessment of the pattern of injuries by hour of the day revealed that while the majority of injuries were reported between 8 AM and 6 PM, there were also appreciable injuries reported during night hours from 10 PM to 3 AM (Figure 8.2). Statistical analysis of occupant injuries showed no significant association ($p=0.481$) between injuries and commuter hours (7-9 AM, 11 AM – 2 PM, 4-6 PM) compared to the intervening hours (9-11 AM, 2-4 PM). Nighttime occupant injuries were found to be more likely on Friday, Saturday and Sunday nights ($RR = 2.26$; $CI = 1.35$-3.78; $p=0.0014$). Pedestrian injuries were not significantly associated with either commuter hours ($p=0.776$) or weekend nights ($p=0.950$).

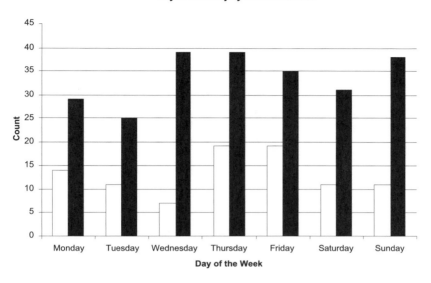

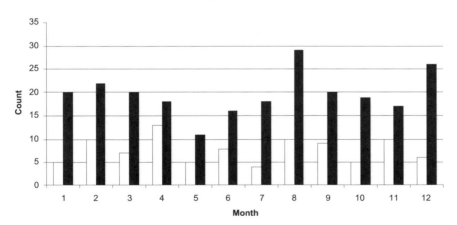

Figure 8.1   Distribution of pedestrian (open bars) and vehicle occupant (closed bars) injuries by (a) day of the week and (b) month of the year

Geographic Analysis

Maps of injuries by location in Boston Chinatown suggest from visual inspection that injuries were not evenly distributed and that the pattern of injury distribution was

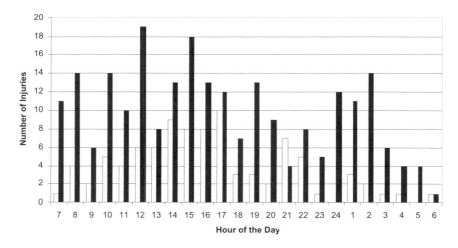

Figure 8.2   Distribution of pedestrian (open bars) and vehicle occupant (closed bars) injuries by hour of the day

relatively consistent from year to year (Figure 8.3). Most injuries occurred along major roadways running through the community, with some intersections exhibiting "clusters" of injury reports in one or more years. A single intersection along the Massachusetts Turnpike (I-90) had the most reported injuries of any intersection in all three years. Three intersections, marked with arrows in Figure 8.3, had two or fewer injuries in two years and clusters of five or more injuries in one year. Other intersections were more stable across the study period. Statistical analysis for the reporting areas designated by the Boston Police Department confirms that occupant injuries (p<0.001) and pedestrian injuries (p=0.039) were significantly associated with location. The pattern of injuries was similar year to year (p=0.261) and the ratio of pedestrian to occupant injuries did not vary significantly between reporting areas (p=0.271).

Video and personal observations were conducted on six occasions at three intersections within the study area between June 17 and October 6, 1997 (Brugge, 1998; Papa, 1997). The intersections were the ones marked with an arrow in Figure 8.3a, the intersection immediately north of that intersection (toward the top of the map) and the intersection immediately West of the second. The videotape study revealed a range of two to 37 illegal turns per two-hour observation period per intersection. "Near miss" events happened from eight to 76 times at the intersections. Potentially hazardous behaviors and infrastructure included: vehicles traveling at high speed, left turns from the far right lane, pedestrians crossing against the light, U-turns, bicyclists and vehicles running red lights, vehicles caught in the intersection during the red cycle of the light, confusing walk signals, lack of lane demarcation, lack of any walk signal unless activated by pedestrians, and walk times as short as 15 seconds. We have not yet been able to associate causes such as these with the injuries analyzed.

1996

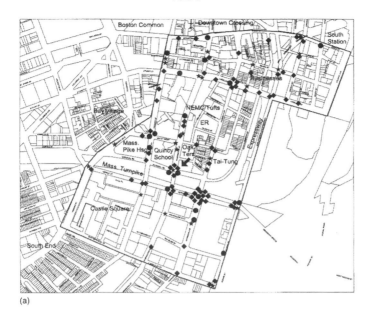

(a)

1997

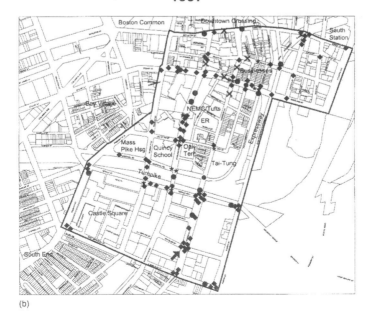

(b)

1998

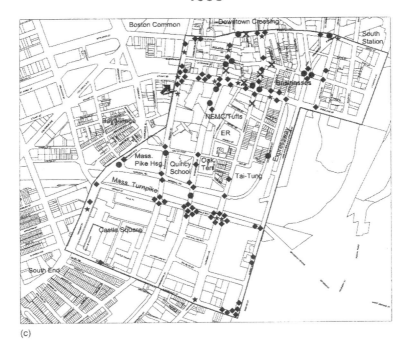

(c)

Figure 8.3   **Distribution of pedestrian and vehicle occupant injuries by geographic location for (a) 1996 (originally published in Brugge et al., 1999), (b) 1997, (c) 1998**

Diamonds are occupant injuries, stars are pedestrian injuries reported in both the BTD and 9-1-1 data bases and circles are pedestrian injuries reported in only the 9-1-1 data base. "X" marks locations at which 24-hour vehicle volume measurements were made. Arrows indicate intersections at which more than 5 injuries were recorded in one year, but not the other two.

24-Hour Vehicle Volumes

For six locations, marked "X" on Figure 8.3(c), uninterrupted 24-hour vehicle volumes were available for a consecutive Friday, Saturday and Sunday in 1999. There were a small number of records of traffic volume that contained evidence of interruption of counts, i.e., sudden drops to zero (Figure 8.4). This could have been due to tampering, damage to the tube or vehicles parking on the instrumentation. The recorded traffic volumes reveal that traffic remained considerable late into the night, dropping off only after 3 AM and rising again by 7 AM. Indeed, for some of the nights measured for the Beach Street location, peak traffic volume was at 2 AM. The circadian traffic patterns at the six sites differed statistically from each other (p<0.001). This was found to be resolvable into two statistically similar subsets consisting of three locations each (p=0.148 and p=0.213, open and closed points in Figure 8.4). It was not apparent to us what caused these two patterns.

Association between Vehicle Volumes and Injuries

Nonparametric correlations were examined between vehicle volume, available for most major intersections, and injuries reported within the intersection. Figure 8.5[1] shows the relationship between total injuries and estimated vehicle volume in the 6-8 AM and 4-6 PM time periods for nine intersection configurations defined as simple (two one-way streets intersecting at right angles) and ten that were complex (most other configurations). The correlation coefficients were $R^2 = 0.589$ (p = 0.010) for simple configurations and $R^2 = 0.104$ (p = 0.397) for complex intersections. For simple intersections, this translates into an increase of between three and five injuries per year for each increase of 1,000 vehicles. Two intersections that were coded as particularly confusing (one-way streets emptying into each other combined with two-way streets) are not shown, however, one of the intersections defined as confusing greatly exceeded all other intersections in terms of injuries normalized by vehicle volume and is the intersection in Figure 8.3 with the largest cluster of injuries in each year.

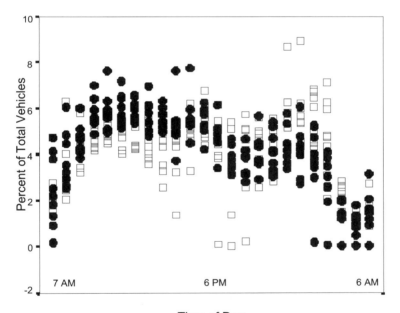

Time of Day

Figure 8.4   Twenty-four hour vehicle volumes, normalized to percent total for six locations in Chinatown (locations marked "X" in Figure 8.3). Closed circles are three of the locations with statistically similar patterns; open squares are the other three locations with a different statistically similar pattern.

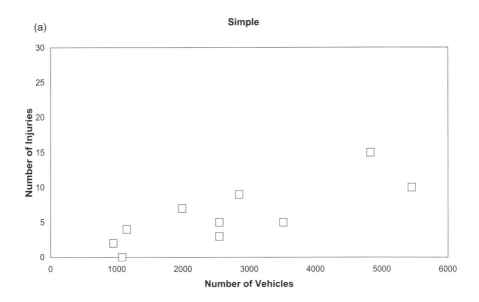

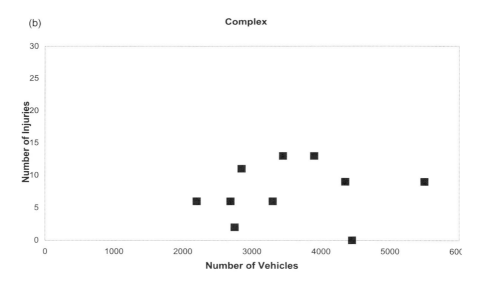

Figure 8.5   Association of modeled vehicle volume at intersections for weekdays at 4:00–6:00 PM and 7:00–9:00 AM with total injuries at (a) simple intersections and (b) complex intersections from 1996–1998

Discussion

This exploratory study was undertaken with the assumption that it would be possible to use available quantitative data about traffic injuries and vehicle volumes to inform future land use and transportation policy in the community and to prompt more immediate safety interventions. Further, it was hoped that our findings would generate avenues of research that could further elucidate the relationship of traffic volume to injuries and that the results for one community would be instructive to other communities. It is necessary first to say something about the limitations to our approach.

Limitations of the Study

The injury databases used were likely to have a number of limitations. First and foremost, it is unlikely that 9-1-1 and/or the Boston Police Department have a report on every vehicle-related injury that occurred over the span of the three-year period investigated. For example, the authors are personally aware of one pedestrian hit by a car within the study area and timeframe. This person left the scene and did not report the injury or seek medical assistance despite painful bruises and scrapes. Other injuries may also have been transported to emergency rooms without placing a call to 9-1-1 and without involvement of police. The availability of an emergency room (marked "ER" on Figure 8.3) in Chinatown could encourage non-EMT transport of injured persons. If this occurred, it would have also led to undercounting of traffic-related injuries. It is possible that injuries occurring closer to the emergency room would be less likely to need to seek 9-1-1 or police assistance.

Another possible problem is that the data may have included reports that were erroneously recorded due to inaccurate reporting or data management errors within the responsible agencies. The larger database kept by the BPD contains, for example, motor vehicle property damage without injury which could be miscoded in either direction. In addition, those 9-1-1 calls that had no corresponding BPD report could have been false or could also have resulted from calls that were inaccurately coded. We were unable to estimate the degree to which these errors occurred, but assume that they were small given the need for accurate record keeping within the police and emergency medical services.

For Chinatown, there was considerable data about traffic available because of the relatively large number of environmental impact reports filed, something that is lacking for many communities (Salmi, 1990). The modeled vehicle volumes at intersections for commuter hours that we used, however, still fail to reflect variation on different days or times of the year and they were based on commuter hour measurements that did not necessarily reflect 24-hour traffic patterns. Further, while the traffic volume data overlapped with the years in which we analyzed injuries, they were not specific to those years and there could have been factors other than the traffic volume in effect during the time in which injury data was collected. The study is limited in accuracy by sample size and design, as well as the lack of information on causes of injury producing crashes.

The limitations discussed above do not undermine, in our opinion, the practical/ applied use of the analysis with respect to policy making or preparing public safety interventions. It is our contention that the analysis presented is inherently more accurate with respect to injuries than other methods commonly used in Boston and Massachusetts since these rely on vehicle volumes alone (Massachusetts Environmental Policy Act, 1972). The study also attempted to contribute to theoretical understanding of traffic injury causation. Our findings in this regard are preliminary, but we think they suggest future areas of research and are suggestive of possible underlying causal factors.

The Meaning of Findings for Chinatown

There are several conclusions that we feel that we can draw with respect to Chinatown. These are:

1. This study was one of the first that responded to the community concerns that there has been and continues to be an historical progression toward worse traffic and more injuries. The construction of the highways, the citing of theater and red light districts and the building of garages, businesses and luxury housing that attract motor vehicle traffic all likely contributed to create the current traffic conditions in the community and rapid new construction currently underway may exacerbate things further still.

2. The high traffic volume that extends into the weekends and late night hours appears to be a contributor to the injuries that follow the same pattern. The lack of statistically significant associations of injuries with most temporal frameworks that we tested (time of day, day of week, month) supports the idea that injuries cannot be assessed at limited "peak" times. We find it intriguing that the pattern of traffic volume over 24-hour periods on the weekend in Chinatown appears to mirror injury distribution over 24-hour periods (compare Figures 8.2 and 8.4). In this regard, it is also noteworthy that injuries were significantly more likely on weekend nights when there are likely more drivers who have been drinking and/or involved in illegal activities associated with drugs and/or prostitution in the Red Light District. Since environmental impact studies in Chinatown have frequently used Friday PM commuter hours (4-6 PM) as "worst case scenarios" they may have failed to account for impacts at other times of the week, day or night when injuries are just as likely to occur (Vanesse Hangen Brustlin, Inc., 1997a; Vanesse Hangen Brustlin, Inc., 1997b).

3. Certain intersections (see Figure 8.3) had greater numbers of injuries consistently over multiple years when compared to other intersections. Together with the almost 24 hours per day, 7 days per week temporal distribution of injuries, these patterns suggest locations and times (including the weekend and late at night) at which to expand intervention efforts (e.g., posting a police detail) and to consider during policy/development decision-making (e.g., redesign of confusing intersections). Added information about causes of crashes would be helpful in designing interventions.

4. There is a need to integrate assessment of transportation impacts from individual developments or other traffic generating sources. The history of Chinatown shows that individual developments and transportation projects frequently contribute only incrementally to traffic volume, but that combined they add up to greater impact. The

city's study of Chinatown acknowledges this and recommends that new traffic impacts be assessed against all planned or approved developments (Boston Transportation Department, 1999).

Negative traffic impacts need to be addressed at both the level of land use and transportation policy and public safety interventions. In the policy arena both vehicle volume and configuration of intersections need to be addressed. This will be challenging in today's development "boom". Safety measures, such as education or police enforcement of traffic laws, are easier to implement and worthwhile, but likely only moderate impacts and do not address underlying causes. Interventions such as those proposed by the Boston Transportation Department (1999), including roadway and sidewalk redesign, changes in signage and signals, and improved enforcement should be ranked by priority and implemented. Long-term planning is needed minimally to prevent increases in vehicle volume and preferably to reduce traffic.

Generalizability of Findings

This study contains lessons for academics, community activists and municipal policy makers. These are:

1. Analysis of total traffic-related injuries allows for micro-scale assessment that would not be possible looking only at fatalities and their relationship to vehicle miles traveled, vehicle speed, seat belts, or population and economic demographics, the most commonly assessed parameters for macro models (Hakim et al., 1991). Fatalities (Mueller et al., 1990; Retting, 1988) are too infrequent to generate the types of patterns that we documented for the microanalysis necessary at the community level.

2. Analysis of injuries provides information not available when vehicle volumes at intersections for limited hours of the day are the sole data. This is mostly relevant to municipal planners and enforcement staff, since most studies in the literature already focus on injuries (Galloway and Patel, 1982; Roberts, et al., 1995; Agran et al., 1996; Mueller et al., 1990; Haddon et al., 1961). Yet, at least in Massachusetts, decision making with respect to transportation policy rests on vehicle volumes and, in particular, delays to motorists, rather than on injuries (Massachusetts Environmental Policy Act, 1972).

3. Our results suggest that it is not reasonable to assume that traffic patterns are "typical" or that they match naive assumptions. Chinatown may or may not reflect the situation in other urban communities as the move toward "24-hour" cities accelerates. At the very least it provides a cautionary lesson against assuming that traffic volume or injury risk is maximum or representative at certain times or locations. Despite being situated in a high commuter district (Downtown Boston), we found that commuter hours on weekdays were not the peak times for traffic injuries. Indeed our finding that weekend nights were at increased risk for traffic-related injuries confirms earlier reports (Galloway and Patel, 1982; Haddon et al., 1961).

4. Many studies (Mueller et al., 1988; Roberts et al., 1995; Agran et al., 1996; Mueller et al., 1990) have been case control approaches that are effective at generating information about the relationship of factors such as density of parked cars, neighborhoods with multifamily dwellings and speed limits to traffic injury risk. We feel that such studies are less well adapted than the method that we used for being a practical approach for informing municipal policy about highly specific risk factors at the micro-scale of individual communities in a way that could effectively target resources to particular sections of roadway.

5. The relationship of vehicle volume to numbers of injuries at intersections is not simple. Pooling all intersections led to a relatively weak association. However, categorizing intersections by level of complexity resulted in a strong association for simple intersections and little association for more complex intersections. We think that it is possible that vehicle volume is a significant factor at simple intersections while the configuration of the intersection dominates for more complex configurations. It would be interesting to test whether or not this finding holds for other communities and larger data sets.

6. Traffic volumes for 24-hour periods may be informative, even if available for limited locations in a community. In our study, 24-hour traffic patterns at a few locations and at very limited times (Figure 8.4) largely mirrored the injury patterns over 24 hours for the whole community (Figure 8.2). Given our limited 24-hour vehicle volume data, we feel that this point is in need of validation before a firm conclusion can be reached.

Conclusions

This study has confirmed that weekend nights are times of increased risk and that Friday commuter hours are not the worst-case scenario for injury risk in Chinatown. We also showed that vehicle volume was strongly associated with risk at simple intersection configurations while intersection configuration may be the primary factor at more complex intersections. These conclusions appear to have immediate implications for land use and transportation policy and for public health and safety interventions. We conclude that communities, city agencies and others would better serve the interests of injury prevention if they included vehicle injury analysis in their decision-making processes.

Note

1   In the original article Figure 8.5a incorrectly plotted the number of injuries on the y-axis as one-half of the actual total. The error is corrected in this version.

Acknowledgments

The authors wish to thank Mike Liu for his comments on the manuscript and the Campaign to Protect Chinatown for inspiring this study and for advocating for the residents of Chinatown.

Thanks to the Boston Transportation Department, particularly Ralph DiNisco, and TAMS Consulting led by David Black, for providing us with vehicle volume data. Thanks also to Tina Zenzola, David Lawrence and Rebecca Reynolds-Ramirez of the Center for Childhood Injury Prevention in San Diego and to H. Patricia Hynes of Boston University for their helpful critiques of the manuscript. Sabine Jean-Louis and Tashiko Tanaka assisted with preparation of the manuscript.

References

Agran, P.F., Winn, D.G., Anderson, C.L., Tran, C. and Del Valle, C.P. (1996), "The role of the physical and traffic environment in child pedestrian injuries", *Pediatrics*, **98**, 1096–1103.

Allard (1982) "Excess mortality from traffic accidents among elderly pedestrians living in the inner city", *American Journal of Public Health*, **72**, 853–4.

Boston Redevelopment Authority (1981), "Chinatown-South Cove District Profile and Proposed 1979-1981 Neighborhood Improvement Plan", Boston Redevelopment Authority.

Boston Transportation Department (1999), "Chinatown transportation study", Boston Transportation Department.

Brown, J. (June 16, 2000), "Philly Chinatown deals with change", Associated Press.

Brugge, D. (1998), "An analysis of the impact of traffic on air pollution and safety in Boston Chinatown", Boston: The Coalition to Protect Chinatown.

Brugge, D., Leong, A. and Lai, Z. (1999), "Can a community inject public health values into transportation questions?", *Public Health Reports*, **114**, 40–47.

Brugge, D., Leong, A. Averbach, A. and Cheung, F. (2000), "An environmental health survey of residents of Boston Chinatown", *Journal of Immigrant Health*, **2**, 97–111.

Calhoun, A.D., McGwin, G., King, W.D. and Rousculp, M.D. (1998), "Pediatric pedestrian injuries: A community assessment using a hospital surveillance system", *Academic Emergency Medicine*, **5**, 685–90.

Chinese Economic Development Council (1975), "Economic Development for Boston's Chinese Community, Phase II, The Acquisition of Title VII-D", Community Development Corporation Planning Grant Proposal.

Durbin, D.R. (1999) "Preventing motor vehicle injuries", *Current Opinion in Pediatrics*, **11**, 583–7.

Fingerhut, L.A. and Warner, M. (1997), *Injury chartbook, Health, United States, 1996-97*, Hyattsville, MD: National Center for Health Statistics.

Galloway, D.J. and Patel AR (1982), "The pedestrian problem: A 12 month review of pedestrian accidents", *Injury*, **13**, 294–8.

Grossman, D.C. (2000), "The history of injury control and the epidemiology of child and adolescent injuries", *The future of children: Unintentional injuries in childhood*, **10**, 23–52.

Haddon, W., Valien, P., McCarroll, J.R. and Umberger, C.J. (1961), "A controlled investigation of the characteristics of adult pedestrians fatally injured by motor vehicles in Manhattan", *Journal of Chronic Disease*, **14**, 655–78.

Hakim, S., Shefer, D., Hakkert, A.S. and Hocherman, I. (1991), "A critical review of macro models for road accidents", *Accident Analysis & Prevention*, **23**, 379–400.

Insurance Research Council (January 31, 2000), "Auto accidents are down, while claims for injuries are up", Press Release.

Lai, Z., Leong, A. and Wu, C.C. (2000), "The Lessons of the Parcel C Struggle: Reflections on Community Lawyering", *UCLA Asian Pacific American Law Journal*, **6**, 1–43.

Langlois, J.A., Keyl, P.M., Guralnik, J.M., Foley, D.J., Marottoli, R.A. and Wallace, R.B. (1997), "Characteristics of older pedestrians who have difficulty crossing the street", *American Journal of Public Health*, **87**, 393–7.

Leong, A. (Winter, 1995/1996), "The struggle over Parcel C: How Boston's Chinatown won a victory in the fight against institutional expansion and environmental racism", *Amerasia Journal*, **3**, 99–119.

Liu, M.C. (1999), "Chinatown's neighborhood mobilization and urban development in Boston", [dissertation] Boston: University of Massachusetts Boston.

Loo, C.M. (1991), *Chinatown: Most time, hard time*, New York: Praeger.

Macpherson, A., Roberts, I. and Pless, I.B. (1998), "Children's exposure to traffic and pedestrian injuries", *American Journal of Public Health*, **88**, 1840–43.

Massachusetts Environmental Policy Act, Mass. Gen. Law nc30, Sect. 61-62H; Stat. 1972, c.781, Sect. 2&3 7/18/1972 as amended.

Massachusetts Turnpike Authority (1993), Air Rights Study.

Massachusetts Highway Department (1996), *South Bay/South Boston Areas Notice of Project Change/Environmental Reevaluation*, Central Artery/tunnel Project, Final supplemental Environmental Impact Statement/Report. Massachusetts Highway Department.

Mueller, A.B., Rivara, F.P. and Bergman, A.B. (1988), "Urban-rural location and the risk of dying in a pedestrian-vehicle collision", *Journal of Trauma*, **28**, 91–4.

Mueller, B.A., Rivera, F.P., Lii, S-M. and Weiss, N.S. (1990), "Environmental factors and the risk for childhood pedestrian-motor vehicle collision occurrence", *American Journal of Epidemiology*, **132**, 550–60.

Palmer. T.C. (August 2, 2000), "Big Dig to pay $6m to victim of car accident", *The Boston Globe*, section 1, col. 16).

Papa, K. (1997), *A field investigation assessing vehicular and pedestrian safety in Boston Chinatown* [thesis], Boston: Boston University School of Medicine.

Rao, R., Hawkins, M. and Guyer, B. (1997), "Children's exposure to traffic and risk of pedestrian injury in an urban setting", *Bulletin of the New York Acadamy of Medicine*, **74**, 65–80.

Retting (1988), "Urban pedestrian safety", *Bulletin N.Y. Academy of Medicine*, **64**, 810–15.

Rivera, F.P., Grossman, D.C. and Cummings, P. (1997), "Injury prevention: First of two parts", *New England Journal of Medicine*, **337**, 543–8.

Roberts, I., Norton, R., Jackson, R., Dunn, R. and Hassall, I. (1995), "Effect of environmental factors on risk of injury of child pedestrians by motor vehicles: A case-control study", *The British Medical Journal*, **310**, 91-94.

Salmi, L.R. and Battista, R.N. (1990), "Epidemiologic assessment of hazardous roadway locations", *Epidemiology*, **1**, 311–4.

Sullivan, C. and Hatch, K. (1970), *The Chinese in Boston, 1970*, Action for Boston Community Development.

U.S. Department of Transportation (1998), *Traffic safety facts 1998: State traffic data*, U.S. Department of Transportation.

Vanasse Hangen Brustlin, Inc. (1997a), *Response to Comments: Millennium Place, Commonwealth Center Site, Boston, MA*, Vanasse Hangen Brustlin, Inc.

Vanasse Hangen Brustlin, Inc. (1997b), *Supplemental Data for the Notice of Project Change EOEA #7113: Millennium Place, Commonwealth Center Site, Boston, MA*, Vanasse Hangen Brustlin, Inc.

Chapter 9

Airborne Concentrations of $PM_{2.5}$ and Diesel Exhaust Particles on Harlem Sidewalks: A Community-Based Pilot Study

Patrick L. Kinney, Maneesha Aggarwal, Mary E. Northridge,
Nicole A.H. Janssen and Peggy Shepard

Introduction

Residents of densely developed urban neighborhoods face a range of environmental risks both indoors and outdoors. Among the outdoor factors of greatest concern to residents of the Harlem neighborhood of New York City (NYC) is the complex mixture of toxic air pollutants emitted in and around the city by mobile sources (e.g., cars, trucks, and buses). Mobile source emissions are of special concern both because of their ubiquitous nature and because emissions occur at ground level in urban street canyons where human activity is greatest. The seemingly disproportionate concentration of diesel emission sources in underprivileged urban neighborhoods such as Harlem, and the potential impacts diesel exhaust particles may have on human health, has in recent years led both to a community-based movement aimed at reducing diesel emissions and a concurrent scientific research agenda directed at understanding the relationships among sources, concentrations, exposures, and human health.

The human health effects of airborne particulate matter (PM) have been examined in numerous recent epidemiological studies (Ostro, 1987; Thurston, et al., 1994; Dockery, et al., 1993; Dockery and Pope, 1994; Pope, et al, 1995; Schwartz, et al., 1993), several of which highlight the special health significance of particles less than 2.5 μm in aerodynamic diameter ($PM_{2.5}$). $PM_{2.5}$ particles are potentially more harmful than larger particles because they can reach deeper into the lower respiratory tract of the lungs. In addition, since they are products of fossil fuel combustion, $PM_{2.5}$ often contain high concentrations of several toxic substances, including acid sulfates, soluble metals, and organic compounds such as polycyclic aromatic hydrocarbons.

Important constituents of $PM_{2.5}$ in NYC are diesel exhaust particles (DEP). DEP aerosols consist of chain aggregates of roughly spherical nuclei comprised largely of elemental carbon (EC). DEP have large surface areas, ranging from 30 to 100 m^2/g, on which a wide range of organic compounds is adsorbed (WHO, 1996). Nearly all diesel particles fall within the $PM_{2.5}$ size range, with mass median diameters ranging from 0.05 to 0.3 μm. Because diesel engines burn fuel more efficiently than conventional spark ignition petrol engines, they offer better fuel economy. Nonetheless, diesel engines emit 10 times more particles per mile than conventional petrol engines and 30–70 times more than engines equipped with catalytic converters (Godlee, 1993).

Both the respirable size and the composition of DEP raise concerns for human health impacts of diesel exhaust exposure. Very few data exist on levels and patterns of human exposures to DEP in urban areas. Especially lacking are data relating spatial variations in source density to variations in ambient DEP concentrations in densely populated urban core neighborhoods. In the case of $PM_{2.5}$, minimal spatial variations exist within or between urban areas in the northeastern United States (Suh, et al., 1997; Thurston, et al., 1992; Burton, Suh and Koutrakis, 1996). This reflects the dominant influence of region-wide sulfate aerosols as major drivers of local $PM_{2.5}$ concentrations, especially during the summer months. In contrast, measures of direct vehicle emissions such as nitrogen oxides and black smoke exhibit greater spatial variations, and these variations have been associated with local traffic sources (Nitta, et al., 1993; Brunekreef, et al., 1997; Nielsen, 1996). The emerging evidence suggests that DEP and other components of $PM_{2.5}$ for which significant local sources exist are likely to exhibit substantial spatial variability in concentrations within urban areas.

Urban sidewalks serve both as pathways for pedestrian movements and as areas of play and recreation for children of many ages. They also are an important locus for congregation and interaction among adults, including the elderly (Jacobs, 1961). These uses are especially prevalent in the urban core neighborhoods of NYC. Risks to children, the elderly, and other vulnerable groups from breathing diesel exhaust and other air pollutants on sidewalks are of special concern.

The present study is a part of an ongoing community-based research and outreach partnership between two academic centers at Columbia University (the Center for Environmental Health in Northern Manhattan and the Harlem Center for Health Promotion and Disease Prevention) and a community-based organization (West Harlem Environmental Action, Inc., or WEACT). The study was designed to generate pilot data on temporal and spatial variations in sidewalk concentrations of $PM_{2.5}$ and EC at street level, and to relate these data to measures of diesel emissions on adjacent streets. In addition, the study represents an emerging model of community-based research in which researchers and community representatives work as full partners in the design, implementation, analysis, and reporting of the study.

Materials and Methods

Community Background and Site Selection

Harlem is located in the northern half of the borough of Manhattan in NYC (Figure 9.1) and is at the center of a large sprawling metropolitan region. NYC has in recent years been out of compliance with the annual National Ambient Air Quality Standard for PM_{10} (50 μg/m^3). Residents of Northern Manhattan are predominantly low-income persons of African-American and/or Hispanic heritage. Air pollution from diesel exhaust has been of special concern to Harlem residents because of the large volume of diesel truck and bus traffic through the community, and because seven of the eight bus depots in Manhattan are located in Northern Manhattan. Nearly two thousand diesel buses are garaged in Harlem, often in close proximity to schools and housing complexes. Two of the major north/south avenues (Broadway and Amsterdam Avenue) that pass through Harlem are principal truck routes for moving goods in and out of Manhattan.

The four monitoring sites for the present study were selected from a total of eight sites in Harlem that had been targeted, in response to community requests, for intensive PM monitoring by the Region 2 office of the United States Environmental Protection Agency (EPA) in the summer of 1996. Community residents and scientists from Columbia University and the EPA selected all monitoring sites jointly at community forums. Site selection was driven primarily by concerns about high traffic volumes and other diesel exhaust sources (e.g., bus depots). Additional criteria included the proximity of important receptor sites (e.g., schools, hospitals, residential complexes), and the need for a 'control' site in a location less impacted by diesel sources.

The four sites chosen for the study of sidewalk PM$_{2.5}$ and DEP concentrations were as follows.

Site 1 (Amsterdam Ave) was on the northeast corner of 125th Street and Amsterdam Avenue, a busy intersection between two heavily traveled roadways in a residential/commercial neighborhood. Eight separate bus routes pass through this intersection. In addition, Amsterdam Avenue is a principal truck route for delivery of goods in and out of Manhattan.

Site 2 (Bus Depot) was on the south side of 133rd Street between Broadway and 12th Avenue. Although traffic volumes are low on 133rd Street, the Manhattanville Bus Depot, on the south side of the street, spans much of the block. The bus depot is equipped with ventilation ducts directed towards 133rd Street. Across the street to the north is a junior high school. One block west (upwind) is a major highway and a commuter rail line linking the northern suburbs with lower Manhattan.

Site 3 (Harlem Hospital) was on the southwest corner of 135th Street and Lenox Avenue, a busy intersection in a residential/commercial neighborhood with fewer local diesel sources than sites 1 and 2. Adjacent to site 3 on the southwest corner of the intersection is a grammar school, while on the northeast corner are located Harlem Hospital and a subway entrance.

Site 4 (Edgecombe Ave) was on the west side of Edgecombe Avenue between 141st and 142nd Streets. This 'control' site was in a quiet residential neighborhood near several schools.

Particle Concentration Measurements

Monitoring and traffic counting was carried out jointly by staff from Columbia University, WEACT, and the University of Wageningen. Each site was staffed by

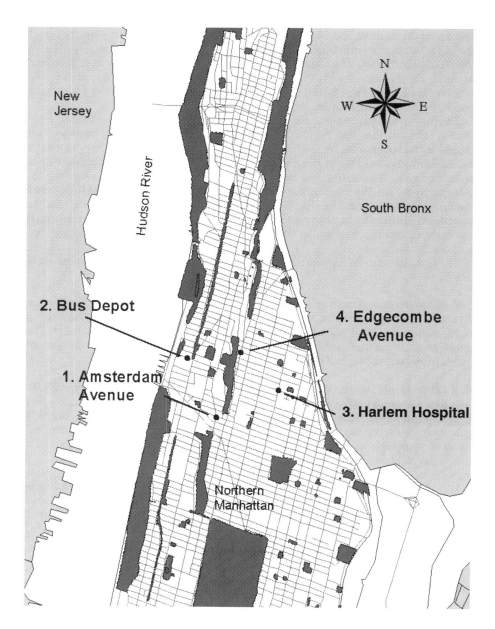

Figure 9.1   Locations of four monitoring sites in the Harlem neighborhood of Northern Manhattan

two to four persons who wore personal particle monitors and, on a subset of days, counted traffic. Although a scientific staff member was present at each site during all sampling events, much of the hands-on work was carried out by members of WEACT's Environmental Leadership Training group (the Earth Crew), a group of 17 paid community interns aged 14 to 18 years. Prior to the start of sampling, scientific staff members assigned to each site were trained in the operation, calibration, and proper placement of the personal samplers by an expert (Ms. Janssen) from the University of Wageningen. The trained scientific staff was responsible, in turn, for oversight of the sampling operations at each site, including the proper physical placement and use by WEACT interns.

At each of the four sites, monitoring for $PM_{2.5}$ and EC was carried out between the hours of 10:00 AM and 6:00 PM on five weekdays in July 1996. July was chosen because of the availability of summer interns and to avoid the heating season when coal and oil furnaces emit EC. We chose to monitor on weekdays for consistency in a small study and to capture typical commercial traffic volumes. The five monitoring days were scattered over a 13-day span.

Air monitors consisted of 4 L/min battery-operated personal sampling pumps (Gillian model Gil-Air 5, Gillian Instrument Corp., W. Caldwell, NJ) attached by flexible tubing to polyethylene filter sampling cartridges (University Research Glassware, Carrboro, NC). The cartridge had an inlet nozzle and a greased impactor plate, which eliminated particles larger than 2.5 μm in aerodynamic diameter from the air stream before collection on the filter.

Pumps were worn at the waist using a belt clip or in a backpack and the sample cartridge was clipped to the shirt collar. Samplers were worn by study staff who sat on folding chairs on the sidewalk facing the flow of traffic. Two identical pump/cartridge sampling assemblies were operated simultaneously at each site (worn by separate individuals), one containing a pre-weighed Teflon filter for gravimetric $PM_{2.5}$ and reflectance analysis and the other containing a quartz fiber filter for EC analysis.

Flow rates were checked by scientific staff prior to and following each air sampling event with pre-calibrated rotameters. Following sampling, cartridges were separated from the tubing and pumps, and were then capped and placed in zip-lock bags for hand transport to the laboratory at Columbia University. At the laboratory, the cartridges were disassembled and the filters were removed in a positive-pressure, particle-free hood by a lab technician. Teflon and quartz filters were placed in individual sterile petri dishes and shipped to external laboratories for $PM_{2.5}$, elemental carbon, and reflectance analyses.

Gravimetric $PM_{2.5}$ Analysis Procedures

Teflon filters were pre- and post-weighed after 24-hour temperature and humidity equilibration in the laboratories of Dr. Petros Koutrakis at the Harvard School of Public Health. A micro-balance connected via serial data port to an IBM-compatible computer, programmed to track mass and tare, was used for weighing. In every batch of 10 samples, the zero, span and linearity of the balance was checked via calibration weights and one filter was randomly chosen for quality assurance (QA) purposes and was weighed by a different individual. $PM_{2.5}$ data have been expressed in μg/m^3.

Elemental Carbon Analysis

The quartz filters were analyzed for elemental carbon by Sunset Laboratory, Inc. (Forest Grove, OR) according to the method of Birch & Cary (1996). The procedure involves heating the sample filter in an oxygen-free helium atmosphere to first remove and measure all organic carbon and then to oxidize and measure the remaining elemental carbon. After all the carbon has been oxidized from the sample, a known volume and concentration of methane is injected into the sample oven, thus calibrating each sample to a known quantity of carbon. Based on the FID response and laser transmission data, the quantities of organic and elemental carbon are calculated for each sample. Elemental carbon data has been expressed in $\mu g/m^3$.

Reflectance Analysis

Following the post-weighing to determine $PM_{2.5}$, Teflon filters were sent to the University of Wageningen, The Netherlands, for reflectance analysis. The blackness of the $PM_{2.5}$ filter deposit was measured using a reflectometer (EEL model #43). Blank filters were used to set reflection to 100%. Reflectance of each sampled filter was measured three times to document homogeneity. The absorption coefficient was calculated using the following formula (ISO 9835):

$$\text{abs coeff } (m^{-1}) = 0.5 \, A * \ln (RO/RF)/V$$

where A= loaded filter area; RO = reflection of field blanks (in percentage); RF = reflection of sampled filters (in percentage); V = Sampled volume of air (m^3). The average of three readings was used to calculate the absorption coefficient, which was then multiplied by 10^5 to make the readings more comprehensible. The reflectance data are expressed as absorption coefficient of the sample filter.

Traffic Counting

Project staff counted traffic for an 8-hr period at each site on at least two air monitoring days using traffic counting boards. Each counting board was equipped with four manually operated digital counters to enable simultaneous counts of diesel buses, diesel trucks, cars, and pedestrians. Counting was carried out in 15-minute active periods alternating with 15-minute rest periods from 10:00 AM to 4:00 PM and in continuous 15-minute blocks from 4:00 PM to 6:00 PM. The two study staff assigned to each traffic counting location took turns counting for the 15-minute blocks. For purposes of reporting, total eight-hour counts were estimated by summing the 4:00 PM to 6:00 PM counts with twice the 10:00 AM to 4:00 PM counts. These daily counts were then averaged across days at each site.

Staff was trained in traffic counting methods by a traffic engineer from Garman Associates, Inc. (Mr. Northridge), who volunteered both time and equipment to this effort. During two training sessions on a busy intersection in Harlem, staff were instructed in the use of counting boards, in the proper traffic lanes and directions to be counted, and in the identification of heavy-duty diesel vehicles (trucks and buses) as distinct from cars and light-duty trucks. All buses were assumed to be diesel powered (during the period of study, all NYC buses used diesel fuel). All trucks larger than pickup trucks, including delivery trucks and "18 wheelers," were counted as diesel trucks. Vans and sport utility vehicles were counted as cars.

At the two four-way traffic intersection (sites 1 and 3), two teams of Earth Crew members sat on diagonal corners in order to count traffic in all directions. One team of two individuals counted traffic moving from W to E and N to S, while the other team counted traffic from E to W and S to N. Counting at sites 1 and 3 occurred on three separate days. At sites 2 and 4, which were in mid-block rather than at intersections, a single team of counters counted traffic in both directions. Counting at sites 2 and 4 occurred on two separate days.

No direct validation of identified traffic counts (i.e., the type of vehicle) was available for the study. Total visual traffic counts (buses+trucks+cars) were validated using an automatic traffic counter for three hours on one day at sites 2 (Bus Depot), 3 (Harlem Hospital) and 4 (Edgecombe Ave). This automated counting was done using pneumatic tubes laid across the road and connected to an automatic data logger.

Statistical Analysis

Simple descriptive statistics were tabulated and plotted to examine the spatial and temporal variations in street-level PM$_{2.5}$ and EC. To assess the relative magnitude of spatial and temporal variations in PM$_{2.5}$ and DEP concentrations, data were analyzed by two-way analysis of variance with site and day as the two main effects.

Results

Cumulative eight-hour traffic counts for trucks, buses, cars, and pedestrians at the four sites are summarized in Table 9.1 and plotted graphically in Figure 9.2. Average total diesel vehicle counts (trucks + buses) varied markedly across intersections, from lows of 61 and 102 diesel vehicles at sites 4 (Edgecombe Ave) and site 2 (Bus Depot) respectively to 2467 vehicles at site 1 (Amsterdam Ave). An intermediate level (927 vehicles) was observed at site 3 (Harlem Hospital). Truck and bus counts correlated closely with one another across sites (Figure 9.2); however, truck counts always exceeded bus counts. Together, diesel trucks and buses represented between 4 and 12 percent of all motor vehicles observed at the four intersections. In addition, car and pedestrian counts tended to correlate with diesel counts, demonstrating that locations with more vehicle traffic of all kinds also had more exposed pedestrians. To validate the traffic counts automated total vehicle counters were installed for three hours at each of three sites. The correlation between the hourly counts by the two methods was 0.995. The percent differences between counts were within plus or minus 5% for 8/9 hours. For the one outlier, the visual counts were 16% high.

Table 9.2 displays eight-hour concentrations of PM$_{2.5}$ and elemental carbon (EC) collected at each site on each day of sampling, as well as averages by site and by day. Average PM$_{2.5}$ concentrations exhibited modest variations across sites, ranging from 36.6 and 38.6 µg/m^3 at sites 3 (Harlem Hospital) and 4 (Edgecombe Ave),

Table 9.1   Mean and range (across days) of daily eight-hour weekday traffic counts at four sites in Harlem

Site	Location	# Days	Diesel Trucks	Buses	Cars	Pedestrians
1	Amsterdam Ave. and 125th St. (Heavy Traffic)	3	1,403 (±34)	1,064 (±67)	18,375 (±1,473)	11,158 (±1,752)
2	West 133rd St. (Bus Depot)	2	75 (±1)	28 (±4)	2302 (±112)	421 (±120)
3	East 135th St. (Harlem Hospital)	3	526 (±80)	401 (±43)	14,229 (±225)	16,760 (±2,620)
4	Edgecombe Ave. (Control)	2	47 (±4)	14 (±0)	1,411 (±190)	1,320 (±240)

respectively, to 45.8 and 47.1 $\mu g/m^3$ at sites 1 (Amsterdam Ave) and 2 (Bus Depot). Further, there was only a modest association between $PM_{2.5}$ concentrations and proximity to local diesel traffic (data not shown). Variations across days in mean $PM_{2.5}$ concentrations were more pronounced than were spatial variations, with daily means ranging from 26.5 $\mu g/m^3$ on day 5 to 53.5 $\mu g/m^3$ on day 4. A two-way ANOVA showed that 73 percent of the variation in $PM_{2.5}$ concentrations was explained by the day effect (i.e., temporal variations) whereas only 14 percent was explained by the site effect (i.e., geographic variations).

In contrast to the situation for $PM_{2.5}$, a strong spatial gradient was observed across sites in EC concentrations, reflecting the importance of local diesel traffic sources (Table 9.2). There was a four-fold difference in mean EC concentrations (1.5 to 6.2 $\mu g/m3$) between the two sites which had the largest contrast in diesel traffic counts (sites 1 and 4). This is shown graphically in Figure 9.3, which plots mean EC concentrations against total diesel vehicle counts at the four intersections. One outlier on this plot is site 2 (Bus Depot), which exhibited elevated EC (and $PM_{2.5}$) concentrations and yet had very low traffic counts. This is most likely due to the impact of the adjacent Manhattanville Bus Depot (with ventilation ducts facing towards the site) as well as the West Side Highway, one block to the west. Thus, although local traffic on 133rd Street itself was very light during the study, the air at the site appeared to be heavily impacted by local diesel and other mobile source emissions.

Variations across days in EC concentrations were much less pronounced than were spatial variations (Table 9.2). This contrasts with the pattern observed for $PM_{2.5}$, where temporal variations were dominant. In a two-way ANOVA (site x day), site-to-site variations explained 76% of the total variation in EC concentrations (i.e., $R^2 = 0.76$) and were highly statistically significant. In contrast, variations across days explained only 6% of the total variations in EC and were not significant. The ratio of EC to $PM_{2.5}$ (i.e., the fraction of $PM_{2.5}$ represented by EC) varied from 0.064 to 0.11 across the five days.

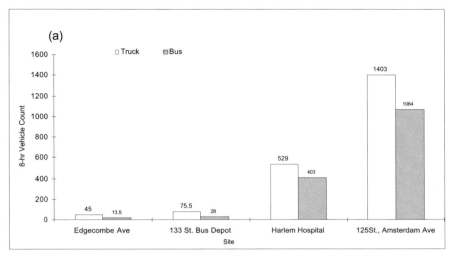

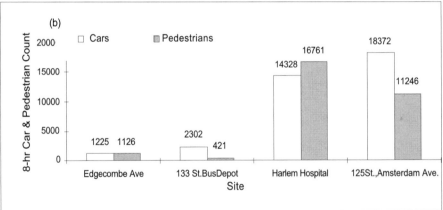

Figure 9.2   Average 10:00 AM to 6:00 PM weekday traffic counts at four sites in Harlem: (a) heavy-duty trucks and buses, (b) cars and pedestrians

The Teflon filters used for measuring PM$_{2.5}$ concentrations were subsequently analyzed by reflectance to determine the absorption coefficient of the particle deposit, a potential surrogate for EC content of the sample. Recall that EC analyses were performed on quartz fiber filter samples collected along side the Teflon PM$_{2.5}$ samples using identical sampling equipment for all sampling events. The scatterplot of EC vs. absorption coefficient (x 100) for the 20 paired samples (four sites for each of five days) indicates a close correspondence between the two measures (Figure 5), with a correlation of 0.95. The regression of EC on absorption coefficient (x 100) yielded a slope of 0.83 µg/m^2 and a non-significant y-intercept. There was no

Table 9.2   Eight-hour average (10:00 AM–6:00 PM) PM$_{2.5}$ and elemental carbon concentrations (µg/m3) at four Harlem sites

Site #	Pollutant	July 17	July 18	July 24	July 25	July 29	Mean(S.D.)
1	PM2.5	40.4	51.7	46.3	58.3	32.0	45.7(10.1)
	EC	7.9	7.6	4.9	7.0	3.6	6.2(1.9)
2	PM2.5	33.0	47.4	56.2	69.1	29.6	47.1(16.4)
	EC	2.8	4.0	4.2	3.3	4.0	3.7(0.6)
3	PM2.5	30.5	37.6	49.7	43.1	22.1	36.6(10.8)
	EC	3.3	2.7	2.8	1.6	1.3	2.3(0.9)
4	PM2.5	33.6	43.4	50.6	43.3	22.4	38.7(10.9)
	EC	1.1	1.4	2.4	1.6	1.1	1.5(0.5)
Mean (S.D.)	PM2.5	34.4 (4.2)	45.0 (6.0)	50.7 (4.1)	53.4 (12.6)	26.5 (5.0)	42.0
	EC (2.9)	3.8 (2.7)	3.9 (1.2)	3.6 (2.5)	3.4 (1.5)	2.5	3.4

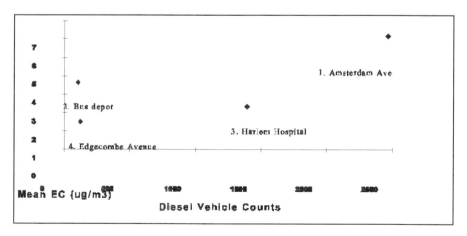

Figure 9.3   Scatterplot of mean elemental carbon concentrations and diesel vehicle counts (heavy-duty trucks and buses) at four monitoring sites in Harlem

evidence that the relationship varied by site. These results suggest that absorption coefficient has utility as a surrogate for fine particle EC concentrations in NYC during summer months.

Discussion

This study demonstrated consistent spatial variations in sidewalk DEP concentrations on the sidewalks of Harlem that appeared to be related to the magnitude of local diesel sources. Spatial variations in sidewalk PM$_{2.5}$, of which DEP forms a part, exhibited less pronounced spatial gradients, due presumably to the influence of regional sulfate aerosols. The observation of spatial variations in DEP exposures implies that health risks associated with diesel exhaust particles may also vary across the community as a function of diesel source density.

Although only a small number of sites and days were monitored in this pilot study, these preliminary results suggest that DEP concentrations are influenced both by vehicular traffic (of which diesel vehicles are assumed to be of special importance) and by point sources such as bus depots where large numbers of diesel vehicles congregate. These basic patterns reinforce concerns that have been raised by community residents about the predominance of both diesel traffic and bus depots in Harlem and other disadvantaged neighborhoods of NYC.

Average concentrations of EC ranged from 1.5 to 6.2 µg/m^3 across the four sites studied, levels that are typical of those reported in other urban areas. We know of no previous studies of sidewalk-level EC concentrations. Annual average outdoor EC concentrations ranged from 3 to 5 µg/m^3 across 10 monitoring sites in the Los Angeles basin in 1982 (Gray and Cass, 1986). Daily 24-hour average values at the Lenox site ranged from approximately 1 µg/m^3 to 17 µg/m^3, with late Fall and early Winter concentrations far exceeding those measured in other seasons. Data collected in 1987 as part of the Southern California Air Quality Study indicated average EC concentrations in summer and fall ranging from 0.10 µg/m^3, at a remote site on San Nicholas Island, to 2.6 µg/m^3 in Azusa, a densely populated community on the northeastern, downwind portion of the basin (Chow, Watson, & Fujita, 1994). The maximum daily EC concentration measured in 1987 in Los Angeles was 5.4 µg/m^3. Thus, EC concentrations observed in the present study were comparable with these levels observed in the 1980's in Los Angeles.

Spatial variations in sidewalk PM$_{2.5}$ exposures were less pronounced and less associated with vehicular traffic than were EC concentrations in the present study. This is consistent with previous studies, which have shown that local PM$_{2.5}$ concentrations in northeastern United States cities are dominated by regional sulfate particles during the summer months (Suh, et al., 1997; Thurston, et al., 1992; Burton, Suh and Koutrakis, 1996). The contributions of local fine particle sources such as diesel exhaust are difficult to discern against the high background levels of regional sulfate aerosol when using a composite particulate metric such as PM$_{2.5}$. Because elemental carbon represents only a portion of the total mass of particles present in diesel exhaust, it is not possible from our data to directly estimate the fraction of PM$_{2.5}$ that was due to DEP. Cass and Gray estimated that elemental carbon represented 59.5 percent of the mass of diesel exhaust particles observed in the Los

Angeles atmosphere (Cass & Gray, 1995). Assuming that the mixes of diesel sources are roughly comparable in the two cities, we can apply this correction factor to the mean EC concentration observed in the present study to calculate the average total mass of DEP. This exercise yields an estimated average total DEP mass of 5.7 $\mu g/m^3$, which is 13.6 percent of the average $PM_{2.5}$ mass we observed.

In order to characterize patterns of exposure to locally generated particles in urban areas, it is critical to measure one or more components of fine particles which are specific to the source in question. In the case of diesel exhaust, EC and filter reflectance appear to represent useful surrogate measures of DEP exposure. It has been estimated that the majority of EC emissions in Los Angeles originate from diesel engines (Gray and Cass, 1986). Several previous studies have reported strong correlations between EC concentrations and diesel vehicle traffic (Delumyea, Chu, and Macias, 1980; Pierson, 1978). This is likely to hold true for NYC and other northeastern United States cities during the summer months when no combustion of oil or coal for space heating occurs. The strong association between EC concentrations and local diesel sources in our study provides support for this idea.

Studies on the health effects of diesel exhaust have until recently focused primarily on cancer outcomes (Bhatia, Lopipero, and Smith, 1998). However, in recent years, attention has begun to focus on understanding the non-cancer respiratory effects of diesel exhaust particles and their possible role in the acute or chronic health effects of airborne particulate matter. There is emerging experimental evidence of irritant and/or immunologic effects of diesel exhaust on the respiratory system (Diaz-Sanchez, 1997; Bayram et al., 1998; Kobayashi et al., 1997; Peterson and Saxon, 1996; Suzuki et al., 1996; Terada et al., 1997). In addition, recent epidemiological studies have demonstrated associations between residential proximity to traffic sources and adverse respiratory outcomes, including asthma hospitalizations among children (Edwards, Walters & Griffiths, 1994), increased respiratory symptoms (Van et al., 1997; Duhme et al., 1996; Wjst et al., 1993), and diminished lung function (Nitta et al., 1993; Brunekreef et al., 1997). Exposure assessment in these studies has included self-reported traffic volumes on residential streets (e.g., high, medium, low), quantitative data on traffic volumes collected by local agencies, and, occasionally, air monitoring data at selected locations. Given the limitations of the exposure data, it is not always possible to uniquely implicate diesel exhaust as distinct from other forms of motor vehicle exhaust in the observed respiratory health effects. However, in one recent study in the Netherlands, chronic respiratory symptoms and lung function decrements in children were associated with local truck traffic density and with black smoke concentrations in schools, whereas no such associations were observed for car traffic, suggesting a specific effect of diesel exhaust (Brunekreef et al., 1997). In addition, the recent experimental studies cited above highlight the role of DEP in enhancing inflammatory and allergic responses in the respiratory system.

New York City is one of four metropolitan areas that lead the United States in annual increase of asthma mortality among 5–34 year olds (Weiss & Wagener, 1990). An investigation of small area variations in asthma hospitalizations in New York City revealed that several sections of Harlem are among those with the highest rates (Carr, Zeitel, and Weiss, 1992). The possible role of diesel exhaust in these alarming asthma statistics has been a prominent concern of Harlem residents in recent years. The present study, while demonstrating spatial variations in diesel exhaust exposures within Harlem, did not address whether exposures in Harlem exceeded those in other areas in New York City or elsewhere, nor whether the observed variations in Harlem were associated with variations in asthma rates.

An interesting result of this study was the high degree of correlation between EC concentrations measured analytically on quartz fiber filters and the simple reflectance-based absorption coefficient measurements of the Teflon filters used for PM$_{2.5}$ analysis (r=0.95; Figure 9.4). These results suggest that absorption coefficient has utility as a surrogate for fine particle EC concentrations in NYC during summer months. A similarly high correlation of 0.96 was found between elemental carbon and black smoke in a recent comparison study conducted in Berlin (Ulrich and Israel, 1992).

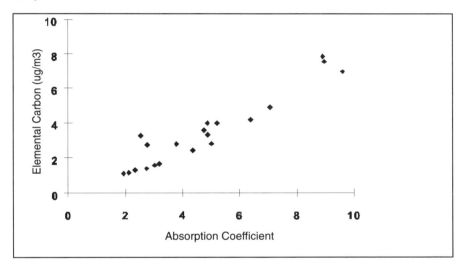

Figure 9.4   **Correlation between co-located elemental carbon concentrations, measured on quartz fiber filters, and absorption coefficient, measured on PM$_{2.5}$ filters**

In addition to providing new scientific data on patterns of exposure to diesel exhaust particles in an urban setting, the present study also demonstrated the feasibility of an emerging model of community-based research addressing environmental health problems in underprivileged communities. In this study, researchers and community representatives worked as full partners in the design, implementation, analysis, and reporting of the data. The study also provided a mechanism for training young people from the community in research methods applied to environmental health problems. It is hoped that this model for community-based research will find application in other settings where there is a natural intersection between community health concerns and public health research needs.

Acknowledgments

The authors wish to thank Luis Benitez, Cecil Corbin-Mark, John Gorzenski, Sergey Nikiforov, Kevin Northridge, and the members of the WE-ACT Earth Crew for their active support and contributions to the success of this study. We especially wish to thank Dr. Bert Brunekreef of the University of Wageningen, The Netherlands, for generously loaning the personal monitoring pumps used in this study.

References

Bayram, H., Devalia, J.L., Sapsford, R.J., Ohtoshi, T., Miyabara, Y., Sagai, M. and Davies, R.J. (1998), "The Effect of diesel exhaust particles on cell function and release of inflammatory mediators from human bronchial epithelial cells in vitro", *Am J Respir Cell Mol Biol*, **18**, 441–48.

Bhatia, R., Lopipero, P. and Smith, A.H. (1998), "Diesel exhaust exposure and lung cancer", *Epidemiology*, **9**, 84–91.

Birch, M.E. and Cary, R.A. (1996), "Elemental carbon based method for monitoring occupational exposures to particulate diesel exhaust", *Aerosol Sciences Tech*, **25**, 221–41.

Brunekreef, B., Janssen, N.A.H., de Hartog, J., Hassema, H., Knape, M. and van Vliet, P. (1997), "Air pollution from truck traffic and lung function in children living near motorways", *Epidemiology*, **8**, 298–303.

Burton, R.M., Suh, H.H. and Koutrakis, P. (1996), "Spatial variation in particulate concentrations within metropolitan Philadelphia", *Environ Sci Tech*, **30**, 400–407.

Carr, W., Zeitel, L. and Weiss, K. (1992), "Variations in asthma hospitalizations and deaths in New York City", *Am J Public Health*, **82**, 59–65.

Cass, G.R. and Gray, H.A. (1995), "Regional emissions and atmospheric concentrations of diesel engine particulate matter: Los Angeles as a case study", in *Diesel Exhaust: A Critical Analysis of Emissions, Exposure, and Health Effects*, A Special Report of the Institute's Diesel Working Group, Health Effects Institute, Cambridge.

Chow, J.C., Watson, J.G. and Fujita, E.M. (1994), "Temporal and spatial variations of PM2.5 and PM10 aerosol in the southern California air quality study", *Atmos Environ*, **28**, 2061–80.

Delumyea, R.G., Chu, L.C. and Macias, E.S. (1980), "Determination of elemental carbon component of soot in ambient samples", *Atmos Environ*, **1**, 647–52.

Diaz-Sanchez, D. (1997), "The role of diesel exhaust particles and their associated polyaromatic hydrocarbons in the induction of allergic airway disease", *Allergy*, **52** (suppl 38), 52–56.

Dockery, D.W. and Pope, C.A. (1994), "Acute respiratory effects of particulate air pollution", *Ann Rev Public Health*, **15**, 107–32.

Dockery, D.W., Pope, C.A., Xu, X., Spengler, J.D., Ware, J.H., Fay, M.E., Ferris, B.G. and Speizer, F.E. (1993), "An association between air pollution and mortality in six US cities", *N Engl J. Med*, **329**, 1753–9.

Duhme, H., Weiland, S.K., Keil, U., Kraemer, B., Schmid, M., Stender, M. and Chabless, L. (1996), "The association between self reported symptoms of asthma and allergic rhinitis and self reported traffic density on street of residence in adolescents", *Epidemiology*, **7**, 578–82.

Edwards, J., Walters, S. and Griffiths, R.K. (1994), "Hospital admissions for asthma in pre-school children: relationship to major roads in Birmingham, United Kingdom", *Arch Environ Health*, **49**, 223–7.

Godlee, F. (1993), "Air Pollution II. Road traffic and modern industry", *Br Med J*, **303**, 1539–43.

Gray, H.A. and Cass, G.R. (1986), "Characteristics of atmospheric organic and elemental carbon particle concentrations in Los Angeles", *Environ Sci Technol*, **20**, 580–89.

Jacobs, J. (1961), *The Death and Life of Great American Cities*, Random House, New York.

Kobayashi, T., Takahisa, I., Tsuyoshi, I., Ikeda, A., Murakami, M., Kato, A., Maejima, K., Nakajima, T. and Suzuki, T. (1997), "Short-term exposure to diesel exhaust induces nasal mucosal hyperresponsiveness to histamine in guinea pigs", *Fund Appl Tox*, **38**, 166–72.

Nielsen, T. (1996), "Traffic contribution of polycyclic aromatic hydrocarbons in the center of a large city", *Atmos Environ*, **30**, 3481–90.

Nitta, H., Sato, T., Nakai, S., Maeda, K., Aoki, S. and Ono, M. (1993), "Respiratory health associated with exposure to automobile exhaust: 1", Results of cross-sectional studies in 1979, 1982 and 1983, *Arch Environ Health*, **48**, 53–8.

Ostro, B.D. (1987), "Air pollution and morbidity revisited: a specification test", *J Environ Econ Management*, **14**, 87–98.

Peterson, B. and Saxon, A. (1996), "Global increases in allergic respiratory disease: the possible role of diesel exhaust particles", *Ann Allergy Asthma Immunol*, **77**, 262–70.

Pierson, W.R. (1978), in T. Novakov (ed) Proceedings: "Carbonaceous Particles in the Atmosphere", Lawrence Berkeley Laboratory, Berkeley, California.

Pope, C.A., Thun, M.J., Namboodiri, M.M., Dockery, D.W., Evans, J.S., Speizer, F.E. and Heath, C.W. (1995), "Particulate air pollution as a predictor of mortality in a prospective study of US adults", *Am J Resp Crit Care Med*, **151**, 669–74.

Schwartz, J., Slater, D., Larson, T.V., Pierson, W.E. and Koenig, J.Q. (1993), "Particulate air pollution and hospital emergency visits for asthma in Seattle", *Am Rev Respir Dis*, **147**, 826–31.

Suh, H.H., Nishioka, Y., Allen, G.A., Koutrakis, P. and Burton, R.M. (1997), "The Metropolitan acid aerosol characterization study: Results from the summer 1994 Washington, D.C. field study", *Environ Health Perspect*, **105**, 826–33.

Suzuki, T., Kanoh, T., Ishimori, M., Ikeda, S. and Ohkuni, H. (1996), "Adjuvant activity of diesel exhaust particulates (DEP) in production of anti-IgE and anti-IgG1 antibodies to mite allergen in mice", *J Clin Immunol*, **48**, 187–99.

Terada, N., Maesako, K., Hiruma, K., Hamano, N., Houki, G., Konno, A., Ikeda, T. and Sai, M. (1997), "Diesel exhaust particulates enhance eosinophil adhesion to nasal epithelial cells and cause degranulation", *Int Arch Allergy Immunol*, **114**, 167–74.

Thurston, G.D., Ito, K., Hayes, C.G., Bates, D.V. and Lippman, M. (1994), "Respiratory hospital admissions and summertime haze air pollution in Toronto, Ontario: consideration for the role of acid aerosols", *Environ Res*, **65**, 271–90.

Thurston, G.D., Ito, K., Kinney, P.L. and Lippmann, P. (1992), "A multi-year study of air pollution and respiratory hospital admissions in three New York State metropolitan areas: Results for 1988 and 1989 summers", *J Expos Anal Environ Epidemiol*, **2**, 429-450.

Ulrich, E. and Israel, G.W. (1992), "Diesel soot measurement under traffic conditions", *J Aerosol Sci*, **23**, S925–S928.

Van Vliet, P., Knape, M., de Hartog, J., Janssen, N.A.H., Harssema, J. and Brunekreef, B. (1997), "Motor vehicle exhaust and chronic respiratory symptoms in children living near freeways", *Environ Res*, **74**, 122–32.

Weiss, K.B. and Wagener, D.K. (1990), "Changing patterns of asthma mortality: identifying target populations at high risk", *J Am Med Assoc*, **264**, 1683–7.

WHO (1996), *Environmental Health Criteria 171: Diesel Fuel and Exhaust Emissions*, World Health Organization, Geneva.

Wjst, M., Reitmeir, O., Dold, S., Wulff, A., Nicolai, T., Loeffelholz-Colberg, E.F.V., Mutius, E.V. (1993), "Road traffic and adverse effects on respiratory health in children", *Br Med J*, **307**, 596–600.

SECTION D:
ENVIRONMENTAL EXPOSURE

Chapter 10

Environmental Justice and Regional Inequality in Southern California: Implications for Future Research

Rachel Morello-Frosch, Manuel Pastor Jr., Carlos Porras and James Sadd

Environmental justice, with its emphasis on public health, social inequality, and environmental degradation, provides a framework for public policy debates about the impact of discrimination on the environmental health of diverse communities in the United States. Indeed, activists, academics, and some decision makers argue that biases within environmental policy making and the regulatory process, combined with discriminatory market forces, result in disproportionate exposures to hazardous pollution among the poor and communities of color. The environmental justice framework also raises the challenging question of whether disparities in exposures to environmental hazards may play an important, yet poorly understood, role in the complex and persistent patterns of disparate health status among the poor and people of color in the United States (Ecob and Davey, 1999; Kawachi and Marmot, 1998; Krieger, et al., 1993; Syme S, Berkman, 1976).

In seeking to redress disparities in exposures to toxics, communities organizing for environmental justice offer environmental health researchers new insights into the junctures of social inequality and public health on one hand, and the political and economic forces that lead to environmental inequality on the other. Emerging research on the broad question of environmental justice attempts to elucidate how socioeconomic and institutional forces create "riskscapes" in which overlapping pollution plumes, emitted by various sources into our air, soil, food, and water, pose a range of health risks to diverse communities, all of which in turn determine inequalities in community susceptibility to environmental hazards. The environmental justice movement has also sparked contentious debates among researchers, policy makers, activists, and industry as to whether environmental discrimination actually exists and why, or whether it is simply the result of other structural forces (Anderton, et al., 1994; Bullard, 1993; Pulido, 1996; Pastor, Sadd and Hipp, 2001; Foreman, 1991). These debates have fueled a surge of academic and scientific inquiry into the question of environmental inequality in the United States over the last two decades.

Research on race and class differences in exposures to toxics varies widely, ranging from anecdotal and descriptive studies to rigorous statistical modeling that quantifies the extent to which race and/or class explain disparities in environmental hazards among diverse communities. Although by no means unequivocal, much of the evidence points to a pattern of disproportionate exposures to toxics and associated health risks among communities of color and the poor, with racial differences sometimes persisting across economic strata (Mohai and Bryant, 1992; Szasz and Meuser, 1997).

Nevertheless, causally linking the presence of environmental pollution with potentially adverse health effects is an ongoing challenge in the environmental health field, particularly in situations in which populations are chronically exposed to complex chemical mixtures (Institute of Medicine, 1999). With few exceptions, researchers examining environmental inequalities have limited their inquiries to evaluating differences in the location of pollution sources between population groups, while placing less emphasis on evaluating the distribution of exposures or, more important, potential health risks. Of special concern has been the need to move beyond chemical-by-chemical or facility-by-facility analysis toward a cumulative exposure approach that accounts for the exposure realities of diverse populations and incorporates concepts of race and class into assessments of community susceptibility to environmental pollutants (Morello-Frosch, Pastor and Sadd, 2001).

We review the evolution of a three-year environmental justice research initiative in Southern California carried out through an academic and community-based collaborative. Our methodological approach entails a regional focus, starting with the premise of previous environmental research that examines the racial distribution of facility siting. We then expand upon this locational approach to look at issues more closely related to health, such as outdoor concentrations of air toxics and associated cancer risks, and then to answer the complex question of temporal trends. Implications of the study results in Southern California for policy making and developing a framework for future research are discussed in the conclusion.

Creating a Regional Collaborative for Environmental Health and Justice

In 1998, the authors, along with other community partners in Southern California, formed an academic–community partnership to address environmental justice issues facing people of color and low-income communities in the Los Angeles Air Basin. (The lead author joined this community-academic collaborative in 1999.) In addition to training, organizing, and policy advocacy, a significant component of this collaborative supported research that would elucidate potential patterns of disproportionate exposures to environmental hazards among diverse communities in the region. Within the collaborative, potential research topics could be proposed by any partner – community or academic – and priorities and project development were decided in a way that was relevant to community organizing and environmental policy making. Although community partners had the most significant influence in the development of the collaborative research agenda, they prioritized basic environmental health research and risk assessment to address some of the persistent methodological challenges in the field of environmental justice research. We have worked toward this goal by making use of advances in air emissions inventories, such as the Toxic Release Inventory (TRI) and ambient air exposure modeling data (U.S. EPA, 1991; Rosenbaum, Ligocki, and Wei, 1999; Rosenbaum et al., 1999). Until recently, there has been a paucity of research in which such environmental health and exposure information have been disaggregated by race and socioeconomic status (U.S. EPA, 1992).

We chose to focus our research efforts on Southern California for several reasons: First, the region has a unique regulatory history in terms of its ongoing struggle to solve some of the worst air pollution problems in the country while still promoting economic growth. Second, Southern California already comprises a majority of people of color and is rapidly becoming a bellwether of demographic and socioeconomic change for the state as well as the nation. Third, a regional focus in environmental justice research is crucial because industrial clusters, transportation planning, and economic development decisions are often regionally rooted. Thus, the equity question is how the social and environmental health effects of such industries are distributed within the regions that host them. Fourth, minority and low-income communities in the region have become increasingly concerned about whether they bear a disproportionate burden of exposures to air pollution and their associated environmental health risks. Thus, our collaborative is connected to community-based strategies for achieving environmental justice and rooted in a region where organizing on various environmental health issues is already happening. This also makes the results of our research directly relevant to ongoing policy efforts of the South Coast Air Quality Management District to address environmental inequality and to a new state legislative mandate, a law that directs California's Office of Planning and Research to coordinate the state's environmental justice initiatives with the federal government and across state agencies, including the California Environmental Protection Agency (California Senate Bill 115, 1999). Finally, the relevance of our work extends beyond Southern California; understanding the patterns in this region may inform studies and policies elsewhere as local, state, and federal policy makers are compelled to consider the equity concerns of diverse communities impacted by environmental health risks from hazardous exposures.

In our research we sought to develop various indicators for assessing environmental inequalities: location of potentially hazardous stationary pollution sources such as TRI facilities and treatment, storage, and disposal facilities (TSDFs), and estimated cancer risks associated with outdoor air toxics exposures. We also sought to use the regulatory tools of risk assessment in a comparative framework to answer scientific and policy questions about what ambient concentrations of certain pollutants might in fact mean for distributions of potential health risks among diverse communities. In short, we wanted to address the ultimate question: Is there environmental inequality in Southern California, and if so, who bears the burden? Our application of traditional regulatory risk assessment in a comparative framework provides a useful policy tool, particularly in situations in which epidemiological data are not available and yet where time-sensitive decisions about disparate impact must be made, such as the judicial and administrative examination of Title VI complaints (42 U.S.C. §§ 2000d to 2000d-7) (Civil Rights Act of 1964).

Evolution of Research Methodology and Results

Locational Studies

Following the lead of early watershed studies on environmental inequality (Mohai & Bryant, 1992; GAO, 1983; United Church of Christ, 1987; Bullard, 1983) our first two studies in Southern California examined the location of TSDFs in Los Angeles and TRI facilities in the entire region. The first study examining TSDFs found significant demographic differences between tracts with TSDFs versus tracts without (Boer et al., 1997). Those tracts hosting a TSDF or located within a one-mile radius of a TSDF had significantly higher percentages of residents of color (particularly Latinos), lower per capita and household incomes, and a lower proportion of registered voters. Logistic regression results (Table 10.1) indicate that communities most impacted by TSDF location in Los Angeles County are working-class communities of color located in predominantly industrial areas. Following previous research (Boer et al., 1997; Been, 1995; Sadd et al., 1999), we found that the relationship between income and TSDF location is curvilinear, following an inverted U-shaped curve in which extremely poor tracts have fewer facilities because of less economic and industrial activity, whereas wealthier residents tend to live in tracts with fewer TSDFs, most likely because of their political power to resist pollution generating activities. This result remained consistent even when the percentages of African American and Latino residents were evaluated as separate groupings (not shown).

Table 10.1   Logistic regression results for association between TSDF location and race/ethnicity, economic, and land use variables

Independent variable	Parameter estimate (t-statistic)
Residents of color (%)	0.03 (6.32)***
Population density	0.00 (0.15)
Employment in manufacturing (%)	0.02 (2.22)**
Per capita income	0.03 (2.59)***
(Per capita income)^2	−0.00 (−2.45)***
Industrial land use (%)	0.03 (7.30)**

$n = 1,636$ tracts. $R^2 = 0.17$. ***$p < 0.01$. **$p < 0.05$.

Our second locational study broadened its regional scope by including the South Coast Air Quality Management District (which includes Ventura, Los Angeles, Orange, San Bernardino, and Riverside counties) and examining the distribution of facilities required to report air emissions to the TRI of the U.S. Environmental Protection Agency (U.S. EPA) (Sadd et al., 1999). The study distinguished between all TRI facilities and those facilities releasing pollutants classified by the U.S. EPA as high priority for reduction and therefore included in the agency's 33/50 program. (The 33/50 program was designed to target 17 priority chemicals, most of them carcinogens, and set as its goal a 33% reduction in releases and transfers of these chemicals by 1992 and a 50% reduction by 1995 [using a 1988 baseline].) Study results indicated that compared with Anglo residents, Latinos have twice the likelihood of living in a tract with a TRI facility with 33/50 releases, followed closely by African Americans. Logistic regression controlling for income, industrial land use, and population density found that the proportion of minority residents was significantly associated with proximity to a TRI facility (Table 10.2). A similar curvilinear relationship with income was also observed in this locational study.

Table 10.2   Logistic regression results for association between TRI location and race/ethnicity, economic, and land use variables

Independent variable	Parameter estimate (*t*-statistic)
Residents of color (%)	0.01 (5.34)***
Population density	−0.00 (0.12)
Employment in manufacturing (%)	0.10 (15.1)***
Per capita income	0.03 (3.50)***
(Per capita income)^2	−0.00 (−3.91)***
Industrial land use (%)	0.05 (10.7)**

$n = 2{,}567$ tracts. $R^2 = 0.17$. ***$p < 0.01$; **$p < 0.05$.

Disparities in Outdoor Air Pollution Exposures and Estimated Cancer Risks

Although our preliminary studies focused on the location of potentially hazardous facilities, we sought to quantitatively assess the implications of outdoor air pollution exposures for potential disparities in estimated individual lifetime cancer risks among diverse communities (Morello-Frosch, Pastor and Sadd, 2001). Making use of a recent modeling analysis undertaken by the U.S. EPA's Cumulative Exposure Project (Rosenbaum et al., 1999; Caldwell et al., 1998; Woodruff et al., 1998; Morello-Frosch et al., 2000), our study combined estimated long-term annual average outdoor concentrations of 148 air toxics, or hazardous air pollutants (HAPs), listed under the 1990 Clean Air Act Amendments (Clean Air Act Amendments of 1990). We combined these data with demographic and land use information from the 1990 U.S. Census and the Southern California Association of Governments. Our study examined a broader scope of air pollutants than previous environmental justice studies, incorporating outdoor HAP concentrations originating from mobile sources (e.g., cars), as well as pollutants from industrial manufacturing facilities, municipal waste combustors, small service industries, and other area emitters. By combining modeled concentration estimates with cancer toxicity information, we derived estimates of lifetime cancer risks and analyzed their distribution among populations in the region.

Estimated lifetime cancer risks associated with outdoor air toxics exposures in the South Coast Air Basin were found to be ubiquitously high, often exceeding the Clean Air Act Goal of one in one million by between one and three orders of magnitude. [In 1990, Congress established a health-based goal for the Clean Air Act: to reduce lifetime cancer risks from major sources of hazardous air pollutants to one in one million. The Act required that over time, U.S. EPA regulations for major sources should "provide an ample margin of safety to protect public health" (Clean Air Act Amendments of 1990).] Figure 10.1 presents source contributions to total air toxics concentrations and total estimated excess lifetime cancer incidence with the effects of background concentrations removed. Background concentrations are attributable to long-range transport, resuspension of historical emissions, and natural sources derived from measurements taken at clean air locations remote from known emissions sources (Rosenbaum et al., 1999).

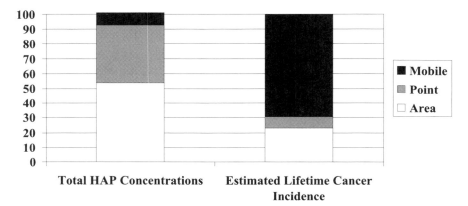

Figure 10.1   Emission source contributions to air toxics concentrations and estimated lifetime cancer incidence in the South Coast Air Basin
Mobile sources include on-road and off-road vehicles, area sources include small manufacturing and non-manufacturing facilities, and point sources include large manufacturing facilities such as TRI sources.

Interestingly, area and point emissions account for over 90% of total estimated HAP concentrations, but mobile sources are the largest driver of estimated excess cancer incidence, accounting for 70% of the estimated excess cancer incidence associated with outdoor HAP concentrations from these three source categories. This difference is consistent with another exposure study conducted recently in Southern California (SCAQMD, 1999) and underscores the importance of distinguishing between exposures versus health risks when assessing emission source contributions to pollution problems. Although, on average, point sources do not appear to

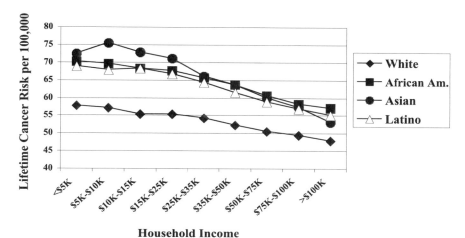

Figure 10.2   Estimated lifetime cancer risks from ambient air toxics exposures by race, ethnicity and income (South Coast Air Basin)

contribute substantially to modeled concentrations and predicted cancer risks, there are several tracts in the South Coast Basin where point source contributions to both concentration and risk estimates are dominant.

Figure 10.2 shows how the racial/ethnic disparities in estimated cancer risks persist across household income strata. The *y*-axis shows a population-weighted individual excess cancer risk estimate for each racial and economic category and the *x*-axis displays nine annual household income categories ranging from less than $5,000 to more than $100,000. As indicated in the figure legend, each line in the graph represents one of four racial/ethnic groups that include Anglos, African Americans, Asians, and Latinos. Asians, African Americans, and Latinos have the highest population cancer risk estimates, with risks nearly 50% higher than that for Anglos. Although risk levels tend to decline for all groups as household income increases, the gap between residents of color and Anglos is fairly consistent across income strata. These preliminary results are likely to be influenced by demographic differences in where population groups reside. Whereas African Americans, Latinos, and Asians are concentrated mainly in the urban core where pollution levels and risks tend to be higher, Anglos are more dispersed, with significant numbers living in less-urban areas where risks are lower.

Table 10.3 presents the multivariate regression models of the association between lifetime cancer risk and race/ethnicity, land use, and economic variables, including the percentage of home ownership, the percentage of industrial, commercial, and transportation land use, median housing value, median household income, and median household income squared. Model 1 uses the percentage of residents of color and model 2 shows a breakdown of the racial/ethnic groups. Multivariate regression results indicate that even after controlling for well-known causes of pollution such as population density, income, land use, and a proxy for assets (home ownership) (Krieger, 1994), race was consistently shown to be positively associated with higher

Table 10.3   Regression results on association between cancer risks associated with air toxics and race/ethnicity, economic, and land use variables

Independent variable	Model 1[a] parameter estimate (*t*-statistic)	Model 2[b] parameter estimate (*t*-statistic)
Residents of color (%)	0.17 (7.03)***	
Population density	0.18 (22.92)***	0.18 (22.67)***
Home ownership (%)	−0.02 (−0.46)	−0.02 (−0.56)
Median housing value	0.09 (5.08)***	0.08 (4.56)***
Median household income	0.26 (4.67)***	0.22 (4.10)***
(Median household income)^2	−0.0007 (−5.48)***	−0.0007 (−4.85)***
Transportation land use (%)	0.53 (6.19)***	0.53 (6.24)***
Industrial land use%	0.27 (5.57)***	0.28 (5.71)***
Commercial land use (%)	0.30 (6.34)***	0.29 (6.05)***
African American (%)		0.17 (5.40)***
Latino (%)		0.13 (4.79)***
Asian (%)		0.28 (5.75)***

***$p < 0.01$. [a]$n = 2,495$ tracts; $R^2 = 0.41$; *F* statistic = 188.3. [b]$n = 2,495$ tracts; $R^2 = 0.41$; *F* statistic = 155.4.

cancer risks. Note that median household income is entered as a quadratic variable. The curvilinear relationship between income and lifetime cancer risk is consistent with the locational studies, following the inverted U-shaped curve in which extremely poor tracts may have lower cancer risks due to low levels of economic and industrial activities, whereas wealthier residents tend to live in tracts with lower cancer risk levels.

Demographic Transition and the Siting of Environmental Hazards

Although these studies suggest that environmental hazards disparately impact communities of color in Southern California, the cross-sectional nature of these results precludes the possibility of assessing the causal sequence of facility siting, that is, whether facilities were sited in communities of color or whether minority residents moved into neighborhoods after facility siting decreased property values and neighborhood desirability. Our subsequent study sought to examine this siting versus minority-move-in hypothesis, which entailed compiling longitudinal data on the siting and location of TSDFs from 1970 to 1990 (Pastor, 2001).

Preliminary results indicate that the proportion of minority residents living within a one-mile radius of a TSDF increased from 9% in 1970 to over 20% in 1990, whereas the increase for White residents was less, from 5% to nearly 8%. Tracts receiving TSDFs between 1960 and 1990 had a higher proportion of residents of color, were poorer and more blue-collar, had lower initial home values and rents, and had significantly fewer homeowners. Moreover, multivariate analysis showed that there was little evidence of so-called minority move-in into areas where TSDFs had been previously sited.

Finally, we sought to examine whether neighborhoods that had undergone drastic demographic transitions in their ethnic and racial composition were more vulnerable to TSDF siting, possibly due to weak social and political networks that could undermine a community's capacity to influence siting decisions. A tract-level variable of ethnic churning was constructed to measure this phenomenon by taking the absolute sum of racial demographic change between 1970 and 1990. Figure 10.3 maps this ethnic-churning variable in Los Angeles overlaid onto the siting of TSDFs during the 1970s and 1980s. The apparent visual correlation between high demographic transition and TSDF siting was tested with simultaneous modeling using a two-stage least-squares regression. Results revealed that this type of demographic transition significantly predicted the siting of a TSDF even after controlling for economic and other demographic indicators (not shown). Thus, in historically or uniformly ethnic areas, siting seems less likely to occur than in locations where the proportion of residents of color is high but split and changing between African American and Latino groups.

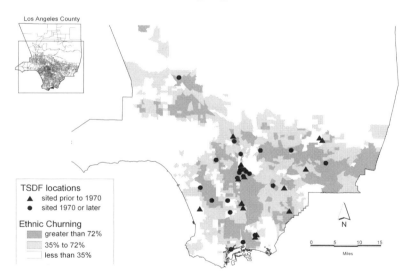

Figure 10.3   High capacity hazardous waste TSDFs and ethnic churning, 1970–1990, southern Los Angeles County, California
Data from 1970, 1980, and 1990 Census. Each category contains one-third of all Los Angeles County census tracts.

Policy Implications of Research Results

Our studies examining environmental inequality in Southern California have consistently revealed a disproportionate burden borne by communities of color, particularly African Americans and Latinos, in the location of TRI and TSD facilities and lifetime cancer risks associated with outdoor air toxics exposures (Morello-Frosch, 2001; Boer, 1997; Sadd, 1999). A longitudinal study further suggests that the disproportionate location of TSD facilities in Los Angeles County has been the result of the siting of facilities predominantly in communities of color and not simply a market-induced move-in of poor residents of color to lower rent areas already affected by environmental hazards (Pastor, 2001). Moreover, communities undergoing rapid demographic transition seem more vulnerable to the placement of TSDFs. This measurement of ethnic churning merits further inquiry, as it may be a crude indicator of a community's capacity to mobilize social networks and politically resist or influence siting decisions.

Although three of our studies were locational, focusing on the siting of potentially hazardous facilities, we were also able to examine the health risk implications of outdoor air toxics exposures attributable to mobile and non-mobile sources. These latter results suggest that air toxics concentrations and their associated health risks originate mostly from smaller area and mobile sources, raising new challenges for policy makers and environmental justice advocates alike in terms of developing regulatory and pollution prevention strategies for these emission sources. Unlike large industrial and waste facilities that traditionally have been the focus of organizing, research, and regulatory attention, mobile and area sources are smaller, more widely dispersed, and diverse in terms of their emissions and production characteristics, making a uniform regulatory approach and community organizing strategy more difficult. Regulatory oversight of small manufacturing and service operations has been minimal because these facilities tend to be the most difficult to control from a technological perspective compared with large point sources that have been the focus of command and control efforts. Indeed, dispersed, small-scale production often turns industry into a moving target, as smaller firms avoid community scrutiny and regulatory responsibility for the social costs and environmental health impacts of production. Small factories are often undercapitalized, short-term operations that do not have the technology or know-how to safely produce, store, and transport toxic inputs and wastes (Mazurek, 1999). Finally, the proliferation of mobile sources may be eroding the previous gains made from stricter emissions standards. Thus, future emissions reduction efforts must better address mobile and area sources with a particular emphasis on how regional economic development, changing land use patterns, suburbanization, and the development of major transportation corridors impact pollution streams and the distribution of health risks among communities of color and the poor.

Equally important, these study results reinforce the need to take a more holistic approach to environmental equity research. As better data become available, future studies should move away from locational and pollutant-by-pollutant analysis and toward a cumulative exposure approach (across pollutants and emission sources) that better answers the question of what disparities in exposure mean for potential inequities in health risks. Of course, the use of risk assessment, even within an equity analysis framework, remains controversial among the public and policy makers alike (Kuehn, 1996; Latin, 1988). We sought to improve the use of risk assessment by using it comparatively to assess the distribution of cancer risk due to outdoor air toxic exposures among diverse communities.

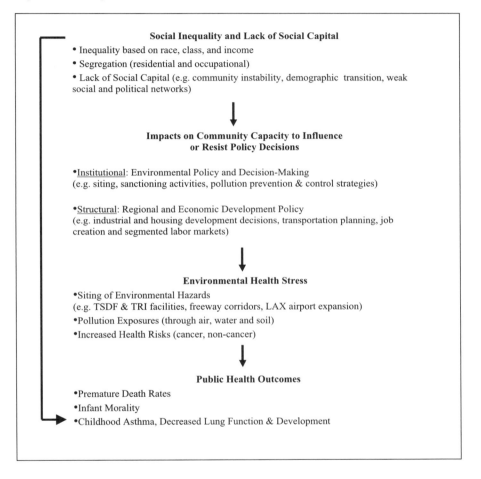

Figure 10.4   Political economy of environmental inequality

Conclusion: A Framework for Future Research

Although risk assessment and statistical analysis can show how inequities in environmental health risks are spread among diverse communities, they shed little light on their origins or the reasons for their persistence. These larger questions necessarily lead us in a new direction in our research to address two overarching issues: *a*) using a social inequality framework (based on race, class and income) to facilitate the integration of knowledge from the fields of economics and sociology in a way that enables researchers to better understand the complex dynamics of environmental inequality (Muntaner, 2000; Boyce, 1999); and *b*) examining the political and economic forces that lead to environmental inequality, which requires consideration of how institutional discrimination (such as occupational and residential segregation) interacts with larger structural forces, including disparities in patterns of economic and regional development. Figure 10.4 proposes such a social inequality framework that could be used to develop future research questions. Patterns of social inequality, segregation, and lack of social capital [such as social networks, cohesion, and a community's ability to mobilize politically (Massey, 1984; Massey, 1993; Massey, 1994) impact a community's capacity to influence or resist environmental policy-making and regulatory enforcement activities (Hill, 1974). Similarly, social inequality diminishes a community's ability to shape regional and economic development activities in systematic ways that would benefit (or at minimum not harm) its residents (Pulido, 1996). The interaction of these institutional and structural processes ultimately places additional environmental stress on communities of color through the placement of potentially hazardous facilities, transportation corridors, and pollutant exposures through various media. Ultimately, the adverse effects of these intersecting processes can be assessed through specific public health outcomes.

Research examining the socioeconomic factors that create environmental inequalities can move policy discussions on environmental justice beyond simply tinkering with the regulatory process and toward addressing how social inequalities and discrimination directly and indirectly impact the environmental health of communities of color and the poor. Preliminary research in this area suggests that disparities in political power and residential segregation affect not only the net costs and benefits of environmentally degrading activities but also the overall magnitude of environmental degradation (e.g., air pollution) and health risks (e.g., individual estimated lifetime cancer risk) (Boyce, 1999; Morello-Frosch, 1997). Community participation is key to developing long-term regulatory, enforcement, and regional development initiatives that are politically and economically sustainable and that protect public health. The challenge for policy makers and researchers alike is to reorient future inquiry to examine how indicators of inequality and political empowerment can promote environmental protection and environmental justice for everyone.

References

Anderton, D.L., Anderson, A.B., Rossi, R.H., Oakes, J.M., Fraser, M.R., Weber, E.W. and Calabrese, E.J. (1994), "Hazardous waste facilities: environmental equity issues in metropolitan areas", *Eval Rev*, **18**, 123–40.

Been, V. (1995), "Analyzing evidence of environmental justice", *J Land Use Environ Law*, **11**, 1–37.

Boer, T.J., Pastor, M., Sadd, J.L. and Snyder, L.D. (1997), "Is there environmental racism? The demographics of hazardous waste in Los Angeles County", *Soc Sci Q*, **78**, 793–810.

Boyce, J., Klemer, A., Templet, P. and Willis, C. (1999), "Power distribution, the environment, and public health: a state-level analysis", *Ecol Econ*, **29**, 127–40.

Bullard, R. (1983), "Solid waste sites and the black community", *Sociol Inq*, **53**, 273–88.

Bullard, R. (1993), *Confronting Environmental Racism: Voices from the Grassroots*, Boston: South End Press.

Caldwell, J.C., Woodruff, T.J., Morello-Frosch, R. and Axelrad, D.A. (1998), "Application of health information to hazardous air pollutants modeled in EPA's Cumulative Exposure Project", *Toxicol Ind Health*, **14**, 429–54.

California Senate Bill 115. Environmental Justice 1999. Government Code § 6504.12 and Public Resource Code §§ 7200–7201.

Civil Rights Act of 1964. Title VII. 42 U.S.C. §§ 2000d to 2000d7.

Clean Air Act Amendments of 1990. § 112 Hazardous Air Pollutants.

Clean Air Act Amendments of 1990. § 112(f) Standard to Protect Health and the Environment.

Ecob, R. and Davey, S.G. (1999), "Income and health: what is the nature of the relationship?" *Soc Sci Med*, **48**, 693–705.

Foreman, C. (1998), *The Promise and Peril of Environmental Justice*, Washington, DC: Brookings Institution.

GAO (1983), *Siting of Hazardous Waste Landfills and Their Correlation with Racial and Economic Status of Surrounding Communities*, Gaithersburg, MD: U.S. General Accounting Office.

Hill, R. (1974), "Separate and unequal: governmental inequality in the metropolis", *Am Pol Sci Rev*, **68**, 1557–68.

Institute of Medicine (1999), *Toward Environmental Justice: Research, Education, and Health Policy Needs*, Washington, DC: Institute of Medicine.

Kawachi, I. and Marmot, M. (1998), "Commentary: what can we learn from studies of occupational class and cardiovascular disease?", *Am J Epidemiol*, **148**, 160–63.

Krieger, N. and Fee, E. (1994), "Social class: the missing link in US health data", *Int J Health Serv*, **24**, 25–44.

Krieger, N., Rowley, D., Herman, A., Avery, B. and Phillips, M. (1993), "Racism, sexism, and social class: implications for studies of health, disease, and well-being", *Am J Prev Med*, **9**, 82–122.

Kuehn, R.R. (1996), "The environmental justice implications of quantitative risk assessment", *Univ Illinois Law Rev*, **1996**, 103–172.

Latin, H. (1988), Good science, bad regulation, and toxic risk assessment. *Yale J Reg*, **5**, 89–148.

Massey, D. and Denton, N. (1993), *American Apartheid: Segregation and the Making of the Underclass*, Cambridge, MA: Harvard University Press.

Massey, D. and Gross, A. (1994), "Migration, segregation, and the geographic concentration of poverty" *Am Sociol Rev*, **59**, 425–45.

Massey, D. (1984), *Spatial Divisions of Labor: Social Structures and the Geography of Production*, New York: Methuen.

Mazurek, J. (1999), *Making Microchips: Policy, Globalization and Economic Restructuring in the Semiconductor Industry*, Cambridge, MA: MIT Press.

Mohai, P. and Bryant, B. (1992), "Environmental racism: reviewing the evidence", *In: Race and the Incidence of Environmental Hazards: A Time for Discourse* (Bryant B, Mohai P, eds). Boulder, CO: Westview, 164–75.

Morello-Frosch, R., Pastor, M. and Sadd, J. (2001), "Environmental justice and southern California's 'riskscape': the distribution of air toxics exposures and health risks among diverse communities", *Urban Aff Rev*, **36**, 551-578.

Morello-Frosch, R.A., Woodruff, T.J., Axelrad, D.A. and Caldwell, J.C. (2000), "Air toxics and health risks in California: the public health implications of outdoor concentrations", *Risk Anal*, **20**, 273–91.

Morello-Frosch, R.A. (1997), "Environmental Justice and California's 'Riskscape': The Distribution of Air Toxics and Associated Cancer and Non-Cancer Health Risks Among Diverse Communities" [PhD Thesis], Berkeley CA: University of California, Berkeley.

Muntaner, C., Lynch, J. and Davey Smith, G. (2000), "Social capital and the third way in public health", *Crit Public Health*, **10**, 107–24.

Pastor, M., Sadd, J. and Hipp, J. (2001), "Which came first? Toxic facilities, minority move-in, and environmental justice", *J Urban Aff*, **23**, 1–21.

Pulido, L., Sidawi, S., Vos, R. (1996), "An archeology of environmental racism in Los Angeles", *Urban Geogr*, **17**, 419–39.

Pulido, L. (1996), "A critical review of the methodology of environmental racism research", *Antipode*, **28**, 142–59.

Rosenbaum, A., Axelrad, D.A., Woodruff, T.J., Wei, Y., Ligocki, M.P. and Cohen, J.P. (1999), "National estimates of outdoor air toxics concentrations", *J Air Waste Manage Assoc*, **49**, 1138–52.

Rosenbaum, A., Ligocki, M. and Wei, Y. (1999), "Modeling Cumulative Outdoor Concentrations of Hazardous Air Pollutants", Revised Final Report. San Rafael, CA: Systems Applications International, Inc. Available: *http://www.epa.gov/Cumulative Exposure/resource/resource.htm* [accessed 12 May 2000].

Sadd, J.L., Pastor, M., Boer, T. and Snyder, L.D. (1999), "'Every breath you take...': The demographics of toxic air releases in Southern California", *Econ Dev Q*, **13**, 107–23.

SCAQMD (1999), Multiple Air Toxics Exposure Study in the South Coast Air Basin – MATES-II. Diamond Bar, CA: South Coast Air Quality Management District.

Syme, S. and Berkman, L. (1976), "Social class, susceptibility and sickness", *Am J Epidemiol*, **104**, 1–8.

Szasz, A. and Meuser, M. (1997), "Environmental inequalities: Literature review and proposals for new directions in research and theory", *Curr Sociol*, **45**, 99–120.

U.S. EPA (1991), Toxic Release Inventory 1987-1990. CD-ROM. Washington, DC: U.S. Environmental Protection Agency.

U.S. EPA (1992) *Environmental Equity: Reducing Risk for all Communities*, Washington, DC: U.S. Environmental Protection Agency.

U.S. EPA. Interim Guidance for Investigating Title VI Complaints Challenging Permits. Available: *http://es.epa.gov/oeca/oej/titlevi.pdf* [accessed 23 June 2001]. Washington, DC: U.S. Environmental Protection Agency.

United Church of Christ (1987), *A National Report on the Racial and Socio-Economic Characteristics of Communities with Hazardous Waste Sites*, New York: United Church of Christ.

Woodruff TJ, Axelrad DA, Caldwell J, Morello-Frosch R, Rosenbaum A (1998), "Public health implications of 1990 air toxics concentrations across the United States", *Environ Health Perspect*, **106**, 245-251.

Chapter 11

Participatory Research Strategies in Nuclear Risk Management for Native Communities

Dianne Quigley, Virginia Sanchez, Dan Handy, Robert Goble
and Patricia George

Introduction

In the early 1990's, a number of community activists and minority researchers began a national movement to combat documented practices of environmental racism that were widespread throughout the United States. Several important studies (UCC, 1987; Bullard and Wright, 1993; Brown, 1994; Bryant and Mohai, 1992) demonstrated that racially diverse populations had a considerably higher proportion of hazardous facilities sited in their neighborhoods than predominately white communities. In addition, these community populations feared the lack of adequate public health protection from environmental contamination, ranging from toxic chemicals, lead poisoning, air pollution, nuclear contamination and a number of other environmental health threats. Unethical and inequitable research practices were highlighted in the relationships between community members and scientific researchers (Russell, 1992; CDC, 1994). Community members were increasingly frustrated by risk assessments, health assessments and epidemiological studies, usually conducted by corporate facilities, federal or state health agencies. In a 1993 published report titled *Inconclusive By Design*; the authors reported environmental health research inadequacies such as; inadequate contact with populations being studied; reliance upon testing techniques entirely inappropriate to types of exposures involved; reliance upon statistical methods which are entirely unsuited to the small and mobile populations residing around waste sites; contracting with researchers who are known to be biased against finding any connection between toxic pollution and disease; and studying the wrong types of illnesses, e.g. focusing on death studies instead of disease studies (i.e. respiratory illnesses or reproductive problems).

Although this report's findings came from the experiences of many minority and other communities facing toxic contamination threats, similar problems exist for communities with nuclear contamination.

Research Inequities and Environmental Injustices in the Nuclear Risk Field

Studies of low-level radiation effects conducted in the fields of exposure assessment, epidemiology and risk assessment often produce findings of uncertainty because of the intrinsic limitations of scientific methods (Wing, 1998; Connor, 1997). Qualitative data of community observations, data collection and narratives of health impacts are frequently dismissed by legal and scientific bodies. Health effects can only be determined by an expert technical elite.

At the same time, these communities are affected by high-risk technologies where the scientific knowledge about their human and environmental impacts is highly uncertain (Wynne, 1992). Low-income, diverse populations in these communities who already suffer a high incidence of many common diseases, are much more vulnerable to the impacts of contamination (Bryant and Mohai, 1992). Another injustice is that exposed community members have no input into decisions about how much exposure they will receive on a yearly basis. Radiation standard-setting processes which determine exposures to workers and communities surrounding nuclear facilities are far removed from those who suffer the exposures (Caulfield, 1989). The environmental health field has been entrenched in these public health inequities for decades (Quigley, 1997; CDC, 1994; Wigley and Schrader-Frechette, 1996; Brown, 1994; Russell et al., 1992) and the victimization continues. To bring justice and equity to this field impacts not just academia and the medical community. Industry and the military have a major stake in the question of whose knowledge of health and environmental impacts is more valid and whose plans for mitigating contamination and its impacts are more legitimate.

Sympathetic public health professionals and community members affected by nuclear contamination from the U.S. Department of Energy (DOE) nuclear weapons complex, from uranium mining and nuclear power facilities cited a number of key issues for social change in various national conferences and published reports (CDC, 1994; EPA, 1996; Quigley, 1994; 1997; Connor, 1997; NIEHS, 1997). Specifically, these issues address the need for equitable relationships between researchers and communities and overall improved public health protection. They include:

1 that community participation be required in all stages of the research process from design, implementation, results, interpretation and dissemination so that technical researchers, federal or state agencies, having potential biases, unethical goals and conflicts of interest, do not exclusively maintain control over the detection, assessment and outcomes of health risk research methods.
2 that community knowledge and observations of disease excesses and environmental abnormalities be integrated into the research process and not be rejected as "anecdotal and subjective".
3 that community members be educated about contamination impacts and be trained to make decisions and conduct community-based research with scientists in understanding and managing complex health issues related to nuclear contamination.
4 that solely quantitative research practices not dominate the assessment and interpretation of radiation health impacts.

This paper has been written to describe a four-year project, the Nuclear Risk Management for Native Communities (NRMNC) Project that sought to apply these principles in a Native community and scientific research partnership dealing with the health impacts of nuclear fallout. Practical methods and strategies for implementing community participation, community-based education, research and strategic-planning are demonstrated. This paper is written primarily for environmental health researchers and community health organizers dealing with environmental health research and risk communication issues in an environmental justice community setting. Specifically, it describes a number of successful interventions as useful models for those working in the nuclear risk field with Native Americans or other small disadvantaged populations in rural settings grappling with environmental health threats.

The Nuclear Risk Management for Native Communities (NRMNC) Project – A Case Study in Utilizing Participatory Research Methods for Dealing with Nuclear Threats in Native Communities

In 1994, President Clinton signed the Executive Order for Environmental Justice requiring all federal health agencies to develop policies to promote environmental justice (Clinton, 1994). In response to this Executive Order, the National Institute of Environmental Health Sciences (NIEHS) at the National Institutes of Health developed a new grant program for "Environmental Equity – Partnerships in Communities" to improve the relationships among community members, scientific researchers and health care providers in resolving environmental health concerns in disadvantaged community settings. This was the first grant program of its kind in the environmental health field that would give substantive multi-year support to scientific - community partnerships for building innovative models for equitable risk communication and research activities. The NRMNC Project received one of the first grant awards under this program, along with a cooperative grant award from the Agency for Toxic Chemicals and Disease Registry (ATSDR) for tribal environmental health education and foundation support. The history of the NRMNC community-tribal-scientific collaboration is presented here along with a discussion of how participatory research theory and methods were conducive to our project design and methods.

Nuclear Contamination and Western Shoshone and Southern Paiute Native Communities

Native communities, primarily in the western US, have been chronically exposed to low doses of radiation for over forty years. This exposure derives from many nuclear activities on Indian land such as uranium mining and milling; uranium conversion and enrichment; and nuclear weapons testing (Churchill and LaDuke, 1992; Eichstedt, 1994; Brugge and Benally, 1998). Human radiation experiments also occurred among Alaskan Natives (ACHRE, 1996). Although Native communities bear a disproportionate burden of risk from those activities compared to the general public, they have little access to the professional and financial resources and expertise to understand this contamination and respond appropriately. Information on exposures and their health effects is often inadequate, incomplete, inaccessible and incomprehensible. Many Native community members view this pollution as another act of cultural destruction from the dominant society.

From 1951 to 1992, 220 of approximately 900 above and below-ground nuclear tests (Church et al., 1990; Thompson and McArthur, 1996) from the Nevada Test Site (NTS) released radioactive fallout over large areas. The tests released primarily radioactive iodine-131, cesium-131, strontium-90, plutonium, tritium and other noble gases. The majority of the radioactive plumes traveled north and east over Native American reservations (Ely, Duckwater, Moapa and Goshute reservation areas) and other small rural communities in Nevada and Utah.

Many Native Americans living in these downwind communities have long been concerned about the effects of this nuclear fallout on their health and environment. Although they have seen excess diseases, particularly cancers, and have perceived decreases in animal herd sizes, poor health in wild animals, and losses in biodiversity; (i.e. wild subsistence crops, such as pine nuts, berries and medicinal plants), there have been no studies of the direct effects of radiation fallout to Native American communities. The risk of high doses of radioactive-iodine to Native Americans has been an important research consideration. Previous studies have established that doses to the Native populations in Nevada were quite high even without an accurate assessment of their special lifestyle risk factors (Church et al. 1990).

The Native American communities face additional public health threats from existing and proposed nuclear facilities. These include (1) *The Nevada Test Site*, a sprawling complex of nuclear testing facilities and volatile radioactive waste storage sites; receiving more than 1 million cubic feet of radioactive waste a year and (2) *Yucca Mountain* being developed as a repository for high-level nuclear wastes; affecting 40 Indian reservations for 30 years or more with transportation and storage risks (Fowler, 1994).

Inadequacies in Traditional Research and Risk Communication Practices in Native Communities with Nuclear Contamination

The most obvious inadequacy of health research in this setting and in other Native communities with nuclear contamination is a dire lack of research. When the NRMNC Project began, the only community study of nuclear contamination to Native communities was a study of birth defects from uranium mining and milling around Shiprock, New Mexico (Shields, 1992). In the past, Native populations have often been neglected in epidemiological studies that restrict participation to homogeneous groups in order to reduce variation in factors not central to the research question. Diverse ethnic populations introduce potential complexities in terms of possible socioeconomic and lifestyle influences on exposure, genetic differences in susceptibility, and on the diagnosis and treatment of disease (Brown, 1994). They introduce these complexities, often with small numbers, which threaten the statistical power of the study to analyze for complexity. Thus the Native American component of uranium miner lung cancer studies has only recently been subject to detailed analysis (Samet et al., 1984). Environmental monitoring of community exposures to contaminants also has largely been neglected (Schleien et al., 1991). The inadequacies in the monitoring of exposures to nuclear workers and uranium miners – which have impeded efforts to characterize the health risks of their occupational exposures – are even more pronounced for Native American populations.

These inherent biases in environmental health research methods magnify the historical neglect of concern for Native communities. Additional inequities include decades of deception by nuclear contractors whose risk communication practices included the marketing of the safety of low-level radiation to populations receiving chronic levels of low dose exposures (Caulfield, 1989; Gallagher, 1993; Fuller, 1984; Pendergrass and Nelson, 1987). With this prevailing opinion of radiation risks from the 1940's to the early 1990's, there was no need for public health officials to study health impacts or educate communities on the effects of radiation and the specific contaminants in their settings. Native community members often went for picnics to watch the bombs explode. Nuclear secrecy and national security interests have impeded the objective assessment of low-level radiation risks for decades (PSR, 1992).

In Southwest Utah, there were several studies of downwinders from the NTS (Kerber et al., 1993 and Stevens et al., 1990) that were limited primarily to studies of schoolchildren in Utah counties and Mormons. Only a handful of Native Americans were included in a study of schoolchildren. Like most case-control and cohort studies at that time, there was no opportunity for community participation and community education in these health studies. The studies were totally technically controlled. Unlike most community studies in radiation health risks, these studies did produce some positive findings but those findings did not lead to any public health policy interventions, as the findings were not considered convincing.

Lastly, a study of exposure assessment to populations in Nevada, Utah and Arizona conducted by the DOE (Church et al., 1990) omitted Native American lifestyles in their dose assessments. This is discussed later in this paper but the DOE claimed that they could not get access to Native communities through their outreach methods, which were limited to a few telephone calls and a questionnaire. This experience is common to Native community members in the Great Basin as they have complained of numerous injustices in public participation and risk communication practices related to local environmental issues. These deficiencies have been highlighted here by Native community activists (personal communication, Zabarte, 1994):

- "Native community members and leaders are lied to about what their participation meant in certain settings; they were not given training or preparation for their role and purpose in providing input; were intentionally confused so external control could be maintained.
- Native input often is appropriated by non-Native people without permission, acknowledgement or recognition of Native contributors or Native culture
- Involvement of Native representatives has not reflected the diversity of tribal communities and interests in public participation forums.
- Native community members and leaders were notified too late or excluded from input into major environmental decisions affecting their communities.

● Native community members and leaders have not been given any decision-making authority in public participation venues; federal agencies or other contractors do what they want without sharing power."

In addition to these experiences encountered by Native community activists in the Great Basin in (1) the siting of nuclear waste facilities (Yucca Mountain), (2) the storage and transportation of nuclear waste at the NTS, and (3) mining, military and land rights issues in Nevada, examples of these deficiencies also exist in current risk assessment studies of the Nevada Test Site (NRAMP, 1996), DOE's exposure assessment studies (Church et al., 1990) and the Southwest Utah epidemiological studies (Kerber et al., 1993; Stevens et al., 1990).

The NRMNC Project and Participatory Research

In 1993, the Western Shoshone National Council, representing a number of tribal reservation communities in the Great Basin area requested the support of the Childhood Cancer Research Institute (CCRI) for investigating their health and environmental concerns. CCRI is a small environmental health education and research institute, which accesses technical and funding support to increase public health protection for communities suffering from nuclear contamination. At the time, CCRI was the only non-profit environmental health organization in the country committed to building community capacity for dealing with radiation health impacts. CCRI had received some limited support for this work through private foundations and had conducted several educational workshops in Native communities near the Sequoyah Fuels nuclear facility in Oklahoma. In responding to the NIEHS grant request in 1994, CCRI formalized its existing collaborative work with Clark University, the Citizen Alert Native American Program (CANAP), Reno, NV, and the Ely-Shoshone Tribe to officially create the NRMNC collaboration. Although both CCRI and Clark University are located in Worcester, MA, CCRI had a national reputation for expertise in building community capacities for dealing with nuclear contamination health impacts. Clark University also offered much experience and expertise with risk assessment and risk management of nuclear risks, as well as expertise in public participation and environmental equity. This expertise was not available locally to these communities and few universities in the country had experience in dealing with nuclear contamination impacts and community capacity-building. Moreover, Native community members had much distrust of local universities where they have stated that experienced both outright racism and scientific elitism. The NRMNC Project also serves Native communities in northeastern Oklahoma and Laguna Pueblo, NM with nuclear contamination issues.

The overall goal of the NRMNC Project has been to build community capacities for managing the health risks of nuclear contamination. As such, community members have a true partnership role in health assessment and health risk management with external scientific researchers and agencies. The NRMNC Project utilizes conventional participatory research (used synonymously with the term, community-based research) strategies to accomplish its environmental health objectives. These features are embedded in the NRMNC project design along with a few other necessary elements for building community capacities and ensuring equitable relationships between communities and researchers. The integration of these principles are reflected here in the following discussion of the four-year progress of the NRMNC Project's community-academic partnership with the Western Shoshone and Southern Paiute communities and Clark/CCRI researchers. At this time, we believe the Project offers important features of a successful model for Native American public participation in health research activities along with holistic approaches for achieving health risk management objectives.

Israel (1998) highlights the need to build on the strengths and resources within the community for health protection. "Community-based research promotes a co-learning and empowering process that facilitates the reciprocal transfer of knowledge, skills, capacity, and power". This is particularly important in working within a Native American setting as health researchers not only have much to learn about Native lifestyles and context of contamination that contrast sharply with non-Native settings, but scientists must also learn a world view that is frequently at odds with reductionist and compartmentalized scientific reasoning. Colorado (1988) stresses that a bicultural research model or a scientific infrastructure recognizing both Indian science and Western science needs to emerge. She describes Native science as holistic, that truth and knowledge necessitate studying the cycles, relationships and connections between things. Native local knowledge is a critical source to tap in the conduct of environmental studies. The Native community members have often lived in those natural environments for centuries and offer a wealth of ecological detail and observations of changes over time (Brush and Stabinsky, 1996; Gadgil, 1993; Pecore, 1992; Posey, 1992; Suzuki and Knudson, 1992). Although there are risks that indigenous knowledge can be exploited, Native community members, as partners in the research process, can negotiate controls over data collection and use of local information by western researchers.

The NRMNC Project collaborators adopted these basic tenets of participatory research, striving to build local knowledge into the research process as well as to transfer critical knowledge about nuclear contamination impacts. They have sought to organize a true partnership with community members, providing the financial and programmatic resources that would facilitate equity in decision-making and control of the project. Additionally, they sought to sustain a long-term public health intervention and to develop a more holistic definition of health research and public health protection, incorporating Native worldviews with western scientific views in project activities.

Due to the scientific complexities of nuclear contamination and the lack of expertise for dealing with nuclear impacts in remote rural areas, a participatory research model that included a partnership between academic scientists and community members seemed most appropriate for this situation.

NRMNC Project Goals and Outcomes for Western Shoshone and Southern Paiute Communities

In order to build community-based capabilities for managing the health risks of nuclear contamination, the Project established four major goals. These goals include

1   providing resources and assistance to Native communities in building a community-based environmental health infrastructure;
2   developing a community exposure profile which provides a summary of technical studies conducted on the site's contamination and a narrative of community experiences and observations of the overall holistic impacts of the site's contamination;
3   implementing an educational program on the contamination impacts of the site through developing a series of educational modules and developing and disseminating educational materials and lastly;
4   developing a community-based hazards management plan for ongoing community and technical interventions in managing the health impacts of the contamination.

GOAL # 1 – Building a Community-Based Environmental Health Infrastructure

In conferences for environmental health in the past several years, federal agencies sponsored the gathering of many community activists from around the country to hear their recommendations for improving environmental health research and public participation (CDC, 1994; EPA, 1996, NIEHS, 1997). In those meetings, there was strong support for the building of community advisory committees. These committees or community boards would be given support to conduct a meaningful oversight role for health research activities. In the NRMNC Project, we built on this concept to develop a community-based environmental health infrastructure.

In the implementation of this goal, the collaborators agreed upon three major objectives. First, in order for community members to be on equal footing with technical researchers, they, too, need resources for their partnership role. Although Clark University takes the lead in applying for and administering federal funding, financial support is provided to the community as well. We try to maintain at least a 50-50 split for grant funding. As such, building infrastructure requires:

● *Sharing Research Funding with the Community.* In 1994, Clark University and CCRI established subcontracts to Citizen Alert Native American Program (CANAP) to carry out their community-based goals. With this funding, CANAP was able to hire staff which were trained by the whole Project team. The budget grew to provide funding for 1.5 staff and various part-time consultants.

● *Recruiting and Training a Community Advisory Committee (CAC) for Shared Decision-making and Control.* A major feature of building a community-based environmental health infrastructure is the recruitment of a community advisory committee. A significant portion of the CANAP Project budget was allocated to the travel costs of bringing eighteen community members, representing nine tribes in a five thousand square mile area to three (two to three-day) workshop meetings a year. The NRMNC collaborators thought it was essential to train a core group of representative community people for a community advisory committee (CAC) who could preside over radiation health issues for the long-term. Early on, CANAP staff members who had much credibility in Native environmental activism in the Great Basin recruited Native community members who had been active in nuclear issues and other environmental problems; who maintained a sense of their Native culture and spirituality or represented tribal councils committed to overcoming local nuclear threats. The recruitment of Native elders also was a priority as they experienced nuclear testing firsthand and would have much local knowledge to offer the research team. In the meetings, CAC members were given time for training and strategic-planning on nuclear risk issues. Significant time was spent on skills building and knowledge sharing among collaborators and this is described more fully in the outcomes of our educational goals.

● *Building Community Control and Shared Leadership – A Four-Year Process.* In terms of sharing decision-making and project control, we adopted shared management procedures with the CAC that included (1) approval of grant applications, their goals and objectives and proposed budgets (2) approval of project publications, research papers and presentations by any community or technical staff of the NRMNC (3) quarterly progress reports on all goals including financial reports (4) the establishment of subcommittees for research, education and management issues where CAC representatives have input into ongoing research activities, the development of educational materials and presentations as well as the facilitation and setting of agendas for CAC meetings, the hiring and terminating of community staff and financial management issues.

The adoption of these shared management features did not happen all at once but evolved over the years. Although the Clark/CCRI staff facilitated the very first CAC meetings, the technical staff learned that it was far more empowering and satisfying to the CAC members to have the meetings facilitated by the CANAP staff. By the end of the second year, the CAC started to ask about budgets and goal setting as these decisions were made primarily between the academic principal investigator and the community-based CANAP co-principal investigator. The staff then began offering more of that information to the CAC and training them on the project operational mechanics. By the third and fourth years, the CAC began slowly taking more and more control as they felt more invested in the Project's activities, leading to the shared control features stated previously. Several factors increased their investment. These included: (1) that the Project was actually gaining visibility and reaching important research and education goals locally (2) that there was hope from potential funders that the Project could continue in a long-term effort and not be a short-term, ineffective waste of their time (3) that the meetings became enjoyable with more participatory activities, field trips and opportunities for social support as well as a sense of themselves as a strong group representing diverse tribal communities facilitating important goals and (4) the fostering of trust and confidence between the CAC and the health researchers as the CAC saw the continued commitment and sincere efforts at education and research by the academic staff who were becoming a consistent presence in their communities . In workshop evaluations, CAC members felt that they were listened to and respected and that NRMNC staff responded to their concerns with changes and improvements in activities. Several community members had commented that they appreciated the humility and apologetic attitudes of the scientists involved when the Native people voiced their disgust with the lack of ethics of western science that led to the poisoning of their land and people and the continued neglect for decades about their health concerns. They appreciated how the physicist had taken the time to give a presentation on how western scientific reasoning can lead to a very narrow view of human and environmental damage and how it differed from their world view.

Additional positive outcomes of building community control and leadership were:

● *The Development of New Training and Occupational Opportunities for Native Community Members:* Training and occupational opportunities for tribal members in isolated rural settings are often limited. As Project activities were conducted in their communities, these job opportunities were more accessible to them and offered networking possibilities regionally and nationally.

● *The Strengthening of CANAP Organizational Stability Through Additional Income and Capacity:* The CANAP organization had to respond to numerous environmental threats to Native communities in the Great Basin area with very limited resources. From 1994 -1998, multiple year funding was helpful to the organization in maintaining financial stability, gaining improved capacity building and a greater capability to attract additional funding. However, it is likely in the future that the CAC of the NRMNC will seek its own management status as an organization.

● *The First Satisfying Experience of Public Participation for Native Community Members in Environmental Research:* Many CAC members have rightfully complained about the public participation processes of previous environmental studies conducted by public agencies or universities summarized earlier in this paper. As such, the CAC members appreciated the broad outreach of this Project to diverse reservations, the community-based support and training, the shared decision-making, the increasing sense of ownership and control and the compensation for travel and time. In their responses to project evaluations, they commented that their experience with serving on the CAC was very positive and that they are very committed to ensuring that the CAC and community staff maintain their funding and community-based control. They unanimously supported the continuation of the project.

GOAL # 2 – Developing a Community Exposure Profile

The purpose of developing a community exposure profile is to produce a written summary of community-based and technical research on contamination impacts by:

1   Conducting interviews and meetings with affected community residents for community experiences with contamination and perceived overall impact on nuclear testing on community life.
2   Conducting technical research on contamination, and compiling and interpreting published technical studies on fallout contamination for a community audience.

Our goal here was to offer communities the "Community Exposure Profile" as a model holistic research product that described baseline quantitative and qualitative impacts of contamination embedded within the community context. This information could then guide community members and technical researchers in setting future health risk management goals together as partners. This blend of technical and community data would help to overcome inaccurate technical assumptions about community exposures, lifestyles, diet, ecology and other site-specific information. It could also facilitate the creation of risk management outcomes that are not solely technical and quantitative but qualitative, holistic and responsive to Native community needs. With this effort, we still acknowledged that quantitative technical analyses are important to conduct, however, they will be strengthened by accurate community information.

This specific goal allows for the fostering of local knowledge and participatory research activities. Additionally, we offered this goal as an alternative to rushing into epidemiological analyses that often produce statistically weak findings and leave community concerns unresolved. Although improved technical analyses may still lead to unresolved negative findings with low statistical power, in the least, community members will have had their own stories of fallout impacts recorded and preserved and will have felt part of the process in understanding the impacts.

In describing the outcomes for this goal, we have divided the sections into those findings which relate more to informing the scientific research process for quantitative objectives and those findings which relate more to the qualitative community research process.

Findings Related to the Scientific Research Process

The Project technical team reviewed numerous documents available on fallout from the NTS. It was not the goal, nor did resources exist, for conducting any rigorous health research activities such as epidemiological analyses or full exposure assessment activities. The technical staff did believe it was important to review reports that existed on fallout impacts, which were often inaccessible both physically and technically to community members. These were then interpreted in an accessible format for the communities. The most important study was the DOE dose reconstruction effort titled "The Off-Site Radiation Effects Review Project (ORERP)" (Church et al., 1990). These technical findings were supplemented by community interview research. We brought out these major points of this study to Native community members:

1 The highlighting of fallout patterns which mostly went northeasterly over Duckwater, Ely, Moapa, Shivwits and Goshute reservations.
2 The omission of Native Americans and their lifestyle (Church et al., 1990).
3 Potentially serious doses from animal thyroid and cow and goat's milk pathways to Native Americans from subsistence activities not included in the ORERP.
4 The NRMNC modeling of doses for eating rabbit thyroids; a child eating a rabbit thyroid several days after a test would receive a dose of 6 rem (Frohmberg et al. 1998).
5 The potential for extra thyroid diseases, leukemias and other cancers in Native populations, which have yet to be studied with dose information provided from

the DOE on exposures to Native communities from external and internal radiation, using the shepherd lifestyle. Information also was provided on the health effects of these doses by reviewing the effects on the Southwest Utah downwinders who had excess leukemias and thyroid cancers based on similar doses (Kerber et al., 1993; Stevens et al., 1990). If the Southwest Utah study findings were taken more seriously then there should have been public health outreach to the tribes long ago.

6   The identification of major research gaps; radiation effects are not well known for many subsistence activities (pine nuts, berries, medicinal plants). Chronic impacts to desert biodiversity and wildlife as well as radiation effects to Native human populations are not well studied.

There is a lack of historical and current environmental monitoring and medical monitoring of fallout impacts. Threats to Native culture from the loss of environmental resources also are not studied.

Findings Related to the Community-Based Research Process on Nuclear Fallout: Building a Local Knowledge Program Through Community Interviews

To date, community-based staff have conducted more than seventy-one community interviews and have transcribed community data. Currently, they are coding, analyzing and summarizing this data in a coordinated effort with the technical staff. They have titled this community research activity as the "Local Knowledge Program" which is providing these findings:

1   Extensive lifestyle, cultural and socio-demographic information on seventy-one community members, primarily elders who were exposed to testing from Duckwater, Ely, Moapa, Elko, Yomba, Battle Mountain, Timbisha, Southfork, Wells in the 1950s.
2   Critical exposure pathway information about Native lifestyles, mobility, diet, housing, subsistence activities; giving more accurate scenarios for potential exposures of Native people in the 1950s.
3   Information on observed increases in diseases and the status and trends of utilization of health care services in the 1950s.
4   Observations of environmental abnormalities and other historical contamination events.
5   Participatory research provides skills training and empowerment to local Native staff, as it is important for Native people to conduct their own research on their people's experiences and culture.

In the NRMNC Project, community interviews have allowed affected residents to voice their feelings about the bombs, to be listened to in a supportive, respectful way and to realize that they have specialized knowledge important to healing their communities. By recalling the time before contamination, they reconnect to a time when they had a richer relationship with their natural environment. Specialized environmental and community knowledge of the past, held by elders, is preserved and disseminated. Some of these cultural learning traditions may be revived by a younger generation if a local knowledge program can continue. Through the interview process, the CANAP staff was able to build good relationships with the community people and conduct one-on-one education and disseminate materials. They have provided a written record of the impact of the NTS on the Native communities and their way of life. The "Local Knowledge Program" has much potential to grow and become a permanent feature of the community's environmental infrastructure. It should be noted that the collection of local knowledge is a serious issue in a research partnership as there are risks of not only the exploitation of that knowledge but the loss of privacy and cultural ownership of information. As such, the CAC is developing internal controls over data collection and use. All community members interviewed will sign releases for the quotes or stories to be used anonymously in reports or publications. Additionally, cultural or spiritual information collected will be maintained in confidential files.

CANAP staff who conducted these interviews often reported that it was the best job that they have ever had. They loved meeting with and listening to their elders and felt the importance of capturing local knowledge. In the Great Basin area, they stated that numerous outside researchers come through and conduct interviews and surveys with their own people and take off with that information, get it published and never get permission to publish the local data or return the published data to the community. They stressed how important it was for them to learn the interviewing and transcription skills and be trained as community researchers so that Native people can conduct their own research on their people's experiences and culture (Sanchez, 1997; George, 1997). They are likely to insist on the community-based research model for any other environmental studies that seek local information.

GOAL # 3 – Implementing Education Modules and Developing Appropriate Educational Materials

Educational outreach has been a major activity of the NRMNC and the educational program was structured to serve several audiences. The Project has stressed a participatory curriculum model incorporating group problem-solving exercises, community mapping, transects and field trips.

In all educational activities, the NRMNC Project required a two-way training process between the technical staff and the community staff, as well as the CAC. The community provided training on their local knowledge and the community-based impacts of the contamination to provide a balance of perspectives between the technical and local knowledge bases. Workshops and materials integrated these sources of knowledge. Community staff facilitated the three-day educational modules. NRMNC collaborators agreed with the important principle of having community facilitation in order to create equity with technical researchers (Israel, 1998). Similar to other community-based projects (Plough and Olafson, 1994; Israel, 1998), the Clark/CCRI researchers learned this important lesson early on as the community did experience our first educational module as an inequitable, unsatisfying experience when we did the facilitation. In future modules, Clark/CCRI researchers, as well as other invited technical presenters, were there to assist the community and their facilitators. Their technical presentations were prepared according to the community's priorities of technical research and were only part of the agenda not the whole agenda. Over time, as the CAC grew in its capacity-building and its ownership of the Project, they demanded more time for group exercises, hands-on learning, and the integration of Native cultural aspects into technical presentations. A significant part of the workshop time has included strategic-planning by the CAC.

The Clark/CCRI teams were responsible for interpreting most of the technical nuclear concepts for the community-based trainers, the CAC, and health care providers; and developing educational materials which summarized technical reports on the site's contamination. Most of this material was taught at "Train-the-Trainer Tutorials" and at educational modules for the CAC and the health care providers. The training materials were then organized into a curriculum workbook for the trainers. The trainers studied and reviewed this material for the implementation of community trainings where they traveled to various Native communities and gave presentations on the impact of the fallout and the work of the NRMNC Project. The trainers also gave presentations in various local and regional tribal events and tribal meetings. These presentations included not only technical information but the community context of contamination and the cultural experience of this contamination. These various components of the educational program and their outcomes are described below.

Outcomes of Two-Way Communication Processes and Capacity-Building Activities

The progress of these educational approaches is described under the heading "Educational Modules". Module is defined here as a series of workshops and presentations within a multi-day period. In all the modules and in the educational materials, we tried to highlight the integration of a two-way process of communication between the community and the researchers. Such processes are highlighted here in the way they led to a deeper learning of each other's values and context.

Education Modules

Train-the-Trainer Tutorials: Five of these trainings were held in the Project's first two and half years. The community staff travelled from both the Nevada and Oklahoma sites to Clark University for week-long trainings and found them to be very worthwhile and productive (feedback from oral and written evaluations). They appreciated the small group intensive training time and the one-on-one attention. Pre and post-testing assessments indicated that they were learning the critical environmental health concepts adequately enough to begin some education in their communities; with their workbooks close by. The drawback of these tutorials was the fact that a significant investment of time and funding went into training some community staff who then left the Project before they actualized their role as community trainers. We noticed however that in Nevada, sometimes due to personal or family stresses, a trainer may leave but will return again, several months or years later. The small size of the training sessions allowed for improved communication between the community trainers and the researchers. The researchers would learn more about how some of their emphases and approaches to education would just not be appropriate for the Native cultural settings. The trainers would elaborate on the daily lives of their people and how some of this technical material could be so far removed from their lives. We were always in a process of trying to link educational terms and activities to something more relevant to the immediate realities of the Native community members.

Community Advisory Committee/Health Care Provider Modules: This activity of the Project was probably one of its most successful features. The community staff conducted excellent recruitment of community advisors. Over eighteen community advisors attended these three-day meetings. The NRMNC Project implemented twelve CAC/health care provider modules in Nevada over a four-year period. These meetings generally were two and one half days long and covered many of these topics designated in the nuclear risk curriculum. Clark and CCRI staff in balance with CANAP staff prepared and presented many of the curriculum topics. However, two to three outside speakers also gave presentations at each module. Slocum et al. (1995) provide a description of many participatory research and training methods utilized in their work in international development, such as life histories, seasonal event calendars, transects and community mapping, NRMNC collaborators successfully incorporated these methods, particularly the community mapping and transects, in our modules and participatory research activities. In one module, we recreated life in Moapa, NV in the 1950s, building a shelter, collecting willows and cooking Native foods. These activities as well as a rabbit skinning in another module were useful to teaching both exposure pathway scenarios and community cultural context of contamination. Whenever possible, Native American technical presenters were invited to assist in teaching technical concepts. Geiger-counters were used to teach nuclear physics concepts.

Two-way communication processes that unfolded between the project team and the CAC were first facilitated by our evaluation processes whereby strengths and weaknesses of our approaches were highlighted in writing or by going around the table and listening to the observations of each CAC member. Within specific workshop presentations, sometimes a topic would trigger many feelings among one or several CAC members and the team would allow the discussion to flow freely so that these important sentiments could get expressed. Quite frequently, we needed to adjust time schedules to foster participant discussions. In lunch and other breaks or in smaller group settings with CAC members, the project team would receive feedback about approaches or content of presentations that were uncomfortable or were effective with the group. The team would then adjust its strategies to be responsive to the group.

Wallerstein (1994), Sissel et al. (1996) and Kiser et al. (1995) all stress the importance of participatory learning by community members in order to improve health conditions. The NRMNC educational activities led to increased capacity building of staff and CAC about nuclear risk issues in order to assist them in meaningful hazard management planning. Generally, participants evaluated the education modules positively. The trainers, health care providers and the CAC members have shown improved understanding of technical radiation health impacts from fallout and health study options through pre- and post-testing assessments. The increase in ownership and control was evidenced through meaningful risk management planning, through an increased interest in setting the workshop agenda topics, conducting module-planning, improved critiquing of studies and presentations and recommendations of effective training methods.

We observed that the Native community members truly gained an understanding of difficult nuclear and health risk methodological concepts through repeated presentations, accompanied by visual graphics and group problem-solving exercises on these topics. The research team in agreement with the CAC, offered group problem solving exercises as a preferred pre and post-assessment tool over written tests which were deemed inappropriate to the Native community members.

The academic researchers benefited from increased environmental and cultural learning on the community context of the contamination and on processes of appropriate research and education in Native communities. The two way communication processes and participatory learning emphases were critical to facilitating this. This was evident in adjustments to the implementation of Project goals, such as the integration of local community knowledge into research papers and presentations and an accommodation within meetings and interpersonal interactions to facilitate communication processes. The technical staff now teaches other colleagues and scientists about the important role of community local knowledge and participatory processes.

Issues in Technical Risk Communication: The community trainers and Clark staff will continue to work on the challenges of technical risk communication; making the technical information accessible on the community level. Clark researchers note that existing technical risk studies on fallout and their findings are unjustly inaccessible to these communities in the way they are designed, written and disseminated (Handy, 2000). Technical risk reports and publications often are not geared to the community members who are affected by the risks but usually are written for other technical scientists. There is often no provision by a public agency or contractor who funded the report to create an interpretation of the findings for the immediate community audience. This burden of risk communication falls to community activists who must find funds to hire experts who can interpret these reports for the community. Much of the work of the technical researchers in the NRMNC Project was focused on interpreting highly technical documents. Many decisions needed to be made about how much technical information gets interpreted; what should be prioritized for community understanding and how to deal with different levels of literacy. We often found that these decisions had to be guided by limited time and limited financial resources. Much of our risk communication material was developed for a high school literacy level.

Local and Regional Community Meetings: After receiving training by the technical staff, the community staff conducted educational outreach which included not only community meetings but many Native gatherings, tribal meetings, and national gatherings. The staff gave over forty-five presentations in four years. We believe that all these educational meetings and materials have not only provided much training for community members but have given much awareness, attention and momentum regionally to the need to increase public health protection from nuclear impacts.

Educational Materials

Numerous educational materials were developed on nuclear risk issues over four years, particularly for the NTS. It is important to note that CCRI and NRMNC are among the first groups in the country to pioneer a community radiation health effects curriculum and develop materials that are accessible to a community audience. Curriculum materials included radiation basics workbooks, radionuclide fact sheets, fact sheets on health risk methodologies and visual guides on site-specific contamination. We also produced several extensive toxicological profiles on contaminants. As stated above, these risk communication materials are an ongoing need for communities affected by contamination; a need that is currently not being met adequately by public health or environmental professionals involved in risk management activities in these communities.

It is important to note that the Project's materials are consistently being requested by technical researchers and Native and non-Native community members across the country who are grappling with nuclear risks. The community researchers also have been invited to local, regional and national meetings and conferences where they present this project model and its findings to date. This broader outreach has contributed to their skills-building and local capacities and provides much validation to their work, as well as assisting the work of other communities.

GOAL # 4 – Developing a Community-Based Hazard Management Plan

As stated earlier, definitions of participatory research require an action plan as the final part of the research process. In this project, such an action plan has been titled "A Community-based Hazard Management Plan". In the field of nuclear risks, risk assessment and risk management generally are quantitative methodologies, determining acceptable levels of exposure with levels of excess cancers such exposures would produce. Plough and Krimsky (1990) write that "in schools of public policy the effective management of environmental and health risks is synonymous with quantitative assessment of problems. Within this orientation, social and cultural context of risk is of marginal concern". Ruckelshaus (1985) offers a definition of risk management that is more inclusive of non-quantitative contexts "risk management in its broadest sense means adjusting our environmental policies to obtain the array of social goods – environmental, health-related, social, economic, psychological – that forms our vision of how we want the world to be."

The NRMNC Project sought to broaden the definition of risk management to include collective decision-making by community members and researchers on developing a plan that responds to the more holistic impacts of contamination; not only its cancer impacts. Project collaborators conducted strategic-planning for future health study options, disease surveillance and community-based activities, such as education, the strengthening of infrastructure and local knowledge.

Outcomes for Developing a Community-Based Plan: Figure 11.1 displays a community-based model for hazards management, which is more holistic and includes qualitative community goals as well as quantitative technical follow-up studies. This actual diagram was developed by the community advisory members. Community members say that they will strive to maintain each of the following components in any health research initiative that is proposed for their communities.

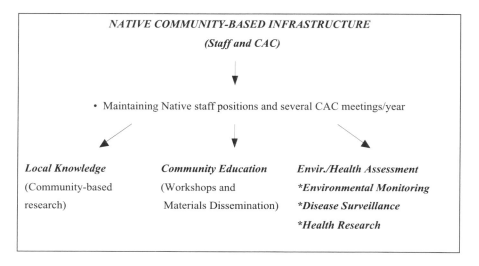

Figure 11.1   Native community-based infrastructure

Implications and Challenges Ahead for Environmental Health Research

The NRMNC Project team acknowledges the good fortune of having secured funding to develop a participatory model for community-based hazards management planning. The new NIEHS grant program on environmental justice started in 1994, as well as private foundation support and ATSDR's commitment to tribal health education, allowed us to build this important collaboration and test these strategies. With new and renewed funding support, we will be able to continue building this model. Few communities with nuclear contamination have had this opportunity. From input of community members, the CAC, Project staff and other Native communities, the Project's participatory strategies are working well and are worth continuing in this setting and replicating elsewhere.

Technical research has been improved by gathering data from the community, particularly in terms of exposure pathways and health outcomes of concern. The NRMNC Project provides a model of power sharing between researchers and community members for common goals. Our relationships are guided by principles of equity in the research process; by respecting each other's knowledge systems and the need to gather, integrate and equitably publish data from both sources. These principles have been successful in various other settings (Sclove et al., 1998; Reardon, 1993; Israel, 1994, 1998). Similarly, in the education process, we are building capacity for community trainers and CAC members so that educational priorities can be equitably determined and educational activities carried out both by technical and community people. In the strategic-planning process, by encouraging capacity-building, local facilitation, two-way communication processes and community ownership of problem-solving, we strive to overcome top-down narrow risk management outcomes and broaden the planning to encompass the meeting of long-term community needs.

These participatory research outcomes are far more preferable to the traditional environmental health approaches whereby a technical team determines a health research methodology, with minimal community accountability and conducts a health study whose findings have little meaning or benefit, and often more detriment, to the community's health protection. Significant funding is expended, the external researchers come and go and the community is left in a hopeless, demoralized state.

Major Challenges of the NRMNC Project

Managing Long-Distance Communications: One of the most difficult challenges in this effort has been overcoming problems created by distance and limited resources. The technical researchers were in Massachusetts, the community co-principal investigator worked between Reno, NV and Duckwater (central Nevada), eight hours apart by car. The community researchers involved were often in Ely, an hour east of Duckwater. CAC representatives stretched from Timbisha, CA to Elko, Nevada about nine hours apart. Communications among team members occurred twice or more weekly by telephone or fax for project planning and assistance. Every sixty to ninety days, the team would be together either on-site in Ely or Moapa, Nevada for CAC modules or for tutorials in Massachusetts. Project planning for the quarters ahead would occur in tutorials, on-site at CAC modules, sometimes on conference calls among the total team. The principal investigator made two separate site visits in addition to the modules. The community researchers were not comfortable with the time-consuming nature of emails or did not yet have the set-up for email in their remote reservations. We will be putting this in place for future projects. With these great distances, the NRMNC Project, unlike similar urban environmental justice projects, cannot be with their partners on a daily basis. Community staff often have to work independently without daily support and direction of on-site supervision. The project lacked an office in Nevada and staff had to work from home. This was hard on all project team members yet some of this is unavoidable in the high deserts of Nevada and Utah. At times, it produced stress in maintaining clear communications, keeping track of all project-related materials and working out minor conflicts and tensions. The principal investigator would them make a special site visit if tensions seemed to be mounting too much.

Distance was also a stress factor in conducting community interviews, community meetings and attending regional events. Both the time it took to do the travel and subsidize the mileage would consume resources that were limited to begin with. These factors must be accounted for in evaluating work performance and goal achievement, everything takes much longer to do in these rural settings. Generally, all project team members were able to adapt to these stresses and still maintain very good communications. Time was spent together professionally and socially in these settings and much trust was gained despite the distance.

Competing Demands: Israel (1998) also writes about common tensions having to do with competing institutional demands. All team members had stressful other institutional demands. The principal investigator was still directing CCRI and trying to conduct a similar effort with Native communities in Oklahoma on resources that were inadequate for the community organizing that was needed. The community co-principal investigator had the responsibility of directing CANAP and giving leadership to defending Native peoples from numerous other environmental threats from military to mining pollution with little funding for other staff and much travel that was required. The need to build more Native leadership in the Great Basin for environmental activism is great. Because of this, the project team understood the need to be accommodating to these other demands and accept unexpected changes in timeliness and deadlines. At times, this was difficult to manage when schedules and tasks needed to be coordinated among various team members during limited time frames. It was essential for all community-based research team members to have flexibility and patience and be resourceful about alternative ways of accomplishing things. This was also true in terms of the NRMNC's trial and error approach to the transfer of technical skills from the technical staff to the community staff. An experimental approach in capacity-building was used with the community researchers/trainers by testing their abilities in communicating technical information to community members through trainings or materials and also in the collection, coding, summary and interpretation of the community interview data.

For the most part, the community staff grew in their capacity in all these areas and was very productive. Sometimes the technical team learned at various stages a need to have stood back or to have intervened sooner with assistance. Often the technical team would have to take back a task that we had hoped the community staff would achieve simply because they did not have enough staff hours to complete it. Sometimes we all decided to forgo some tasks that none of us had time to do (additional trainings, fact sheets, writing and dissemination activities and grant development). It is important to note that the CAC members, too, had various other institutional demands that affected their ability to give time to the Project. They were often serving on boards of tribal organizations (schools, hospitals, environmental groups) within their local communities or regionally and nationally. Some were tribal officials who had many responsibilities and travel schedules to juggle. This was a major reason why they needed to ensure that their participation in the Project was meaningful and not a waste of their very valuable time.

These issues were the major challenges within our community-scientific partnerships. The NRMNC still has to confront the scientific challenges of implementing epidemiological and exposure assessment analyses. In doing so, it will need to provide scientific interpretation and credibility to local knowledge data and overcome the problems of small numbers of cases, lack of medical records, and the prevailing biases of radiation health sciences which lead to a dismissal of positive findings with low statistical power. While the technical researchers struggle with those long-term issues, the community will have at least made gains in its environmental health protection for the long-term. Staff and a core group of community members will have the skills to oversee environmental health activities. The community will have been educated on radiation health impacts and the community interviewing and educational meeting programs will have allowed them to express their betrayal and fears, find answers to some of their questions and offer them an opportunity to have their voices heard and their talents used in protecting their environmental health in the future. They are much more prepared to confront the technical deceptions of nuclear contractors and demand more full and honest accountability. They will have the skills to access resources for their long-term goals in environmental health by maintaining and expanding their local knowledge and by requiring any external environmental researchers seeking to work in their communities to abide by their participatory approaches.

Some Key Ingredients of the Project's Progress

As the NRMNC is providing participatory support to Native communities in other areas of the country, we have been able to determine some features in the Nevada setting that helped this work proceed more quickly. The fact that a functioning, trusted Native environmental organization, namely, CANAP, already existed and offered the leadership of the community co-principal investigator, (also the director of CANAP) made a world of difference to the success of this work. The importance of this has been highlighted by other researchers (Israel, 1998; Levine et al, 1994). Many Native communities do not have such a functioning organization or the personnel experience in community building and education. This will slow participatory efforts down, particularly if a community has strong traditions of paternalism and hierarchical relationships. Also important has been the unity and savvy experience of the Native community representatives on the CAC. They all believed in the importance of the health organizing and demonstrated that commitment together without much tension or divisiveness among them. This too was critical. Many communities, Native and non-Native alike, will suffer a tension between political organizing, which comes more naturally to activists, than health organizing. Health education and research require a sensitivity, tolerance and patience that is sometimes difficult for the political activists that have had to fight facility contractors for decades in court and on the streets. In some communities, where there is scarce community participation and resources for environmental protection, the two priorities can come into conflict - the political work can seem much more urgent and is usually crisis-oriented vs. the commitment to the slow process of capacity-building, education and research. Divisiveness can result over the conflicting agendas and the work can be slowed.

The skilled members of the CAC also can be credited with keeping the researchers honest and accountable. From the beginning, the CAC made sure to inform the Clark/CCRI staff of their complete distrust of and cynicism about outside researchers and their disdain for a scientific worldview that led to the radiation poisoning of their people. Fortunately, the researchers did not get defensive but admitted to the limits of their scientific traditions and acknowledged the betrayal and victimization of the dominant society. An openness in communication developed between the community and researchers that kept the tendencies in check of those of us from western traditions to dominate the discourse and direction. This teaching of cultural sensitivity by the CAC to the researchers kept a level of harmony between the two cultures so the Project could move forward.

The NRMNC Project utilized participatory evaluation processes that included a four-year evaluation by the CAC of conditions before and after the activities of the Project. In small break-out groups and then with the larger group, we sought to have the CAC and staff rank the project's progress in the key areas: building infrastructure, conducting research, education and hazard management activities. Ford et al. (1998) have developed methods for community-based evaluation, whereby stakeholders conduct their own community-based evaluation and monitoring. Such techniques include trend lines for community monitoring; depicting changes and improvements in priority areas of community sustainability concerns over project year periods. Rankings of priorities by villagers also were charted, listing major issues on a scale of 1–10 and how these priorities change over time.

In the NRMNC Project evaluation, the community co-principal investigator began the evaluation exercise with a Western Shoshone and Southern Paiute timeline, which starts with time immemorial as a long black line stretching into the past and then utilizing different colors, she depicted smaller lines of the major changes in the last several hundred years; the invasion and occupation of the United States, the forming of reservations, the changes in lifestyle, Native children forced off to boarding schools, the Nevada Test Site, the introduction of electricity and so forth, ending in the NRMNC Project as a line heading upward. The timeline has been very effective for setting the project into the context of strengthening Native culture from the recent past into the future. For the specific project interventions, the CAC reported that previously nearly none of these interventions existed and were enthusiastic about the progress of the project. However, they still identified a need for more resources, particularly for the community-based infrastructure, staff support and training. They commented that more work was still needed to build the bridge in communicating an understanding of technical risk concepts. They strongly support the community-based research and educational activities.

Throughout the four years, every NRMNC education module was evaluated using written participant evaluation forms and oral group feedback. The NRMNC community and technical staff diligently worked to respond to criticisms of our workshops. Some typical criticisms were "too technical, use more visuals", "agenda too crammed - too many facts to absorb", "prefer to have break-out groups", "have a Native facilitator summarize the major technical terms", "more topics on Native culture". The CAC complimented the project staff in making great strides in improving the workshops since the first year. In evaluating our total progress for over four years (that is, the productivity of the team in conducting research, producing educational materials, consistently convening the CAC meetings and raising additional funding), the CAC generally had been grateful to the staff. They often thanked the technical team for their hard work and commitment to Native issues. That commitment was perhaps one of the most key elements to the building of trust between the community and the scientists.

One last key ingredient important to the project's success was the support of the Ely-Shoshone tribe whose health director sits on the CAC and helps to oversee the

Project. The tribe manages one of the funding sources to the Project and will manage future grant support to the project. Tribal support is a crucial element in making the project successful; particularly for providing legitimacy to the project's work and accessing federal funding for future projects.

Acknowledgments

The authors gratefully acknowledge the support of the Great Basin NRMNC Community Advisory Committee with this article; the ongoing support of the Ely-Shoshone Tribe, Ely, NV; Citizen Alert Native American Program, Reno, NV, the Childhood Cancer Research Institute and Clark University, Worcester, MA for their sponsorship of the NRMNC Project. The NRMNC Project is grateful to these funding sources for their support of this Project; a grant R25 ES 08206–01, "Environmental Justice – Partnerships in Communication" from the National Institute of Environmental Health Sciences (NIEHS) and CERCLA with a cooperative agreement through the Agency for Toxic Substances and Disease Registry (ATSDR) Tribal Health Environmental Education Activities; the National Center for Environmental Health (NCEH) of the Centers for Disease Control (CDC), the Ruth Mott Fund, W. Alton Jones Foundation, the Ben and Jerry's Foundation, the Public Welfare Foundation and the North Shore Unitarian Veatch Foundation.

References

Advisory Committee on Human Radiation Experiments (1996), *Final Report*, Washington DC, Federal Advisory Committee.

Brown, P. (1994), *Environmental health and environmental justice*, Working Papers Series of the Working Group on Society and Health, Boston, MA: Tufts/New England Medical Center.

Brugge, D. and Benally, T. (1998), "Navajo Indian Voices and Faces Testify to the Legacy of Uranium Mining", *Cultural Survival Quarterly*, Spring.

Brugge, D., Benally, T., Harrison, P. (Jr.), Austin, M.G. and Fasthorse-Begay, L. (1997), *Memories Come to Us in the Rain and the Wind: Oral Histories and Photographs of Navajo Uranium Miners and Their Families*, Boston: Department of Family Medicine and Community Health, Tufts School of Medicine.

Brush, B.S. and Stabinsky, D. (eds) (1996), *Valuing Local Knowledge: Indigenous People and Intellectual Property Rights*, Island Press, Boston, MA.

Bryant, B. and Mohai, P .(1992), *Race and the Incidence of Environmental Hazards: A Time for Discourse*. Westview Press, Boulder, CO.

Bullard, R.D. and Wright, B.H. (1993), "Environmental Justice For All: Community Perspectives On Health and Research Needs", *Toxicology and Industrial Health*, **9**, 821–41.

Cancian, F. and Armstead, C. (1992), "Participatory Research", *Encyclopedia of Sociology*, **3,**1427–32.

Caulfield, C. (1989), *Multiple Exposures*, Michelen House, London.

Centers for Disease Control, proceedings from "Community, Tribal, Labor Involvement in DOE Public Health Activities" Conference, Atlanta, GA, February 1994.

Chambers, R. (1994) "Participatory Rural Appraisal (PRA): Challenges, Potentials and Paradigms", *World Development*, **22**.

Church, B. et al. (1990), "Overview of the Department of Energy's Off-Site Radiation Exposure Review Project (ORERP)", *Health Physics*, **59**.

Churchill, W. and LaDuke, W. (1992), "The Political Economy of Radioactive Colonialism", in Annette M. Jaimes (ed.), *The State of Native America*, South End Press, Boston, pp. 241–66.

Clinton, W.J. (1994a), *Executive Order No. 12898: Federal Actions to Address Environmental Justice in Minority Populations and Low-Income Populations*, Federal Register, 59:7629, February 11.

Colorado, P. (1988), "Bridging Native and Western Science", *Convergence, 21*, 49–68.

Connor, T. (1997), *Burdens of Proof: Science and Public Accountability in the Field of Environmental Epidemiology with a Focus on Low Dose Radiation and Community Health Studies*, Energy Research Foundation, Columbia, SC.

Eichstaedt, P.H. (1994), *If You Poison Us: Uranium and Native Americans*, Red Crane Books, Santa Fe.

Eisenbud, M. (1996), *Environmental Radioactivity*, Academic Press, Orlando, Florida Environmental Protection Agency.

Final Report of the Federal Facilities Environmental Restoration Dialogue Committee (1987), Washington, DC.

Ford, R., Lelo, F. and Rabarison, H. (1998), *Linking Governance and Effective Resource Management: A Guidebook for Community-based Monitoring and Evaluation*, Clark University, Massachusetts and Egerton University, Kenya.

Fowler, C. (1991), "Native Americans and Yucca Mountain", A Revised and Updated Summary Report on Research Undertaken Between 1987–1991 for State of Nevada Agency for Nuclear Projects and Nuclear Waste Project Office.

Fuller, J. (1984), *The Day We Bombed Utah*, New American Library, New York.

Friere, P. (1970), *Pedagogy of the Oppressed*, Seabury Press, New York.

Frohmberg, E., Goble, R., Sanchez, V. and Quigley, D. (2000), "The Assessment of Radiation Exposures to Native Communities from Nuclear Weapons Testing in Nevada", Society for Risk Analysis, March.

Gadgil, M. et al. (1993), "Indigenous Knowledge for Biodiversity Conservation", Ambio, May, **22**(2–3).

Gallagher, C. (1993), *American Ground Zero*, MIT Press, Cambridge, MA.

George, P. (1997), "Working Towards Community Health", W. Shoshone Defense Project Newsletter, Fall/Winter.

Hall, B. (1981), "Participatory Research, Popular Knowledge, and Power: Personal Reflection", *Convergence, 3*, 6–19.

Handy, D. (2001), "The Language of Environmental Management: Environmental Justice at Nuclear Facilities in Native Communities", Master's Thesis, Clark University, Worcester, MA, Spring.

Israel, B., Schultz, A.J., Parker, E. and Becker, A. (1981), "Review of Community-based Research: Assessing Partnership Approaches to Improve Public Health", *Annual Review of Public Health, 19*,173–202.

Israel, B., Checkoway, B., Schultz, A.J. and Zimmerman, M.A. (1994), "Health Education and Community Empowerment: conceptualizing and measuring perceptions of individual, organizational and community control", *Health Education Quarterly, 21*,149–70.

Kerber, R., Till, J., Simon, S., Lyon, J., Thomas, D., Preston-Martin, S., Rallison, M., Lloyd, R. and Stevens, W. (1993), "A Cohort Study of Thyroid Disease in Relation to Fallout From Nuclear Weapons Testing", *JAMA*, **270**, 1076–2082.

Kiser, M., Boario, M. and Hilton, D. (1995), "Transformation for Health: A Participatory Empowerment Education Training Model in the Faith Community", *Journal of Health Education*, November/December, **26**.

Levine, D.M., Becker, D.M., Bone, L.R., Hill, M.N., Tuggle, M.B. et al. (1994), "Community-academic health center partnerships for underserved minority populations", *JAMA*, **272**, 309–11.

National Research Council (1990), *Health Effects of Exposure to Low-Levels of Ionizing Radiation -BEIR V*, Report of the National Academy of Sciences, Washington, DC.

National Institute of Environmental Health Sciences (1997), Environmental Justice and Community-Based Prevention/Intervention Research Grantee Meeting, *Advancing the Community-Driven Research Agenda Conference Report*, October 27–29, Research Triangle Park, NC.

Nevada Risk Assessment/Management Program (NRAMP) (1996), "DRAFT Preliminary Risk Assessment of DOE Sites in Nevada", Harry Reid Center for Environmental Studies, UNLV, Las Vegas.

Pendergrass, G. and Nelson, L. (1987), *The Mushroom Cloud and The Downwinders*, Forlagat Futurum, Denmark.

Pecore, M. (1992), "Menominee Sustained Yield Management", *Journal of Forestry*, **90**.

Plough, A. and Olafson, F. (1994), "Implementing the Boston Healthy Start Initiative: a case study of community empowerment and public health", *Health Education Quarterly*, **21**, 221–34.

Plough, A. and Sheldon, K. (1990), "The Emergence of Risk Communication Studies: Social and Political Context", in *Readings in Risk*, Glickman, T. and Gough, M., Resources for the Future, Washington, DC.

Posey, D. (1982), "The Journey to become a Shaman", *Journal of Latin American Literature*.

Quigley, D. (1997), "Meeting Community Needs: Improving Health Research and Risk Assessment Methodologies", Conference Proceedings, Worcester, MA: Childhood Cancer Research Institute, Sept. 20–22, 1996.

Quigley, D., Sanchez, V., Proctor, D., Goble, R., Handy, D., Frohmberg, E., Townsend, K. and Stierwalt, M. (1996a), "Participatory Approaches To Managing the Health Risks of Nuclear Contamination", *Subsistence and Environmental Health*, Fall, USDOE, Washington, DC.

Reardon, K. (1995), "Creating University/Community Partnerships that Work: Lessons From the East St. Louis Action Research Project", *Metropolitan Universities: An International Forum*, Spring, 47–59.

Ruckelshaus, W. (1985), "Risk, Science and Democracy", *Issues In Science and Technology*, **1**(3).

Russell, D., Lewis, S. and Keating, B. (1992), *Inconclusive by Design: Waste, Fraud and Abuse in Federal Environmental Health Research*, Boston, MA: The National Toxics Campaign Fund and Chesapeake, VA, Environmental Health Network.

Samet, J.M., Kutvirt, D.M., Waxweiler, R.J. and Keyes, C.R. (1984), "Uranium Mining and Lung Cancer in Navajo Men", *New England Journal of Medicine*, **310**,1481–4.

Sanchez, V. (1997a), "Nuclear Risk Management for Native Communities", Western Shoshone Defense Project Newsletter, Spring, Crescent Valley, NV.

Sanchez, V. (1997), "Nuclear Risk Management for Native Communities Update", Citizen Alert Newsletter, July.

Sclove, R. (1995), "Putting Science to Work in Communities", *The Chronicle of Higher Education*, **41**, B1–B2.

Schleien, B., Ruttenber, J. and Sage, M. (1991), "Epidemiological Studies of Cancer in Populations Near Nuclear Facilities", *Health Physics*, **61**.

Shields, L., Wieser, W.H., Skipper, B.J., Charlay, B. and Benally, L. (1991), "Navajo Birth Outcomes in the Shiprock Uranium Mining Area", *Health Physics*, **63**, 542–51.

Sissel, P.A. and Horn, M.D. (1996), "Literacy and Health Communities: Potential Partners in Practice", *New Directions for Adult and Continuing Education*, Summer, **70**.

Slocum, R., Wichhart, L., Rocheleau, D. and Thomas-Slayter, B. (1995), *Power, Process and Participation - Tools for Change*, Intermediate Technology Publications London, UK.

Stevens, W., Thomas, D., Till, J., Lyon, J., Kerber, R., Simon, S., Lloyd, R., Elghany, N.A. and Preston-Martin, S. (1990), "Leukemia in Utah and Radioactive Fallout from the Nevada Test Site", *JAMA*, **264**.

Suzuki, D. aand Knudson, P. (1992), *Wisdom of the Elders*, Bantam Books, New York.

Thompson, C.B. and McArthur, R.D. (1996), *Health Physics*, **71**, 470–76.

United Church of Christ (UCC) Commission for Racial Justice (1987), *Toxic Wastes and Race in the United States: A National Study of the Racial and Socioeconomic Characteristics of Communities with Hazardous Waste Sites*, New York: United Church of Christ.

United States Census (1990), US Census Bureau, Washington, DC.

Wallerstein, N. (1994), "Introduction to community empowerment, participatory education and health", *Health Education Quarterly*, **21**, 141–8.

Wigley, D.C. and Schrader-Frechette, K. (1996), "Environmental Racism and Biased Methods of Risk Assessment", *Risk: Health, Safety and Environment*, **7**, 55, Winter.

Wing, S. (1998), "Whose Epidemiology, Whose Health?", *International Journal of Human Services*, **28**, 241–52.

Wynne, B. (1992), "Risk and Social Learning: Reification to Engagement", in Krimsky, S. and Golding, D. (eds), *Social Theories of Risk*, Praeger, Westport, CT.

Zabarte, I. (1996), Personal communication, Memorandum re: "Native American Sovereignty and Nuclear Waste Issues".

Chapter 12

Social Responsibility and Research Ethics in Community-Driven Studies of Industrialized Hog Production

Steve Wing

Most environmental health research has been conducted in relation to problems identified by governments, industries, health professionals, and the scientific community. These institutions have some degree of prestige and power; they have played an active role in developing environmental health science itself, and their members are seldom forced to live with serious environmental contamination. In contrast, communities of low income and people of color seldom have had access to researchers; they have been underrepresented in the research professions (St. George et al., 1997), they have been used as test subjects for biomedical research (Thomas and Quinn, 1991), and they sometimes have had no choice but to live and work in the presence of contaminants (Brown, 1995). Environmental health research that takes as its starting point the experiences and concerns of communities of low income and people of color raises numerous questions regarding methodology (the formation of study hypotheses, research design, analysis, interpretation, and communication of findings) as well as ethical issues related to the role of professionals and academic and government institutions, responsibilities for communication, respect, collaboration, protection of human subjects, and protection of the communities in which research is conducted.

In this article I describe environmental health studies of industrial swine production facilities conducted by a community-driven research and education partnership. I use these examples to explore ethical issues that arise in community-driven research conducted in the setting of gross inequalities between powerful institutions and communities exposed to environmental injustices.

Industrial agriculture in general, and pork producers in particular, have strong ties to government and academic institutions (Thu, 2001). Researchers can face ethical and legal dilemmas that arise from conflict between groups that create and permit industrial operations and their contaminants, and the communities living with the industries and contaminants. Recognizing the distinction that epidemiologists have drawn between biomedical research focused on individuals and public health research conducted from a population perspective (Rose, 1989), I conclude that community-driven research involves analogous ethical dimensions regarding autonomy and risk of harm to entire communities, not simply to individual research subjects whose welfare is the traditional domain of institutional review boards (IRBs).

Background

In the early 1990s, news stories appeared in rural Halifax County in northeastern North Carolina (Economic Development for Tillery, 1991; Schwebke, 1992) announcing that the historically underdeveloped southeast region of the county was slated for 17 new industrialized hog production facilities that would bring economic development to a predominantly African-American and low-income population.

Public reaction was slow to emerge. Most rural residents of this area are familiar with raising hogs on family farms. However, citizens soon began to learn that industrialized production operations are nothing like family farms. Far from being independent businesses, confined animal feeding operations (CAFOs) are generally owned by or run under contracts with large corporations that control the animals, feed, veterinary supplies, and management plans (Thu, 1998). If the operation is run under contract, the contractor owns the buildings, equipment, land, and waste but not the animals. Some CAFOs raise hogs from birth to market weight, whereas others are designed for only one stage of an animal's life: birth to weaning, weaning to about 40 pounds, or 40 to about 250 pounds, the weight at which hogs are typically slaughtered. The corporate integrator trucks its hogs between CAFOs that are specialized for growing animals of each size.

Swine CAFOs house thousands of hogs in close confinement in large buildings (Figure 12.1). Subtherapeutic doses of antibiotics are used to control infection and promote growth. Large ventilation fans exhaust dusts and gases that pose health risks to the animals and workers. Animal waste falls through slats in the floor and is washed into cesspools called lagoons. There the waste undergoes anaerobic decomposition; the remaining liquids are subsequently sprayed on nearby fields (Figure 12.1).

The rapid growth of industrialized hog production in North Carolina occurred between the middle 1980s and the late 1990s (Furuseth, 1997). As hog production in the state expanded from less than three million to approximately 10 million hogs per year, the number of operations shrank dramatically as smaller independent family farmers were replaced by industrial-style operations. At the same time, hog production, which had previously been distributed across the state, became concentrated in eastern North Carolina (Furuseth, 1997). Expansion of industrial operations occurred under regulatory controls strongly influenced by hog producers and other agribusiness interests in the North Carolina General Assembly. State legislation was enacted to prevent local and county governments from zoning agriculture, and state universities closely allied with agribusiness concerns provided research support (Cecelski and Kerr, 1992).

As citizens of Halifax County began to learn about industrialized hog production, many became deeply concerned about local impacts of such "economic development." They worried about air pollution and noxious odors. They feared that groundwater could be contaminated in an area with sandy soils and high water tables where most residents depend on private wells for drinking water. They learned of the potential for surface water pollution from spray field runoff and lagoon failures. They were concerned about loss of independent family farmers and the land that they had farmed, and they were concerned about the vitality of their churches, schools, and communities. They felt they had been targeted for this kind of "economic development" because their primarily African-American, low-income communities lacked political power (Wing et al., 1996).

The Concerned Citizens of Tillery (CCT), a grassroots organization in southeast Halifax County, worked with county officials to develop an intensive livestock ordinance that would impose stricter environmental controls than state regulations. In that effort, and in the course of providing assistance to other communities in the path of corporate pork production, CCT sought support from environmentalists, social activists, and researchers who could help document economic, social, environmental, and public health issues affecting communities living with swine CAFOs (Wing et al., 1996). Although university scientists had conducted many studies related to agricultural technologies, veterinary health, and health of agricultural workers, relatively little research had addressed environmental, social, and health concerns of communities affected by industrial hog production.

Environmental Injustice in North Carolina's Hog Industry

The siting of a landfill for polychlorinated biphenyls (PCBs) not far from Tillery in predominantly African-American Warren County, North Carolina, in 1982 is often cited as an event that introduced the term "environmental racism" to a national audience (Bullard, 1994). Ten years later, CCT and other community-based organizations in eastern North Carolina were beginning to see industrial hog production as an environmental justice and public health issue. During 1982–1997, leading hog-producing areas experienced greater loss of family farms than did other areas of North Carolina (Edwards and Ladd, 2000). This raises concerns for rural communities because family farms keep money in local economies and help maintain local businesses and services. Biologic and chemical contaminants from swine CAFOs, including bacteria, viruses, nitrates, hydrogen sulfide, and endotoxins, threaten community health when they contaminate air, aquifers used for drinking water, and streams and rivers used for subsistence fishing and recreation (Cole et al., 2000). Ironically, any health effects occurring from these exposures would be difficult to detect by examining medical records because the communities affected most have little access to medical care. Residents also distrust local health departments and other medical care institutions because of a history of segregation, exclusion, and prejudice (Gamble, 1993; Wing, 1998).

A Community-Driven Research Partnership

Noxious odors – so severe that residents who can afford it sometimes leave their homes to spend especially bad nights in motels – prevent neighbors of CAFOs from enjoying their homes and the outdoors. Odorant chemicals can penetrate clothing, curtains, and upholstery, affecting people long after plumes of emissions pass and subjecting them to possible ostracism at school or in public. One study suggested that hog odors can affect the mental health of nearby residents (Schiffman et al., 1995); another suggested that neighbors experience respiratory effects similar to those seen among workers in the confinement buildings (Thu et al., 1997). Mothers in eastern

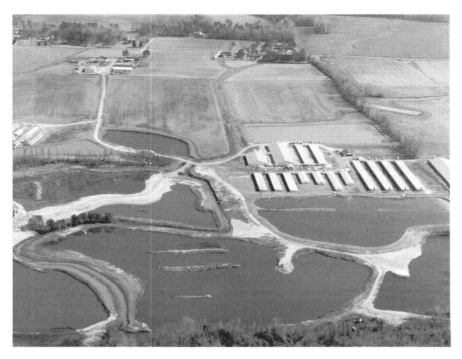

Figure 12.1   Confined animal feeding operations in eastern North Carolina showing fecal waste pits in the foreground, confinement structures (left and right middle), spray fields, and neighboring homes

North Carolina report that their asthmatic children experience episodes of wheezing in the presence of strong plumes from nearby hog operations.

I met numerous residents of low-income, African-American communities who told me that industrial hog operations were increasingly being located in their communities. In one area residents had marked locations of churches, schools, and hog operations on a large map to demonstrate the proximity of African-American communities to swine CAFOs. However, when residents spoke to journalists and government officials about discriminatory patterns in the siting of these facilities, they were frustrated by responses that community observations were anecdotal and did not prove any consistent pattern. African-American and white neighbors of swine CAFOs, frustrated by lack of action from local governments, kept diaries to document odors and health problems, took photographs of waste spills and rotting hog carcasses, and wrote to state and federal officials.

In late 1996, a partnership formed by CCT with the Halifax County Health Department and the University of North Carolina (UNC) School of Public Health received funding from the National Institute of Environmental Health Sciences' (NIEHS) Environmental Justice: Partnerships for Communication program (Wing et al., 1996). Along with environmental justice education and outreach to communities and medical providers, we were funded to conduct research that, using official records, could quantify systematically the extent to which hog CAFOs and their potential impacts on health and quality of life disproportionately affected communities of low income and people of color (primarily African Americans) in the state. Our aims were to evaluate data for local communities, to consider possible alternative explanations for observed patterns, and to consider data on household water source (well or municipal), because groundwater contamination is an important public health concern.

Although data analyses were conducted at the university, the study questions originated in the exposed communities. Community members participated in evaluating data quality through their knowledge of local CAFOs. In consultation with our community partners, we made decisions about how to define the study population and data sources, how to choose and define variables for the analysis, and how to interpret results. We augmented our statistical analyses with maps and charts. And we found that hog CAFOs were far more common in poor communities and communities of people of color, that this concentration was more extreme for integrator-owned or contracted CAFOs than for independent operations, and that the pattern was explained only partly by differences in population density. Furthermore, we found that hog operations were concentrated in areas where most people depend on household wells for drinking water (Wing et al., 2000).

Reactions to the Environmental Justice Study

We were invited to present our findings at an environmental justice session sponsored by the NIEHS during the annual meeting of the Society of Toxicology in March 1999. The North Carolina General Assembly recently had passed a moratorium on construction of new hog CAFOs (except those using "new technologies"), the governor's office was developing a plan to address environmental problems from the lagoon and spray field system, and industrial hog producers were in the news because of waste spills and impacts of nutrient loading on fish, shellfish, and a recently discovered toxic dinoflagellate, *Pfiesteria piscicida*. The CCT had worked in partnership with numerous grassroots groups and traditional environmental organizations to educate the public about effects of industrial hog production and to provide organizational support to local affected communities. To support these efforts and contribute to the ongoing policy debate, we decided to release information about our findings to the press in conjunction with my presentation at the national meeting. The release was coordinated with the UNC News Service, which routinely prepares stories about topical research when it is publicly presented or published. Several major state newspapers ran stories on our findings.

I immediately received calls from representatives of industry groups who wanted to explain to me how the pork business is run. In their view, it was just good business to select the cheapest land for hog CAFOs – and that just happened to be areas that were rural, poor, and disproportionately African American. I soon learned that one of the industry representatives who called me was a member of the UNC Board of Governors. In early April I received an invitation to appear before the House Agriculture Committee of the North Carolina General Assembly. I was pleased by their interest and excited about the opportunity to address a group of policy makers interested in our findings. However, when I told CCT Executive Director Gary Grant about the invitation, he explained that the committee included a number of hog producers, was friendly to agribusiness concerns, and was probably not very pleased with our research. I asked Gary to appear with me before the committee.

The UNC-Chapel Hill Associate Vice Chancellor for Government Relations set up a meeting to discuss my impending appearance at the General Assembly with the Associate Dean of the School of Public Health. The administrators stated that they did not want to tell me how to present our research, but they were clearly concerned that I make a good impression at the legislature, which, after all, votes on UNC appropriations. Meanwhile, in Tillery, at the weekly meeting of the Open Minded Seniors, one of CCT's most active member organizations, Gary Grant announced that I had been called to the General Assembly to present our findings on environmental justice, and that I was not likely to be warmly received. Many members of the group were interested in attending the session to support Gary and me as we presented our research. About 30 CCT members traveled to Raleigh to attend the meeting of the House Agriculture Committee on 27 April 1999.

The Associate Vice Chancellor accompanied me to the hearing. The Open Minded Seniors had filled most of the public seating when we entered the hearing room; a couple of dozen lobbyists, staffers, environmentalists, activists, and other spectators stood at the back of the room. After staff members finished setting up the slide projector and providing water for the committee members, the CCT members were the only African Americans remaining in the room. Some committee members had a few technical questions about my presentation, such as why we didn't use more recent income data, and made other remarks about the business logic of locating hog CAFOs in poor areas. Committee members also wanted to know whether state funds had been used for our research. Next, Gary Grant spoke about the policy implications of our work and the urgent need for the North Carolina General Assembly to help citizens of eastern North Carolina living with air and water pollution from hog CAFOs. At one point the Open Minded Seniors began to applaud, which prompted the committee chair to use his gavel to quiet the room with the statement that applause was not permitted. Despite this admonition, the Open Minded Seniors had made their support for us clear to all present.

At the end of the hearing, I spoke cordially with the committee chair and a number of spectators, including one industry lobbyist.

Then another industry lobbyist who introduced himself by handing me his business card approached me. He refused my offer to shake his hand, demanded a copy of our full report, and said that if I did not send him one immediately I would be facing a lawsuit. I was startled by his hostility but shrugged it off as an overreaction.

The Rural Health Survey

In addition to the environmental justice study, we were also involved in more traditional health effects research. In the fall of 1998, with support from the North Carolina State Health Department, we initiated a survey of rural residents in eastern North Carolina. Reports of odor problems and respiratory effects had been coming in from hog CAFO neighbors across eastern North Carolina, and the State Health

Department was interested in obtaining more information. To our knowledge, only one small study, from Iowa, had been published on respiratory health effects among swine CAFO neighbors (Thu et al., 1997). In consultation with our community partners and staff from the State Health Department, we designed a survey to compare health and quality of life of residents of three communities, one in the neighborhood of a hog CAFO, one in the neighborhood of a dairy operation that used a liquid waste management system, and a third with no intensive livestock production.

Design and Conduct of the Health Survey

Designing the study presented a number of challenges. Our environmental justice analyses were, by then, confirming the observations of community members that hog CAFOs are disproportionately located in low-income and African-American communities. We would need to ask for the participation of people whose past experiences led them to distrust health departments, medical providers, universities, or researchers. The relationships with community-based organizations that we had established in our environmental justice project would be essential for collecting reliable data and establishing a high response rate in defined populations in the three areas. At the same time, we knew that to avoid potential biases that could be introduced by community participation in areas divided between those with negative feelings about the hog industry and those whose livelihood depends on the industry, we would need to insulate the data collection process from peer pressure or leading questioning. Quantification of individuals' exposures to hog CAFO emissions, a key component in establishing dose–response relationships, would be extremely expensive; furthermore, even if we could afford to make environmental measurements, it was not clear which of the many hazardous agents present in odorous plumes are most relevant to health effects. Clinical confirmation of symptoms would also be desirable; however, severe responses to air pollution episodes are too uncommon to evaluate statistically in small populations, and poor access to medical care could lead to underestimation of problems. We debated carefully whether it would be ethical to conduct a study if we could not measure exposures and outcomes sufficiently well to detect a health effect if one existed, recognizing that our design would be constrained by funding that could be provided by the State Health Department. Our decision to proceed was influenced by evidence from previous studies and by community members and state officials who felt an urgent need for respiratory health data from North Carolina.

We developed a structured symptom questionnaire based on previous studies and input from eastern North Carolina residents who helped us use culturally appropriate language. We used the same questions in each of the three communities, and included no questions about odor, hogs, or livestock because one community had no livestock. We chose three communities with similar demographic characteristics according to census data. In each community, we conducted a household census, noting each occupied dwelling on a map and assigning a code to the residence (Wing and Wolf, 2000).

We collaborated with a community-based organization in each area. Community members helped us locate roads and houses, and they served as community consultants during the data collection. Trained interviewers from UNC visited households in each area, accompanied by a community consultant who made the initial introduction of the researcher. Interviews were conducted without the presence of the community consultant unless the participant requested that the consultant remain. The interviewer read aloud, and provided the study participant with a copy of, an "Agreement to Participate" that explained that the study was about environmental exposures and health of rural residents. Participants were assured that their responses would be kept confidential and that their name would not be written on the questionnaire, although a link would be maintained between their address and responses. UNC's IRB gave us permission to obtain oral consent because we used no interventions or sensitive questions, and because a signed consent form would have been the only record of a person's name.

In the two livestock communities, interviewing teams visited households nearest the CAFOs first and then visited households in order, moving away from the CAFO, until they reached our target sample size of 50, with one adult in each household interviewed. Data collection took place in January and February 1999. We completed 155 interviews, with a refusal rate of 14%. Respondents were 92% African American and 65% female, and 27% were 65 years old or older (Wing and Wolf, 2000).

In mid-April 1999, before submitting our report to the State Health Department, we invited members of the three community-based organizations to a meeting to discuss our initial findings. We obtained input from community members and responded to questions and concerns about excesses of respiratory and digestive symptoms that had been reported by hog CAFO neighbors compared with residents of the other communities. Community members decided at this meeting that they did not want the names of their communities to be included in our report. We therefore removed from our report any data on numbers of households, population size, race, and income characteristics of the census block groups in the study. These characteristics had been used to match communities in the study, but the figures could have been used by others to deduce the identities of the communities. We also removed from the report any exact information about the size of the hog and cattle CAFOs, which had been derived from Department of Water Quality permit data, and replaced the numbers with approximate figures. At the end of April, we submitted a draft report to the State Health Department. Our analyses showed that the frequency of miscellaneous symptoms such as muscle aches and vision and hearing problems was similar in the three communities. In contrast, residents near the hog CAFO reported increased numbers of headaches, runny noses, sore throats, excessive coughing, diarrhea, and burning eyes. They also reported many more occasions when they could not open windows or go outside even in nice weather. The report was reviewed by State Health Department staff, the chief statistician for the State Center for Health Statistics, the chair of the UNC Department of Epidemiology, and others. Our final report incorporated their comments.

The Pork Industry Response

The State Health Department issued a press statement releasing our report to the public on 7 May 1999. Later that day, attorneys for the North Carolina Pork Council wrote to my coauthor, Susanne Wolf, and me requesting that we:

... make available for copying by this office any and all documentation in your possession (or that you are aware of in the possession of other State agencies or State personnel) that contain, represent, record, document, discuss, or otherwise reflect or memorialize the results of the Study or any conclusions or recommendations that you or any local, state or federal agency might draw from the Study or any other matter discussed in the Report, including, without limitation, the studies of the three communities referred to in the Release; any notes or other records from any site visits or interviews made during the course or as a part of the Study; any sampling, testing or other analysis that was performed as a part of the Study; any calculations, research, or other work papers that reflect any analysis that you or others made from or using the data collected as a part of the Study; any contracts or other similar documents that define the Study or any having to do with payment for the study; the identities of all persons who worked on or contributed to the Study (including persons interviewed); and any other documentation that were generated as a part of or in the course of the Study.

This request was made under the North Carolina Public Records Statute, which defines a public record as all:

...documents, papers, letters, maps, books, photographs, films, sound recordings, magnetic or other tapes, electronic data-processing records, artifacts, or other documentary material, regardless of physical form or characteristics, made or received pursuant to law or ordinance in connection with the transaction of public business by any agency of North Carolina government or its subdivisions.

The North Carolina Public Records Statute does not protect documents collected in the course of research involving human subjects and requires public officials, defined to include university faculty, staff, and graduate assistants who work for pay, to turn over records in a timely manner. The letter also stated that attorneys for the Pork Council would evaluate whether any of our statements were defamatory. Finally, the letter stated:

...it is imperative that we be given access to those documents no later than Wednesday, May 12. If we are not granted access to those documents in a timely manner, we have been directed to prepare an action for filing in the appropriate division of the General Court of Justice, pursuant to N.C. Gen. Stat. §132-9, for an order compelling disclosure or copying of those records and to seek such other remedies as are available for those statutes.

The Pork Council request raised a number of concerns. First, I was obligated to protect the confidentiality of participants. My name and contact information appeared on the Agreement to Participate that had been given to each participant. Although we did not record participants' names, we did have maps of the locations of their homes linked to their responses by a randomly assigned study number. Even without the maps, information about participants, including age, race, sex, occupation, industry, number in household, water source, and responses to questions about health status, was certainly sufficient to deduce which individuals from a particular area were in the study in these sparsely populated rural communities.

Breach of confidentiality was a concern not only from a legal and ethical standpoint. The community trust upon which our research depended would be seriously compromised as well, potentially destroying valued professional and personal relationships and threatening the continuation of research into exposures and health of neighbors of swine CAFOs. Given my professional and institutional position, I could not expect a second chance. Furthermore, if I violated my agreement with participants I could be branded, across the state and in other regions where there is a growing network of communities affected by corporate swine production, as untrustworthy.

The pork industry responded not only to the university but also to our federal funders. Shortly after receiving the letter from the Pork Council attorney, I received a message from the official at NIEHS in charge of the environmental justice grant program: "I've had a request to put together a summary of your project. Do you have any relevant health effects data available? I have been asked to do this ASAP so any help you can provide will be greatly appreciated." He further explained that "this request has to do with a congressional inquiry" and that "we may have to provide records under the Freedom of Information Act." I interpreted this as an effort of the industry to challenge federal support for our research, and responded by sharing with NIEHS the letter from the Pork Council attorney and suggesting that material from our annual report be used to respond to the request. There were no further requests from NIEHS.

Although the primary purpose of the Pork Council's request appeared to be harassment and intimidation, the request related to an important and legitimate part of scientific inquiry: the ability to replicate findings and evaluate evidence independently. In fact, I had recently conducted an independent reevaluation of environmental health effects using data from a study that had been designed and conducted with funding from industry (Wing et al., 1997a; Wing et al., 1997b; Wing et al., 1997c). Just as some community members in that case were concerned about conclusions from an industry-funded study, now an industry group was concerned about findings from a study that was conducted with community participation. To evaluate the quality, internal consistency, and analytical methods in our rural health survey, the industry would need to be able to conduct an independent reanalysis. The need to protect confidentiality would have to be considered in relation to a scientific culture in which reanalysis is essential and in relation to power inequalities between industry and the exposed communities.

The university attorney, who had been copied on the Pork Council attorney's letter, explained to me that North Carolina law required us to turn over all documents related to the study as quickly as possible. Because this would have violated our agreement with study participants, I consulted with the chair of our IRB and other university officials. One administrator told me that if I refused to turn over documents as directed by the university attorney, the university "would call the SBI [State Bureau of Investigation] and have me arrested for stealing state property." We discussed withholding documents on the grounds that their release would have a chilling effect on future research, and on grounds that we would be violating the confidentiality promised in the Agreement to Participate. The administrators were not hopeful that these arguments would be accepted, and in any case deferred to the university attorney on making a final decision.

In June, the university attorney agreed to release records to the Pork Council, including computerized files of individual responses, interviewer training instructions, draft copies of our report, other statistical tabulations, and study related correspondence, including electronic mail messages of all project staff. To protect confidentiality of the participants and the communities, the university attorney agreed that we should withhold any information that could lead to disclosure of where the study was done, including maps, driving instructions, and any references in our communications or study materials to locations or names of persons that would identify locations in the study. We reasoned that no individuals could be identified, even with information in the survey, unless the locations of the survey were known. Staff members and I spent considerable time in assembling and redacting documents. In the presence of the rural health survey project director and other staff, an attorney for the Pork Council reviewed the documents and copied many of them. They continued until August to request information that we had withheld and then ceased to express interest.

In July 1999, I was invited by the State Health Department to present findings of our study at a conference on the public health impacts of intensive livestock operations. The conference was held at North Carolina State University in Raleigh, which has the Animal and Poultry Waste Management Center, a veterinary school, and other programs related to industrial agriculture. A number of pork producers attended the conference and posed hostile questions after my presentation. Later, I was approached by an assistant professor from another UNC-system institution, who told me, "I have been conducting research on neighbors of hog operations, but I'm afraid that if I have to deal with legal problems like yours, I'll never get tenure. So I've decided to drop my research for now."

The Sustainable Hog Farming Summit

In the fall of 2000, I accepted an invitation to speak about our environmental justice and public health research at a conference being organized by a coalition of independent farmers, environmentalists, and grassroots organizations billed as the "Sustainable Hog Farming Summit." The conference was scheduled for January 2001 in New Bern, North Carolina. On 8 December, I was copied, along with the Dean of the School of Public Health and the UNC Chancellor, on e-mail correspondence from the UNC Associate Vice Chancellor for Government Relations. Staff in the UNC system president's office had written to the Associate Vice Chancellor:

> We have received several questions and complaints from legislators and others –received through different offices in the University – about the Sustainable Hog Farming Summit announced for Thursday, January 11, 2001 at New Bern.... Five faculty members at three different UNC institutions show on the Summit agenda as program participants (moderators or panelists). I've been asked whether those faculty members are representing themselves or the universities where they are employed, are attending on university time or their own, and whether they are paying their own expenses or is someone else (presumably meaning the university or the conference sponsors).

During 15 years on the UNC faculty I had presented research at scores of meetings but had never before been asked to account for myself in this way. The associate vice chancellor described a senior member of the North Carolina Senate who "had concerns about Carolina's [UNC's] 'involvement' with the program." She also described a conversation with two Pork Council lobbyists "whom I consider to be friends" and reported that "they are fully cognizant of the fact that we cannot and will not censure our faculty." I responded to the administrators by explaining that I was appearing as a university employee to present my research, and that I would be funded by our environmental justice research and education grant.

Social and Ethical Responsibilities of Researchers

Environmental health research can influence conflicts between communities of low income or people of color and the institutions that derive benefits (profits, federal and state funding or services, avoidance of wastes) from the activities and policies that burden these communities. Researchers, most of whom work in relatively privileged institutions, are placed in situations of conflicting loyalties if they conduct research in collaboration with, or on behalf of, communities burdened by environmental injustices. These conflicts can threaten the self-interest of researchers and may raise social and ethical issues that do not typically arise in research projects that respond to the agendas of institutions.

Principles of Research Design

Before addressing some of these conflicts as they apply to our case, it is important to be clear that researchers performing community-driven environmental health research should not encounter conflicts over the logic used to design research. Our scientific culture values expert opinion and standardized, replicable techniques overlay opinion and observation. Because observations of community members do not "count" in the scientific literature used by policy makers and courts, researchers can maximize their service to communities by devising standardized procedures, including data collection and measurement techniques, that comport with professional standards, even as we may need to change those standards to improve science. First among our considerations should be to conduct studies that have the sensitivity to detect an effect if one exists. The ability to detect no effect when one does not exist is also important, although in the case of community-driven environmental health, researchers must carefully distinguish "no effect" for a specific biologic end point from "no effect" in an ecologic context that encompasses social, psychologic, and economic impacts.

The challenge for researchers is to work with community members to frame questions, and design procedures to produce answers, that respect community concerns by investigating them with the best technical approaches possible, including newly devised methods to enhance community input and analyze data. Results of these investigations will be useful to communities burdened by environmental problems because such research can address topics that could not be investigated without the technical resources of institutions, and because the findings can be used in situations where community observations are not valued. Rather than facing a conflict between standard procedures and alternatives that are acceptable to the community but viewed as "unscientific" by scientists, both researchers and community members benefit from negotiating the use of rigorous methods.

Responding to Government, Industry, and the Media

In responding to concerns and inquiries from the state legislature, university administration, and federal granting agency, I might have distanced myself from the communities living with hog CAFOs and their allies. Instead, I kept them informed. This strategy had two effects. First, I maintained the trust of the communities who had been instrumental in identifying research questions, conducting fieldwork, and educating the public about our findings. This trust would continue to be essential if we were to address additional research questions. Second, the communities responded by appearing at the legislative hearing, giving advice on acceptable means of responding to the public records request, helping to identify external legal support, and providing strong encouragement and support. If I had backed away from the community under institutional pressure, not only would I have compromised relationships essential to conducting high-quality research, our research partnership would have lost support of an outside constituency at the very time when it was most needed.

Some academics are reluctant to interact with the media. They feel that their findings are misrepresented and misunderstood and that interviews take considerable time and have little potential to influence scientific publications or grant funding, the criteria that matter most for career advancement. However, community-driven researchers have responsibilities regarding publication of scientific findings, making those findings public in appropriate ways, and participating in processes involving the media and policy makers (Sandman, 1991; Viel et al., 1998). Environmental health findings can help exposed community members protect themselves, can motivate participation in democratic processes, and can influence public opinion and policy makers. Researchers have an obligation to be involved in targeted efforts to inform affected communities about research results as well as to participate in activities that have a wider audience (Sandman, 1991). These activities must be conducted in partnership with affected communities.

Researchers have a responsibility to report findings of studies even when they can be expected to produce negative reactions from industry, government, or universities. Publications are a key goal of researchers seeking to compete for positions and grant funding in an entrepreneurial environment. However, when research sheds light on institutional discrimination, environmental contamination, or health effects that could create legal problems for institutions that provide jobs and funding to researchers, researchers may be motivated to withhold or delay publication, or to provide benign interpretations even when there is evidence of harm. Such actions fail to meet responsibilities to research participants, exposed communities in the study area and elsewhere, policy makers, and researchers working on the same or related problems.

Respecting Interests of Individuals and Communities

Our experiences with the public records act request have similarities with cases of other researchers whose records have been subpoenaed in lawsuits involving large corporations (Fisher, 1996; Picou, 1996a; Traynor, 1996; Picou, 1996b; Picou, 1996c). Tobacco, oil, and pharmaceutical industries have sought and obtained research records that university investigators had assumed would be protected by confidentiality requirements. Furthermore, it cannot be presumed that university administrators will take a strong advocacy role in protecting research records or faculty members (Fisher, 1996; Picou, 1996a). Our compromise, revealing responses but not locations of the respondents, was based on the assumption that both pieces of information would be required for deductive disclosure of the identity of participants through age, sex, race, occupation, and household characteristics. This compromise was accepted by the university attorney despite the concern that the university might have to go to court to protect the identity of communities. However, given the complexities of deductive disclosure from a statistical as well as an ethical standpoint, it is inappropriate for a researcher and an attorney, especially under threat of litigation, to make the final decision about release of data. Researchers and institutions faced with similar decisions should consult a panel, possibly an IRB or a committee of an IRB that includes a statistician, community members, and others experienced in protection of human subjects.

A more fundamental problem is that IRBs are concerned only with protecting individual research participants. In our research, we were also concerned with pro- tecting the communities where the research was conducted. The presence of industrial hog operations has split communities between those who depend on the industry for income and those whose quality of life and health have been adversely affected (Snell, 2001). In some areas, community members have been fearful of participating in research because of the influence of the hog industry in local affairs. One resident told us, "If you want to do a survey in this community, you'd better finish on the first day, because you won't be able to come back." We were also advised not to call the sheriff's department if we had trouble on the road. Several community members who have publicly opposed the industry told me that they have been followed and threatened, and that they carry weapons for their own protection. In 1998, attorneys for a hog grower wrote to Elsie Herring, a North Carolina woman who had requested help from local and state public health officials regarding spraying of hog waste that drifted onto her and her mother's homes and cars (Herring, personal communication). The attorneys threatened to sue Herring and impose a restraining order if she persisted in her requests for assistance. "If you violate any such restraining order," the letter stated, "we will ask the court to put you in prison for contempt." At the Sustainable Hog Farming Summit, Herring reported that the grower blocked passage of her car on the road to her mother's house, and that he entered her mother's home without invitation, shouted at her mother, and shook her as she sat in her chair. Herring's mother was in her 90s.

On 11 September 1995, Dana Webber reported in the *Wilmington Star* (Webber, 1995) that two residents of Duplin County, North Carolina, who had publicly opposed industrial hog production, became concerned for their jobs after representatives of Murphy Farms, then the largest hog producer in the world, contacted their supervisors. Although both left their jobs, "not solely because of Murphy's intimidation tactics," one of the workers said, "It's a mind game. This pork industry has got people scared thinking that they're so big and strong and that we can't do without them." According to Webber, "Duplin County officials contend that people in the county have complained to them about the kind of intimidation tactics [the workers] describe."

In this adversarial climate, the very choice of research topics almost invariably involves taking sides, whether it is research on environmental health or waste management technology. Human subjects are not the only ones at risk in public health research; community organizations that cooperate with researchers, community consultants who facilitate contacts between researchers and human subjects, family members, and others may reasonably fear intimidation and threat. Furthermore, communities that host facilities widely known for repellent odors may fear stigmatization if their identities are known. Researchers working on environmental health issues in the area of environmental injustice need to consider not only their obligation to individual human subjects but also their social responsibilities to entire communities (Rose, 1989; Coughlin, 1996).

Conclusions

Most researchers are accustomed to full-time employment with health insurance, pension benefits, and wages that afford housing in neighborhoods with access to clean water, sewerage, adequate schools, and medical facilities and that are free from major sources of environmental contamination. For us, antagonism from an industry that is threatened by environmental health research, or the question of support from our own institutions, can be very disturbing. However, these problems pale in comparison with the situations of people who live every day in a contaminated environment, unable to enjoy their homes and neighborhoods, unable to sell their property (if they are owners), fearful for their own health and the health of their family members. Although I have focused on the perspectives of an epidemiologist working on community-driven research, it is important to emphasize that researchers may choose to walk away from pollution and conflict; most community members who live with discrimination, pollution, and conflict have no choice but to accept or to fight injustice.

Acknowledgments

This research was supported by the National Institute of Allergy and Infectious Diseases Grant Program on Research Ethics 1T15 AA149650 and by National Institute of Environmental Health Sciences grant R25-ES08206-04 under the Environmental Justice: Partnerships for Communication program.

References

Brown, P. (1995), "Race, class, and environmental health: a review and systematization of the literature", *Environ Res*, **69**, 15–30.
Bullard, R. (1994), "Environmental justice for all", in Bullard R, ed., *Unequal Protection: Environmental Justice and Communities of Color*, San Francisco:Sierra Club Books; 3–22.
Cecelski, D. and Kerr, M.L. (1992), "Hog wild", *South Expo* **20**, 9–15.
Cole, D., Todd, L. and Wing, S. (2000), "Concentrated swine feeding operations and public health: a review of occupational and community health effects", *Environ Health Perspect*, **108**, 685–99.

Coughlin, S.S. (1996), "Environmental justice: the role of epidemiology in protecting unempowered communities from environmental hazards", *Sci Total Environ*, **184**, 67–76.

Economic development for Tillery (18 December 1991), The Circular [Scotland Neck, NC], 3.

Edwards, B. and Ladd, A. (2000), "Environmental justice, swine production and farm loss in North Carolina", *Sociol Spectrum*, **20**, 263–90.

Fisher, P.M. (1996), "Science and subpoenas: when do the courts become instruments of manipulation?", *Law Contemp Prob*, **59**, 159–67.

Furuseth, O. (1997), "Restructuring of hog farming in North Carolina: explosion and implosion", *Prof Geogr*, **49**, 391–403.

Gamble, V.N. (1993), "A legacy of distrust: African Americans and medical research", *Am J Prev Med*, **9**, 35–38.

Picou, J.S. (1996a), "Compelled disclosure of scholarly research: some comments on 'high stakes litigation'", *Law Contemp Prob*, **59**, 149–57.

Picou, J.S. (1996b), "Toxins in the environment, damage to the community: sociology and the toxic tort", in Jenkins, P.J. and Kroll-Smith, S. (eds), *Witnessing for Sociology: Sociologists in Court 211*, Westport, CT: Praeger, 212–24.

Picou, J.S. (1996c), "Sociology and compelled disclosure: protecting respondent confidentiality", *Sociol Spectrum*, **16**, 209–37.

Rose, G. (1989), "High-risk and population strategies of prevention: ethical considerations", *Ann Med*, **21**, 409–13.

Sandman, P.M. (1991), "Emerging communication responsibilities of epidemiologists", *J Clin Epidemiol*, **44**, 41S–50S.

Schiffman, S., Sattely Miller, E., Suggs, M. and Graham, B. (1995), "The effect of environmental odors emanating from commercial swine operations on the mood of nearby residents", *Brain Res Bull*, **37**, 369–75.

Schwebke, S. (19 August 1992), "Hog firm buys land near Tillery", *The Daily Herald* [Roanoke Rapids, NC], 1.

Snell, M. (March/April, 2001), "Downwind in Mississippi: the struggle to keep a community from going to the hogs", *Sierra*, 22–6.

St. George, D., Schoenbach, V., Reynolds, G., Nwangwu, J. and Adams-Campbell, L. (1997), "Recruitment of minority students to U.S. epidemiology degree programs", *Ann Epidemiol*, **7**, 304–10.

Thomas, S. and Quinn, S. (1991), "The Tuskegee Syphilis Study, 1932 to 1972: implications for HIV education and AIDS risk education programs in the black community", *Am J Public Health*, **81**, 1498–1504.

Thu, K. (2001), "Agriculture, the environment, and sources of state ideology and power", *Cult Agric*, **23**, 1–7.

Thu, K., Donham, K., Ziegenhorn, R., Reynolds, S., Thorne, P., Subramanian, P., Whitten, P. and Stookesberry, J. (1997), "A control study of the physical and mental health of residents living near a large-scale swine operation", *J Agric Safety Health*, **3**, 13–26.

Thu, K., Durrneberger, E. (eds) (1998), Pigs, Profits, and Rural Communities, Albany, NY: State University of New York Press.

Traynor, M. (1996), "Countering the excessive subpoena for scholarly research", *Law Contemp Prob*, **59**, 119–48.

Viel, J., Wing, S. and Hoffmann, W. (1998), "Environmental epidemiology, public health advocacy, and policy", in Lawson, A., Biggeri, A., Boehning, D., Lesaffre, E., Viel, J. and Bertollini, R. (eds), *Disease Mapping and Risk Assessment for Public Health,* Chichester, England: Wiley & Sons, 295–9.

Webber, D. (11 November 1995), "Two critics say hog industry leaned on their bosses", Wilmington Star [Wilmington, NC], 1B.

Wing, S., Grant, G., Green, M. and Stewart, C. (1996), "Community based collaboration for environmental justice: south-east Halifax environmental reawakening", *Environ Urban*, **8**, 129–40.

Wing, S. (1998), "Whose epidemiology, whose health?", *Int J Health Serv*, **28**, 241–52.

Wing, S., Cole, D. and Grant, G. (2000), "Environmental injustice in North Carolina's hog industry", *Environ Health Perspect*, **108**, 225–31.

Wing, S., Richardson, D. and Armstrong, D. (1997a), "Reply to comments on 'A reevaluation of cancer incidence near the Three Mile Island'", [Letter], *Environ Health Perspect*, **105**, 266–8.

Wing, S., Richardson, D. and Armstrong, D. (1997b), "Response: Science, public health and objectivity: research into the accident at Three Mile Island", *Environ Health Perspect*, **105**, 567–70.

Wing, S., Richardson, D., Armstrong, D. and Crawford-Brown, D. (1997), "A reevaluation of cancer incidence near the Three Mile Island nuclear plant: the collision of evidence and assumptions.", *Environ Health Perspect*, **105**, 52–7.

Wing, S. and Wolf, S. (2000), "Intensive livestock operations, health, and quality of life among eastern North Carolina residents", *Environ Health Perspect*, **108**, 233–8.

SECTION E:
LESSONS AND CONCLUSION

Afterword

H. Patricia Hynes and Doug Brugge

The studies featured in this edited volume were chosen for three primary reasons. All were undertaken in the *spirit of collaboration* between community and university partners, albeit that some collaborators worked in varying degrees of close and consistent partnership while others worked more like consultants for their community partners. Each case study included here employed *sound science* methods, tools and designs that were discussed and, in some cases, modified and improved by community input. Finally, the studies' results were *intentionally beneficial* to community participants and to the process of community research in one or more ways: through the relevant and actionable knowledge gained in the research process; as an intervention to reduce environmental exposure and risk; as evidence that generated further credibility for and investment in community projects and community-university partnerships; or as a basis of reflection and insight into the challenges of research partnerships which arise across boundaries of privilege and power, from differing ideas of expertise, and often out of opposing historical experiences of research.

Embedded within the criteria that guided our selection of studies are principles of community-collaborative research, principles that we endeavor to employ in our own work and that we also saw at work in varying degrees in the case studies featured in this book. We have adapted these principles from others' foundational work (see Israel et al., 1998; Minkler and Wallerstein, 2003), and re-formulated them in the light of our own working experience in community-university research partnerships within environmental health. They are meant to be guides that inspire and enlighten collaboration rather than fundamentalist prescriptions that rigidify partnerships. They include the following:

- The community partner brings strengths, assets, and expertise to the collaboration as well as vulnerability to the environmental risks that are the research focus of the partnership.
- The research process is equitable and collaborative, involving community partners, to the extent feasible, in problem definition, design of study, data collection, interpretation and dissemination of results, and application of results for action.
- The community-university collaboration promotes learning, consciousness, and capacity building among all partners involved, and works to address the social inequalities among the members.
- Community partners are fairly compensated for their contribution to the work of the research partnership.

- Research is undertaken for the goal of creating knowledge that is instrumental in education, action, and social change.
- Environmental health research acknowledges the health impacts of inequality, including the social, economic, and cultural determinants of ill health, and endeavors to reduce inequality as well as environmental risk through the opportunity of collaborative research.
- All partners receive the research results and participate, to the degree they elect, in the discussion, interpretation and dissemination of results, including reports and publications.
- Community-university research partnerships require generous time and personal commitment, and they generally benefit from sustained, long-term collaboration. These realities need to be acknowledged and supported by the partners' respective employers and funding organizations.

It's no coincidence that most community-university collaborations in environmental health have been undertaken with low-income communities and communities of color. The disproportionate burden of environmental pollution and risks, including those treated in this book – lead poisoning, asthma and poor housing conditions; traffic injuries and diesel exhaust; vacant land, abandoned housing, and crime; air toxics and radiation; and unsafe working conditions, is borne by those who also lose health, quality of life and years of life to the harmful impacts of inequality by race and ethnicity, economic status, gender, and other forms of discrimination. This central thesis of environmental injustice has been borne out in study after study.

Neighborhoods with high percentages of poor people have higher levels of infant mortality, increased risk of avoidable deaths, and a greater chance that they will bear a disproportionate burden of the environmental costs of contemporary society (Diez-Roux, 2002). Yet, the phenomena of communities opposing multi-family and affordable housing joined with suburbanization and the growth of gated communities have combined to place poor people further away from the non-poor. This economic isolation reinforces the consequences of poverty, including poor health, and allows the non-poor to ignore the problems of poverty or even to deny the existence of the poor (Massey, 1996).

Race and racial segregation are consistently implicated in higher rates of illness, disparities in diagnosis and treatment, greater exposure to toxic substances, poorer services, and fewer resources. More highly segregated African Americans tend to live in higher poverty census tracts with lower quality of medical care, more discriminatory care, and greater social inequality, all of which are associated with higher stress and higher blood pressure (Polednak, 1996). A study of 1990 exposures found that African Americans were breathing air with higher total modeled air toxics concentrations than Whites in every large metropolitan area in the United States; moreover, the more highly segregated the area, the higher the air toxics levels (Lopez, 2002). In an update using 2000 data, this relationship between segregation and air toxics exposure was found to extend to Hispanics and Asians as well as to Blacks and to describe a pattern of disproportionate exposure by race and ethnicity in metropolitan areas regardless of size.

The growing literature on social determinants of health makes a compelling case for the role of other related social factors in significantly affecting the health of individuals within a community. These factors include discrimination; poverty and length of time in isolated, marginalized communities; unemployment; poor nutrition, housing, and transportation; deprivation in early childhood; lack of control over one's life; and poor social relations. Researchers in the field of social inequality have concluded that health disparities within populations are most commonly caused by environmental factors. These include the social environment (e.g., gender, income, race, unemployment/status in work and society); the built environment (housing quality, proximity to locally undesirable land uses); and the physical environment (pollution). Life expectancy is lower for people who are poorer, lower in the workplace hierarchy, or less educated, and for those who suffer more stress, have less control over their lives, or experience discrimination. Health, they conclude follows a social gradient, and policy initiatives to improve health and healthful living conditions must strive to reduce the burden of inequality (Marmot and Wilkinson, 1999; Wilkinson and Marmot, 2003).

Community-collaborative research in environmental health will consistently be confronted with socially caused inequality and its health consequences, no matter what the particular research questions. Because of this, community-collaborative research is challenged to generate meaningful and constructive knowledge and interventions that improve environmental health and that also strive to reduce discrimination and inequality. Beginning with the research process and team, the partners can acknowledge their diversity and the varying levels of privilege, power and decision-making. This, after all, is the local social ground upon which a multicultural working team will make decisions on research questions and design, data collection, analysis and interpretation, publication and dissemination, and action and advocacy. University partners can encourage and seek opportunities for people from low-income communities and communities of color to pursue higher education so as to build the social resources of communities diminished by structural inequality and ill health. Finally, the findings of the research process can be used to advocate within the public sector for policy change – in environmental standards, building codes, zoning, health programs, and workplace practices; within the funding sectors to invest in public interest community-based partnerships and intervention programs proven to be successful in reducing risk and disparities; and within academia and the research sector to promote racial and ethnic diversity in research and teaching.

Science has traditionally employed convenient dichotomies, such as "hard" and "soft," to construct a bias for basic, abstract, theoretical, often solitary, and so-called value free science, deeming it superior and more rigorous intellectual research than that of applied, integrated, and value-centered research. In our opinion, community-collaborative research, with its commitment to equitable collaboration, to sound science, and to actionable knowledge is more challenging and more rigorous for its ambition to join social justice to the enterprise of science. Some of the rigors have been alluded to within the studies we featured in this collection. These include: achieving adequate sample size in communities abused by and distrustful of research and researchers; accounting for interactions from the many factors in discriminated communities that contribute to ill health; designing alternative models to the standard intervention study in which the control receives no intervention; and identifying potential bias when working within an informed (versus blinded) and value-centered research context.

The studies featured in this book are among the first generation of community-collaborative research in environmental health. We look forward to the growth and maturation of more equitable partnerships, enhanced and improved science methods and designs, and more strategic policy outcomes that promote environmental and social justice as they prevent environmental exposure and risk. We hope that this book contributes to the next generation of this work.

References

Diez-Roux, A. (2002), "Invited commentary: places, people, and health," *American Journal of Epidemiology*, **155**, 516–19.

Israel, B.A., Schulz, A.J. and Parker, E.A. (1998), "Review of community-based research: Assessing partnership approaches to improve public health," *Annual Review of Public Health*, **19**, 173–202.

Lopez, R. (2002), "Segregation and black/white differences to air toxics in 1990," *Environmental Health Perspectives*, **110** (Supplement 2), 289–95.

Marmot, M. and Wilkinson, R. (eds) (1999), *Social determinants of health*, New York: Oxford University Press.

Massey, D. (1996), "The age of extremes: Concentrated affluence and poverty in the twenty-first century," *Demography*, **33**, 395–412.

Minkler, M. and Wallerstein, N. (eds) (2003), *Community-based participatory research for health*, San Francisco, CA: Jossey-Bass, a Wiley Imprint.

Polednak, A. (1996), "Segregation, discrimination and mortality in U.S. Blacks," *Ethnicity and Disease*, **6**, 99–105.

Wilkinson, R. and Marmot, M. (eds) (2003), *Social determinants of health: The solid facts*, Geneva: World Health Organization.

Index

The index covers all parts of the text, including notes, n, figures, f, and tables, t.